K

The Epidemiology of Schizophrenia

For the first time in one volume, an international team of leading researchers and practitioners have come together to provide a comprehensive, contemporary, epidemiological overview of this multifaceted and mysterious disorder and address some of the age-old questions it raises. What is the genetic contribution to schizophrenia? Do pregnancy and birth complications increase the risk for schizophrenia? Is the incidence of schizophrenia decreasing? Why is the rate higher among immigrants and in those born in cities? Controversial issues such as the validity of dimensional classifications of schizophrenia and the continuum between psychosis and 'normality' are explored in depth. Separate chapters are devoted to topics of particular relevance to schizophrenia such as suicide, violence and substance abuse.

Drawing together the findings from the social, genetic, developmental and classical epidemiology of schizophrenia, this text will prove an invaluable resource for both clinicians and researchers.

Robin M. Murray is Professor of Psychiatry at the Institute of Psychiatry in London and heads the largest psychiatric research department in Europe. He has co-authored eight books and over 500 research publications and is on the editorial board of numerous journals. He was President of the Association of European Psychiatrists (1994–96).

Peter B. Jones is Professor of Psychiatry, University of Cambridge. He is on the editorial board of *Psychological Medicine.*

Ezra Susser is Chair of the Department of Epidemiology at the Joseph L. Mailman School of Public Health, Columbia University and Head of the Epidemiology of Brain Disorders Department at the New York State Psychiatric Institute, New York. He is on the editorial board of *International Journal of Epidemiology* and *Public Health Reports.*

Jim van Os is Professor of Psychiatric Epidemiology in the Department of Psychiatry and Neuropsychology, University of Maastricht, the Netherlands. He is on the editorial board of *Acta Psychiatrica Scandinavica* and *European Psychiatry.*

Mary Cannon is Senior Lecturer and Wellcome Trust Advanced Research Fellow in the Division of Psychological Medicine at the Institute of Psychiatry, London. She is on the editorial board of the *British Journal of Psychiatry.*

The Epidemiology of Schizophrenia

Edited by

Robin M. Murray
Institute of Psychiatry, London, UK

Peter B. Jones
University of Cambridge, UK

Ezra Susser
Columbia University and
New York Psychiatric Institute,
New York, USA

Jim van Os
University of Maastricht, the Netherlands

and

Mary Cannon
Institute of Psychiatry, London, UK

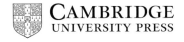

CAMBRIDGE
UNIVERSITY PRESS

PUBLISHED BY THE PRESS SYNDICATE OF THE UNIVERSITY OF CAMBRIDGE
The Pitt Building, Trumpington Street, Cambridge, United Kingdom

CAMBRIDGE UNIVERSITY PRESS
The Edinburgh Building, Cambridge CB2 2RU, UK
40 West 20th Street, New York, NY 10011-4211, USA
477 Williamstown Road, Port Melbourne, VIC 3207, Australia
Ruiz de Alarcón 13, 28014 Madrid, Spain
Dock House, The Waterfront, Cape Town 8001, South Africa

http://www.cambridge.org

First published 2003

Printed in the United Kingdom at the University Press, Cambridge

Typeface Minion 10.5/14pt   *System* QuarkXPress™   [S E]

A catalogue record for this book is available from the British Library

Library of Congress Cataloguing in Publication data

The epidemiology of schizophrenia / editors Robin M. Murray . . . [et al.].
     p. cm.
  Includes bibliographical references and index.
  ISBN 0 521 77540 X (hb.)
   1. Schizophrenia – Epidemiology.   I. Murray, Robin.

  RC514 .E425 2002
  362.2′6 – dc21   2002017390

ISBN 0 521 77540 X hardback

Contents

I   The social epidemiology of schizophrenia

II   The developmental epidemiology of schizophrenia

Contributors

Jane Boydell
Wellcome Trust Research Training Fellow in
Clinical Epidemiology
Division of Psychological Medicine,
Institute of Psychiatry, Kings College
London, UK

Michaeline Bresnahan
Assistant Professor
Columbia University, Department of
Epidemiology, New York, USA

Alec Buchanan
Senior Lecturer and Honorary Consultant
Psychiatrist
Department of Forensic Psychiatry,
Institute of Psychiatry, Kings College
London, UK

William Carpenter
Professor of Psychiatry and Pharmacology,
University of Maryland School of Medicine
and
Director, Maryland Psychiatric Research
Center, Baltimore, MD, USA

Mary Cannon
Senior Lecturer and Wellcome Trust
Advanced Research Fellow
Division of Psychological Medicine,
Institute of Psychiatry, Kings College
London, UK

Tyrone D. Cannon
Staglin Family Professor of Psychology,
Psychiatry and Human Genetics
Departments of Psychology, Psychiatry and
Human Genetics, University of California,
Los Angeles, CA, USA

Alastair G. Cardno
Senior Lecturer
Department of Psychological Medicine,
University of Wales College of Medicine,
Cardiff, UK

David Castle
Professorial Fellow
Mental Health Research Institute &
University of Melbourne, Australia

Mary Clarke
Consultant Psychiatrist
St John of God Hospital, Co. Dublin,
Ireland

Timothy L. Gasperoni
Graduate Student
Department of Psychology, University of
California, Los Angles, CA, USA

Anton Grech
Consultant Psychiatrist
Victoria, Gozo, Malta

Heinz Häfner
Professor Emeritus
Central Institute of Mental Health,
Mannheim, Germany

Hannele Heilä
Senior Researcher
National Public Health Institute,
Department of Mental Health and Alcohol
Research, Helsinki, Finland

Matti O. Huttunen
Senior Researcher
Department of Mental Health and Alcohol
Research, National Public Health Institute,
Helsinki, Finland
and
Docent, Department of Psychiatry,
University of Helsinki, Finland

Sonia Johnson
Senior Lecturer in Social and Community
Psychiatry
Royal Free and University College Medical
Schools, London, UK

Peter B. Jones
Professor of Psychiatry and Head
Division of Psychiatry, University of
Cambridge, Cambridge, UK

Robert E. Kendell
Professor Emeritus
Department of Psychiatry, University of
Edinburgh, Edinburgh, UK

Glyn Lewis
Professor of Psychiatric Epidemiology
Division of Psychiatry, University of Bristol,
Bristol, UK

Jouko Lönnqvist
Research Professor, Director
Department of Mental Health and Alcohol
Research, National Public Health Institute,
Helsinki, Finland

John McGrath
Director
Queensland Centre for Schizophrenia
Research, Queensland, Australia

Paulo Menezes
Professor Doutor
Departmento de Medicina Preventiva,
Facultade de Medicina da USP, São
Paulo-SP, Brazil

Preben Bo Mortensen
Professor, Head of Centre
National Centre for Register-based Research,
Faculty of Social Sciences, University of
Aarhus, Aarhus, Denmark

Robin M. Murray
Professor of Psychiatry
Division of Psychological Medicine,
Institute of Psychiatry, Kings College
London, UK

Eadbhard O'Callaghan
Professor of Biological Psychiatry
University College Dublin
and
Director, Stanley Foundation Research
Centre, Cluain Mhuire Family Centre, Co.
Dublin, Ireland

Kenneth G. D. Orr
Consultant Psychiatrist
Fremantle Hospital and Health Service,
Fremantle, Western Australia

Michael J. Owen
Professor and Head of Department
Division of Psychological Medicine,
University of Wales College of Medicine,
Cardiff, UK

Peter A. Phillips
Research Fellow in Mental Health Nursing
Department of Psychiatry and Behavioural
Sciences, Royal Free and University College
London Medical Schools, London, UK

Isabelle M. Rosso
Postdoctoral Fellow
Department of Psychology, University of
California, Los Angeles, CA, USA

Pak Sham
Professor of Psychiatric and Statistical
Genetics
Department of Psychological Medicine, and
Social Genetic and Development Psychiatry
Research Centre, Institute of Psychiatry,
Kings College London, UK

Ezra Susser
Professor of Epidemiology and Psychiatry,
and Head of the Department of
Epidemiology, Mailman School of Public
Health, Columbia University
and
Head, Department of Epidemiology of
Brain Disorders
New York State Psychiatric Institute, New
York, USA

Michele Tansella
Professor of Psychiatry
Department of Medicine and Public Health,
Section of Psychiatry, University of Verona,
Verona, Italy

C. Jane Tarrant
Specialist Registrar
Department of Psychiatry, University of
Nottingham, Nottingham, UK

Graham Thornicroft
Professor of Community Psychiatry and
Head, Health Services Research Department
Institute of Psychiatry, Kings College
London, UK

Theo G. M. van Erp
Graduate Student
Department of Psychology, University of
California, Los Angeles, CA, USA

Jim van Os
Professor of Psychiatric Epidemiology
Department of Psychiatry and
Neuropsychology, Section of Social
Psychiatry and Neuropsychology, Maastricht
University, Maastricht, the Netherlands
and
Visiting Professor
Division of Psychological Medicine,
Institute of Psychiatry, London, UK

Vijoy Varma
Columbia University, Division of
Epidemiology, New York, USA

Hélène Verdoux
Professor
Service Universitaire de Psychiatrie,
Bordeaux, France

Elizabeth Walsh
Clinical Lecturer in Forensic Mental Health
Section of Forensic Mental Health, Division
of Psychological Medicine, Institute of
Psychiatry, King's College London, UK

Stanley Zammit
MRC Clinical Training Fellow
Division of Psychological Medicine,
University of Wales College of Medicine,
Cardiff, UK

Preface

The aim of this book is to weave together the diverse threads of epidemiological research in schizophrenia into a single volume that captures the new and exciting themes that have been emerging over recent years. Diverse topics are juxtaposed to expose synergy and to reveal new avenues of work, while the power of the epidemiological method runs throughout the book. The sections correspond to different subdisciplines within epidemiology: social, genetic and developmental epidemiology, with additional sections for special and emerging issues relevant to the epidemiological study of schizophrenia. Despite the multiple authorship, we have tried to maintain a unified approach to epidemiological thinking throughout the book. Authors were asked to concentrate on findings that have been established through robust epidemiological investigation.

The book provides an overview of the current state of epidemiological knowledge and research in schizophrenia and is intended as a reference for those involved in research about schizophrenia or in clinical work with individuals who suffer from schizophrenia. We have placed much emphasis on findings that may elucidate the causes of this complex illness. No previous training in epidemiology is assumed and a glossary of epidemiological terms is included at the back of the book. The editors are based in the UK, the USA and the Netherlands and are all engaged in schizophrenia. We are very fortunate in having gathered together a talented and internationally respected group of contributors and we thank them for their enthusiastic participation.

The editors

Foreword

Schizophrenia may be the leading unsolved disease afflicting humans. Ranked fourth among causes of disability worldwide, the disease syndrome is associated with an immense financial burden for clinical care and living support across the 50 or so years that the average patient is identified as ill. Secondary costs in lost productivity, homelessness and entanglement with law enforcement are also high, but the most poignant burden of illness is experienced by patients and their families. Subtle impairments in information processing and neurointegrative function are often present from birth, curtailing achievement and social engagement years before hallucinations, delusions, disorganized thought and behaviour make public the presence of illness and the need for treatment. Erosion of the fundamental building blocks of human experience lead to a reduced level of functioning and quality of life. Stigma further pains and isolates the person who suffers from this illness. The picture is also complicated by low drive and restricted affect in many patients, and dysphoric mood and suicide in others. Patients are at increased risk for drug abuse, and intense nicotine consumption causes additional health problems. Although illness manifestations, treatment response, course pattern and functional outcome are quite variable, most life stories reflect serious adverse effects of schizophrenia.

Treatment remains a part-way technology. Antipsychotic drugs and supportive and educationally oriented psychosocial therapies reduce psychotic symptoms and relapse rate, but no treatment is documented as efficacious for primary negative symptom and cognitive impairments. Little wonder that the long-term disease effects were modified little during the 20th century. Neither cure or prevention is yet in sight. Investigation of this illness syndrome is especially challenging because human behaviour is complex, the human brain is the most difficult organ system to manipulate and access experimentally, tissue pathology is not yet determined, and model systems (including animal preparations) are partial and difficult to validate. Finally, it is not yet known whether one disease or many resides in the schizophrenia syndrome.

This view of schizophrenia issues a clarion call for epidemiology.

Substantial progress in understanding schizophrenia aetiopathophysiology is dependent on discovery of cause. It is here that the aetiological discipline of epidemiology provides the most compelling data. Skewed distribution of cases in identified populations has led to discovery of risk factors that, in turn, now organize the search for specific aetiological variables. The range of inquiry is necessarily broad, for increased risk for schizophrenia is associated with geography, season of birth, migration, urbanization, gestational insult, birth complications, physical and social developmental patterns and, of course, genes. There are also interesting comorbid groupings relating schizophrenia to violence, suicide, drug abuse and reduced lifespan. These studies in schizophrenia are profoundly important in understanding this disease (or diseases), but methodology and concepts in psychiatric epidemiology are not well understood by the nonspecialist. There has been considerable recent accumulation of knowledge in this field, and the time is right for a succinct and critical presentation of concepts, methods and facts regarding the epidemiology of schizophrenia.

Murray, Jones, Susser, van Os and Cannon have organized a text that is both thorough and readable. For the student of schizophrenia, it will provide a contemporaneous review and critical interpretation of the rich data generated in epidemiological investigations. For the generalist and the informed lay reader, it is plainly presented and highly informative. Each chapter stands on its own but is carefully integrated and cross-referenced with other chapters. With a distinguished group of authors, it is especially pleasing that the writing styles and chapter organization are consistent, providing seamless transitions from topic to topic. I found this text generously informative and believe that both the serious and the casual student of schizophrenia will profit from time spent with this book.

William Carpenter

Part I

The social epidemiology of schizophrenia

Introduction

Social epidemiology studies the link between the social environment and the development and distribution of diseases in populations (Kaufman and Cooper, 1999). Research into social and behavioural determinants of health and illness is an area of interest for both sociologists and social epidemiologists. This section provides an introduction to some design and conceptual issues in social epidemiology and detailed discussion of temporal and geographical variations in the incidence, course and outcome of schizophrenia, with particular emphasis on issues of urbanization and migration.

Epidemiologists are very familiar with individual-level effects or risk factors such as birth complications, smoking or substance misuse. However Bresnahan and Susser in Chapter 1 emphasize the importance of societal-level effects (such as racism or level of socioeconomic development) in elucidating disease trends and mechanisms. The use of age–period–cohort effect analyses and life-course approaches to epidemiology are also included.

One of the central tenets of schizophrenia epidemiology is that the (narrowly defined) disorder appears to occur with equal incidence worldwide. However some variation in incidence rates between the developed and developing world has been noted for broadly defined schizophrenia. Bresnahan and colleagues examine this issue in Chapter 2 but recognize that the question of variation in incidence will remain unresolved 'while we await incidence rates based on rediagnosis using modern diagnostic systems'. On the other hand, there is 'clear and convincing evidence' currently available for more favourable course and outcome of schizophrenia in developing countries. This finding is 'remarkable' in view of the scarcity of treatment options in the developing world. Bresnahan and colleagues conclude that some aspect of the cultural circumstances in developing countries may provide a more therapeutic context for recovery.

Is schizophrenia disappearing? In Chapter 3 Bresnahan and colleagues investigate whether the incidence of schizophrenia has been declining over the past few decades. They consider that the apparent decline appears to reflect mainly period effects, pointing again to the role of social environment. Is schizophrenia becoming less severe? Bresnahan and colleagues also examine time trends in course and outcome of schizophrenia and find that improvements in outcome from the beginning to the end of the 20th century are modest. As the authors point out, this is surprising in view of the dramatic impact of antipsychotic medication on symptoms. Unfortunately, the data used to detect changes in outcome are unsystematic and do not yield insight into possible explanatory factors.

In Chapter 4, Boydell and Murray examine urban birth and migration as risk factors for schizophrenia. They conclude that there is 'substantial' evidence that urban birth and/or upbringing are associated with an increased risk for psychosis and that this effect may be increasing. The high rate of schizophrenia and psychosis among migrant groups, particularly first- and second-generation African-Caribbean immigrants in the UK, has been the subject of much discussion and debate over the past few years. Boydell and Murray examine the many possible reasons why 'urban birth' and 'migration' may increase the incidence of schizophrenia. Although there are no clear answers at present, the authors conclude that social and psychological aetiological factors are likely to be important. It seems as though researchers into schizophrenia will have to pay more attention to the social environment in the future to help to solve these unanswered questions.

REFERENCE

Kaufman JS, Cooper RS (1999) Seeking causal explanations in social epidemiology. American Journal of Epidemiology 150, 113–120.

1

Investigating socioenvironmental influences in schizophrenia: conceptual and design issues

Michaeline Bresnahan and Ezra Susser

Division of Epidemiology, Columbia University, New York, USA

The investigation of socioenvironmental influences began early in the history of schizophrenia research. As far back as the 19th century, reports emerged that insanity was more common among the lower social classes, and early in the 20th century this association was reported specifically for the diagnosis of schizophrenia. The association between low social class and schizophrenia was later confirmed by the classic study of Hollingshead and Redlich in New Haven in the 1950s (Hollingshead and Redlich, 1958). They suggested that the relation was causal: lower social class increased the risk of schizophrenia. This view was shortly disputed, however, in another classic study by Goldberg and Morrison (1963). Relying upon national registry data to establish occupation of father at birth, Goldberg and Morrison found that fathers of patients had a social class distribution similar to the population as a whole. Despite decades of work and further exceptional contributions (Link et al., 1986; Dohrenwend et al., 1992; also see Table 1.1), the matter is still not entirely resolved; however, the weight of evidence suggests that socioeconomic status has at most a modest effect on risk of schizophrenia. Therefore, while social class provided an early foothold in the examination of socioenvironmental influences in schizophrenia, no clear findings have emerged.

Nonetheless, emanating from this initial concern with social class, researchers have extended investigations to a broad range of socioenvironmental influences in schizophrenia. This section addresses socioenvironmental influences that are an active focus of current research and appear to have an impact on schizophrenia. The chapters to follow deal in turn with socioeconomic development (Ch. 2), time trends (Ch. 3), and urbanicity and immigration (Ch. 4). What ties these together is that, in each domain, social environment is likely to be a significant contributing factor to any observed variation in schizophrenia morbidity. In addition, they represent societal influences that cause populations to differ from one another, but they may not account for differences between individuals within a given population.

Table 1.1. Social class of origin and risk of schizophrenia

Study	Study description	Paternal social class	Diagnosis	Finding
Goldberg & Morrison (1963) England/Wales	Psychiatric Register; first admission (1956) ($n = 369$) Compared with population statistics	Paternal occupation at birth General Register Office (I–V) Comparison: 1931 Census of Occupied Men ages 20–44	Register diagnosis	Social class distribution of fathers of patients at birth similar to that of the population as a whole
Turner and Wagenfeld (1967) Monroe County, New York	Psychiatric Register, all first contact (1960–63) diagnosed with schizophrenia having no prior psychiatric hospitalization ($n = 214$) Compared with population statistics	Paternal occupational score (1–7) for last/current/usual job, and job when patient was 16 Comparison: 1950 County Census occupations, age and sex adjusted	Register diagnosis	Paternal occupation when patient was 16 years and usual occupation over-represent the lowest prestige categories compared with expectation
Wiersma et al. (1983) the Netherlands	Incident treated cases (Schizophrenia $n = 34$) Compared with random sample of general population	Paternal status on occupational scale (1–5/6)	ICD-9 schizophrenia (295)	Paternal occupation tended to be higher than expected based on the population sample; the relationship was not linear
Castle et al. (1993) Camberwell, UK	Camberwell Cumulative Psychiatric Case Register (1965–84), first contact ($n = 128$) Matched nonpsychotic patients in the Register ($n = 128$)	Paternal occupation at birth medical records or Birth Record data, General Register Office (I–V). Occupations dichotomized (nonmanual/ manual)	RDC criteria, schizophrenia	Patients were twice as likely to have fathers in manual occupations than nonpsychotic matched psychiatric patient controls
Jones et al. (1994) UK	1946 British Birth Cohort (cases, $n = 30$; stratified random sample of cohort; $n = 5362$)	Paternal occupation at birth General Register Office (I–V)	DSM-III-R schizophrenia	Social class at birth not associated with later risk of schizophrenia; a nonsignificant trend towards higher social class increasing risk reported

Study	Sample	Diagnostic criteria	Measure of social class	Result
Done et al. (1994) UK	1958 British Birth Cohort (cases, n = 40; controls 10% of sample with no history of psychiatric admission)	PSE, CATEGO	Paternal occupation at birth General Register Office (I–V)	Social class of origin significantly higher for preschizophrenics than for controls
Makikyro et al. (1997) Finland	1966 Finnish Birth Cohort (cases, n = 76; n cohort = 11 017)	DSM-III-R schizophrenia	Paternal occupation at birth (I–V)	Incidence of early-onset (<23 years) schizophrenia higher than expected in the highest social class (I) compared with lower social classes (II–V)
Timms (1998) Sweden	1963 Stockholm Cohort of residents born in 1953; cases (n = 71) hospital admissions for Stockholm County (1969–83), i.e. cohort ages 16–30; n cohort = 15 117	ICD-8 schizophrenia; Inpatient Register Diagnosis	Parental occupation at member age 10 from population register; classification used by National Central Bureau of Statistics (1–5) trichotomized	Low parental social class at patient age 10 not related to risk of schizophrenia; middle-class parental status related to increased risk of schizophrenia compared with working class (nonsignificant)

Notes:

Studies appearing in the table include incident cases of diagnosed schizophrenia, and individual measures of parental social class (occupation). Studies excluded from the table do not meet all three inclusion criteria. For example, Hollingshead and Redlich (1958) was not included because the measure of social class combined education occupation and residence; Lapouse et al. (1956) not included because measure of class was based on residence. See text for diagnostic criteria.

Societal influences have rarely been addressed in recent reviews of schizophrenia epidemiology. Of course, neither societal nor individual social experience are considered as alternatives to biological causation; they are, however, often antecedent and account for patterns of biological exposures.

In order to appreciate and understand fully the range of epidemiological studies represented, it is helpful to be familiar with certain central concepts in the epidemiology. Epidemiological studies of socioenvironmental influences often address questions framed by contrasts (Schwartz and Carpenter, 1999). Why do some individuals in a population develop disease and not others? Why is the rate of disease higher/lower in one population compared with another? Why is the rate of disease changing over time? How does experience in each stage of life build on risk arising from earlier experience? These questions all fall squarely within one of the key missions of epidemiology: to identify determinants of disease. The strategies that can be used to answer each of these questions are quite different, however, and focus attention on distinct effects. As these differences are often overlooked and have important implications, we draw attention to them here.

Effects at the level of the individual

Why do some individuals develop schizophrenia and not others? This question pertains to individuals. To answer this question, we focus on variation between individuals in hypothesized risk factors. Thus, we establish both the exposure and disease experience for individuals under study within a given population, using such strategies as cohort and case-control studies. When there is evidence of association between exposure and disease, effort is directed at determining if the connection is causal (Schwartz and Susser, 2001).

In searching for determinants in this way, the natural focus is on factors that vary between individuals within the population at hand. For example, we hypothesize that prenatal exposure to influenza is a risk factor for schizophrenia. This hypothesis is testable in a population when some individuals are exposed and some are not. We then compare the proportion of those exposed to prenatal influenza who develop schizophrenia with the proportion of those not exposed to prenatal influenza who develop schizophrenia.

This much is well known to most schizophrenia researchers. There are two constraints to the approach, however, that are not widely recognized. First, when there is no interindividual variation in a factor, it cannot explain why some people within a population get disease and not others. A factor that is ubiquitous in a given population will not contribute to individual variation of risk in that population even if it can and does contribute to disease (Schwartz and Carpenter, 1999). For example, in an ethnically homogeneous population, there may be little variation between individuals in skin complexion; therefore, complexion may not be identified as a determinant of individual risk for skin cancer within this population. Paradoxically, this could occur within a population consisting wholly of individuals whose complexion puts them at extremely high risk (e.g. a Nordic population). A number of individual factors that are of compelling interest in schizophrenia research may be ubiquitous within samples commonly studied (e.g. poverty, race), with the result that their effects are undetectable.

An intriguing example of an ubiquitous exposure are childhood vaccinations. In the field of psychiatry, interest in the impact of vaccines has surfaced in the context of childhood autism. Recently, hypotheses have been advanced relating the MMR (measles, mumps and rubella) vaccine to autism. Because this vaccination is ubiquitous in most developed countries, it is extremely difficult to examine the impact of vaccines on differences in risk for autism within one of these populations.

Second, the relationship of exposure to disease necessarily varies across populations. Because disease causation is multifactorial, whether or not a given factor causes disease will depend upon the presence of other factors (i.e. cofactors in disease causation). The presence of these other factors will clearly vary between populations. Consequently, there is no expectation that individual risk factors identified in studies of individual level effects will be exactly the same from population to population, nor is there an expectation that the magnitude of relative risk pertaining to the risk factor will be the same from population to population. For example, if prenatal influenza acts as a risk factor for schizophrenia only in conjunction with adverse postnatal exposures, the association of influenza and schizophrenia will be affected by the prevalence of these postnatal cofactors in the population. Despite this caveat, one generally does expect some consistency across studies in different populations, and the lack of it is a source of concern or interest.

Studies of individual risk factors for schizophrenia are vital, and in subsequent chapters we will see that they have made important contributions in schizophrenia research. It is equally important, however, to investigate the role of societal level factors in the causation of schizophrenia.

Effects at the societal level

Usually the investigation of societal effects begins with the question: Why is the rate of disease higher/lower in one population compared with another? This question contrasts populations rather than individuals within populations, focusing on differences in the rates of disease between populations. With the shift in focus from individual to societal level effects, the range of substantive questions has changed (Rose, 1992; Schwartz, 1994; Schwartz and Carpenter, 1999).

The critical contribution of contrasting populations, rather than individuals within populations, is to draw attention to factors with meaning residing at the societal level. Contextual factors such as stage of socioeconomic development are defined at the societal level: individuals within a society share the experience of living in a 'developed' or 'developing' country. Similarly, average individual income in a society, although constructed from an individual factor, describes a milieu or societal characteristic: individuals living in the population share the experience of living in a low-income or high-income society. Societal racism (political, economic and social) is also definable at the group level. The association of societal measures of the degree of contextual racism with rates of schizophrenia in groups of minorities living in different societies may illuminate the impact of a broad group-level phenomenon. Investigations of differences between populations are particularly crucial to identifying and describing these sorts of factor as determinants of rates of disease.

Sometimes the distinction between an individual- and population-level factor is obvious; however, in other instances it is not. It is important to clarify the distinction or delineate levels in order to avoid mistaken inference. An example particularly germane to schizophrenia research is the impact of 'treatment'. There is definitive evidence that within given populations modern treatments (e.g. medications, family interventions) reduce the risk of relapse in patients with schizophrenia. From this evidence, however, it cannot be inferred that a society with more highly developed treatment systems – even including the most effective treatments – will have lower rates of relapse among patients with schizophrenia. In fact, for reasons that remain unclear, the course of schizophrenia is substantially better in societies with the least developed treatment systems (Ch. 2). Some have speculated that treatment systems lead to segregation and enhanced stigma on a societal level, and that they interfere with reintegration. Therefore, 'treatment' has a different meaning at societal and individual levels. This distinction is often overlooked.

It is possible to conduct studies where both individual and societal level effects are examined at the same time. For example, in a multisite study conducted in several countries, it would be possible to consider both individual income and mean societal income/level of socioeconomic development in the same analysis. The impact of societal level factors on individual processes, and their interaction with individual level factors to affect individual processes, can be examined. With notable exceptions (van Os et al., 2000), there are still few examples of such analyses in schizophrenia research.

Sometimes studies contrast populations when seeking to identify individual effects. It is always risky to make comparisons at one level and inferences at another. Nonetheless, differences between populations can provide important indirect evidence for the impact of individual factors that do not vary within a given population. In the example described above, skin complexion was confined to a very narrow range in a hypothetical population. A comparison of this population with another ethnically dissimilar population may yield a comparison of two populations of wholly different complexion (e.g. Nordic versus Ugandan). This comparison might contribute important information about complexion as a determinant of skin cancer. Migrants studies, most often used to isolate genetic from environmental causes of disease, may also uncover the causal contribution of ubiquitous environmental exposures. Systematic first- and second-generation differences between rates in immigrant populations in the country of destination and population rates in the country of origin provide nonspecific evidence for environmental determinants. Higher rates of schizophrenia among African-Caribbean immigrants than found in countries of origin are consistent with a number of possible mechanisms including discrimination stress, a potential ubiquitous exposure among immigrants (Ch. 4). Unfortunately, migrant populations are not always available for study.

Age–period–cohort effects

Why is the rate of disease increasing/decreasing within a population over time? Contrasting the same population at different points in time is akin to comparing different societies. Instead of comparing the rate in one society with that in another, the rate of disease in the same society is being compared at one time with another.

In spite of the apparent similarities between these comparisons, there are important differences. Dynamic socioenvironmental influences are the leading suspect as a cause of secular trends. The time periods analysed are generally too brief to capture significant shifts in population genetics. In comparisons between populations, however, population genetic differences are more likely to play a role alongside socioenvironmental factors.

Another important distinction is in the analytic techniques. Time is continuous, whereas populations are categorical. The differences over time are measured in change. Moreover, change over time can be measured in three dimensions: historical period, age and cohort (usually birth cohort defined by year of birth). The view of rate change is different in each of these metrics. Disentangling the three time effects is essential for interpretation of secular trends; for understanding the literature on change in schizophrenia incidence, it is helpful to understand how these dimensions are differentiated.

Period effects

Period effects capture the point-in-time experience of a population, i.e. specific historical conditions such as an economic depression or war. Increased rates of suicide during economic depression or decreased rates of suicide in wartime are examples of period effects. Similarly, a change in the diagnostic system in use during the period of measurement will be reflected as a period effect. Thus, the incidence rate of schizophrenia should be higher in years when a broader definition of disease is in use, and lower in years when a narrower definition of disease is in use (e.g. rates of schizophrenia in 1960 versus 1990). Secular trends attributable to artifact (i.e. changes in diagnostic criteria, changes in ascertainment) are often subsumed in period effects.

Age effects

Age effects reflect the varying susceptibility to disease over the life cycle. In schizophrenia, peak risk for onset occurs during young adulthood. Because age structures risk, the underlying age structure of a population will affect overall rates. A population that is 'younger' (i.e. where a greater proportion of individuals are in their young adult years) will be expected to have higher overall incidence rates than a population that is 'older' (i.e. where a greater proportion of individuals are in ages of lower risk of onset). In studies of schizophrenia trends, the principal reason for interest in age effects is based on their capacity to introduce artifact or confounding in trend analyses. When the age structure of the population changes, the overall population rates will change. Age stratification and age standardization are used to address these problems.

Generational effects

Generational effects or cohort effects capture the effect of cumulative experiences in population groups, usually defined by birth year. Trends based on the disease experience of birth cohorts reflect the unique group experience of being in utero in a given year, experiencing childhood during a given historical period and adulthood during a specific period. Therefore, the cumulative experience of people who are 30 years old in 1960 is different from people who are 30 years old in 1990. When this causes a difference in disease rates, it is a generational effect. If the investigator is interested in the impact of childhood exposures, individuals who are 30 years old in 1960 are the same as people who are 5 years old in 1935. When there is evidence of generational shifts in rates over short periods of time (measured in birth years), differences arising from fetal or infant experience are implicated.

Discriminating age–period–cohort effects

For interpretation of secular trends, it is essential to separate these component effects: period, age and cohort. This represents a first step to developing hypotheses and investigating the causes of the rate changes (Susser, 1973). It can be difficult, however, to disentangle these effects. Figures 1.1 and 1.2 are graphical displays that allow visual discrimination of these effects.

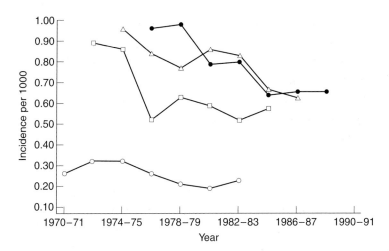

Fig. 1.1.   This graph shows age-stratified incidence of schizophrenia by calendar year. These period data for four age groups (male aged 16–17 (○), 18–19 (□), 20–21 (△) and 22–23 (●) years) are taken from Suvisaari et al. (1999). The study followed individuals born from 1954 to 1965 over the period from 1970 to 1991 for schizophrenia. In this figure, we see a period effect with generally declining rates over time in all age groups except the 16–17 year olds, and age effects with ages 16–17 years at lowest risk and ages 20–21 and 22–23 years at highest risk.

Age–period confusion is common. For example, risk of drug use varies with age, adolescents and young adults being at highest risk. At the same time, the availability of illicit substances varies over historical period. A period effect owing to the increased availability of illicit drugs could be masked by a change in the age structure in the population. If adolescents and young adults decrease as a proportion of the population from one historical period to another, this will produce a countervailing trend towards reduced drug use. A comparison of historical period within age groups would expose the period effect.

Age–cohort confusion can also occur. For example, when a generation particularly inclined to drug use enters adolescence, it will at first appear that there is a high rate of drug use among adolescents. This would suggest an age effect. However, following this generation as they age will reveal their proclivity to drug use. As the generation grows older, they will have higher rates at every age than the preceding or subsequent generations examined at the same age. A comparison of birth years within age groups would expose the cohort effect.

Discriminating between period and generation effects can be illuminating in understanding disease processes. The classic example of a Gordian knot was posed by trends in tuberculosis mortality (Susser, 1973). As the rates of tuberculosis declined over time (1880 to 1930), a steady increase in risk with age was observed

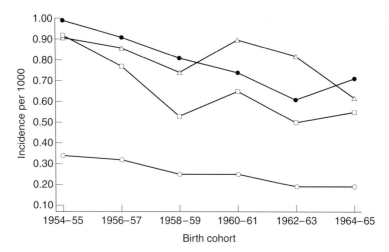

Fig. 1.2.   This graph shows age-stratified incidence of schizophrenia by year of birth. The data for four age groups (males aged 16–17 (○), 18–19 (□), 20–21 (△) and 22–23 (●) years) are taken from Suvisaari et al. (1999). This study followed individuals born from 1954 to 1965 over the period from 1970 to 1991 for schizophrenia. In this figure, we see a cohort effect in the general decline in incidence over birth years – with each age group trending downwards – and the age effect with ages 16–17 years at lowest risk, and ages 20–21 and 22–23 at higher risk.

in later historical periods. The shift from younger age at maximum risk to older age at maximum risk over historical periods may have led some to conclude that, while tuberculosis was on the wane, it had become more lethal to the elderly. Analysing trends by generation, however, revealed that in each generation the peak in rates occurred between 20 and 30 years of age, and that over each succeeding generation rates were declining in an orderly fashion. The disease had not undergone a metamorphosis, nor had the elderly developed a peculiar susceptibility to the disease; instead, experience had changed over successive generations. Understanding this also pointed to early life experience as crucial to risk for the disease.

Graphical display analysis is useful in visually discriminating period and age, or chort and age effects. Data displayed as in Fig. 1.1 discriminates period and age effects, and data displayed as in Fig. 1.2 discriminates cohort and age effects. However, there are limitations to assessing these three effects simultaneously.

Period, age and cohort effects may all be influential in a given secular trend, as is made obvious in the example of tuberculosis. Using ordinary graphical displays, it is not possible to control two while examining the third. Thus, in Figure 1.1, while examining period trends we control for age but not for cohort effects; and in Figure 1.2, while examining cohort trends we control for age but not for period effects. Statistical methods have been developed to examine the three effects simultaneously (e.g. Holford, 1983; Clayton and Schifflers, 1987). However, these methods require additional complex assumptions. Notwithstanding its limitations, graphical display still provides a direct and understandable method of analysis (Case, 1956).

Life-course effects

The structure of age–period–cohort trends emerges from the multitudes of individual life-course effects. Life-course effects capture the longitudinal component of human biological as well as social exposures and existence to the point of disease or risk assessment. Individual life-course effects are framed at each given age within a unique historical period, creating an experience set that is particular to each generation.

Evidence and reason suggest that socioenvironmental factors influence health risk over the lifespan, contributing as early as the prenatal period to adult disease (Kuh and Ben-Shlomo, 1997; Marmot and Wadsworth, 1997; Davey Smith et al., 1997). Evidence for prenatal and childhood exposures contributing to risk of adult disease is perhaps more well known in psychiatry than other fields of study. For example, prenatal nutritional and viral exposures have been linked to risk of schizophrenia, and childhood neglect, abuse and loss have been linked to risk of adult depression. The notion that many prenatal and childhood exposures are socially patterned is also widely accepted. From this starting point, the individual progresses through time, accumulating risk associated with age and historical period.

The relative importance of prenatal, childhood and adult experience in shaping risk for disease, and the importance of cumulative experiences, may vary with specific diseases. Studies at the individual level, for example, indicate that childhood social status and related childhood pulmonary exposures are relatively more influential in tuberculosis, whereas adult social status and adult behaviour are more influential in lung cancer (Davey Smith, 2001). In the case of cardiovascular mortality, there is evidence for independent risk attached to socioeconomic adversity during different phases of life, and for the accumulation of risk associated with socioeconomic adversity (Davey Smith et al., 1997). For this reason, a longitudinal view of individual development is necessary to identify critical periods, to develop a schema for understanding the accumulation of risk and to translate 'vulnerability' to disease into a more specific set of risk factors. This was described by G. Davey Smith in 2001:

Human bodies in different social locations become crystallized reflections of the social experiences within which they have developed. The socially patterned nutritional, health and environmental experiences of the parents and of the individuals concerned influence birthweight, height, weight and lung function, for example, which are in turn important indicators of future health prospects. These biological aspects of bodies (and the history of bodies) should be viewed as frozen social relations . . .

REFERENCES

Case RA (1956) Cohort analysis of mortality rate as an historical or narrative technique. British Journal of Preventative Social Medicine 10, 159–171.

Castle DJ, Scott K, Wessely S, Murray RM (1993) Does social deprivation during gestation and early life predispose to later schizophrenia? Social Psychiatry and Psychiatric Epidemiology 28, 1–4.

Clayton D, Schifflers E (1987) Models for temporal variations in cancer rates, II: age–period–cohort models. Statistics in Medicine 6, 469–481.

Davey Smith G (2001) The uses of 'Uses of Epidemiology'. International Journal of Epidemiology 30, 1146–1155.

Davey Smith G, Hart C, Blane D, Gillis C, Hawthorne V (1997) Lifetime socioeconomic position and mortality: prospective observational study. British Medical Journal 314, 547–552.

Dohrenwend BP, Levav I, Shrout PE et al. (1992) Socioeconomic status and psychiatric disorders: the causation–selection issue. Science 255, 946–952.

Done DJ, Crow TJ, Johnstone EC, Sacker A (1994) Childhood antecedents of schizophrenia and affective illness: social adjustment at ages 7 and 11. British Medical Journal 309, 699–703.

Goldberg EM, Morrison SL (1963) Schizophrenia and social class. British Journal of Psychiatry 109, 785–802.

Holford TR (1983) The estimation of age, period and cohort effects for vital rates. Biometrics 39, 311–324.

Hollingshead AB, Redlich FC (1958) Social Class and Mental Illness. New York: Wiley.

Jones P, Rodgers B, Murray R, Marmot M (1994) Child developmental risk factors for adult schizophrenia in the British 1946 birth cohort. Lancet 344, 1398–1402.

Kuh E, Ben-Shlomo Y (1997) A Life Course Approach to Chronic Disease Epidemiology. Oxford: Oxford University Press.

Lapouse R, Monk MA, Terris M (1956) The drift hypothesis and socioeconomic differentials in schizophrenia. Mental Diseases 46, 978–986.

Link BG, Dohrenwend BP, Skodol AE (1986) Socio-economic status and schizophrenia: noisome occupational characteristics as a risk factor. American Sociological Review 22, 288–292.

Makikyro T, Isohanni M, Moring J et al. (1997) Is a child's risk of early onset schizophrenia increased in the highest social classes? Schizophrenia Research 23, 245–252.

Marmot MG, Wadsworth MEJ (eds.) (1997) Foetal and early childhood environment: long-term health implications. British Medical Bulletin 53, 1–227.

Rose G (1992) The Strategy of Preventive Medicine. Oxford: Oxford University Press.

Schwartz S (1994) The fallacy of the ecologic fallacy: the potential misuse of a concept and the consequences. American Journal of Public Health 84, 819–824.

Schwartz S, Carpenter KM (1999) The right answer for the wrong question: consequences of type III error for public health research. American Journal of Public Health, 89, 1175–1180.

Schwartz S, Susser E (2001) What is a cause? In Psychiatric Epidemiology: Concepts and Method, Susser E, Bromet E, Morabia A, Schwarz S, Gorman J (eds.).

Susser M (1973) Causal Thinking in the Health Sciences. London: Oxford Medical Publications.

Suvisaari JM, Haukka JK, Tanskanen AJ, Lonnqvist JK (1999) Decline in the incidence of schizo-phrenia in Finnish cohorts born from 1954 to 1965. Archives of General Psychiatry 56, 733–740.

Timms D (1998) Gender, social mobility and psychiatric diagnoses. Social Science and Medicine 46, 1235–1247.

Turner RJ, Wagenfeld MO (1967) Occupational mobility and schizophrenia: an assessment of the social causation and social selection hypotheses. American Sociological Review 32, 104–113.

van Os J, Driessen G, Gunther N, Delespaul P (2000) Neighbourhood variation in incidence of schizophrenia. Evidence for person–environment interaction. British Journal of Psychiatry 176, 243–248.

Wiersma D, Giel R, deJong A, Slooff CJ (1983) Social class and schizophrenia in a Dutch cohort. Psychological Medicine 13, 141–150.

Geographical variation in incidence, course and outcome of schizophrenia: a comparison of developing and developed countries

Michaeline Bresnahan[1], Paulo Menezes[2], Vijoy Varma[1] and Ezra Susser[1]

[1]Division of Epidemiology, Columbia University, New York, USA
[2]Department of Preventative Medicine, University of São Paulo, Brazil

Schizophrenia was not identified as a discrete illness until the dawn of the 20th century and was once widely considered a 'disease of civilization'. Later evidence suggested that at least some cases of schizophrenia could be identified in any community at whatever level of development, but the incidence rate of schizophrenia in developing countries is still largely a matter for bold speculation based on minimal data. In the meantime, strong evidence has emerged for a surprising result: the course of schizophrenia is more benign in the developing countries, where treatment options are minimal.

In this chapter, we review the evidence for differences in incidence as well as course of schizophrenia between developing and developed countries. Present day researchers often prefer the more neutral designation of 'low-income' versus 'high-income' countries, which does not imply any universal continuum of economic development. For clarity, however, we retain the term used in the literature we review.

Incidence

In a recent review of schizophrenia incidence studies, the annual incidence rates ranged from 0.04 to 0.58 per 1000 (Eaton, 1999). Because the observed variation is likely to result in part from differences in the methods of individual studies (Bresnahan et al., 2000), its meaning with respect to geographic distribution is unclear. Systematic patterns of variation are obscured by these and other artifacts.

Here we have chosen to examine variation across sociocultural settings by comparing developing and developed countries. This approach is promising, in view of the high contrast between the sociocultural environments in these two settings. In addition, the division has been shown to have predictive value for studies of outcome.

Is the incidence of schizophrenia different in developing and developed countries? Our capacity to answer this question is constrained by the small number of studies conducted in developing countries. The total developing country evidence is slim and includes four published incidence studies (Jablensky et al., 1992; Hickling and Rodgers-Johnson, 1995; Bhugra et al., 1996; Mahy et al., 1999) based on first treatment contact and direct assessments in a defined population. The study locations include rural and urban Chandigarh, Trinidad, Barbados and Jamaica (Table 2.1). (One additional incidence study conducted in Madras (Rajkumar et al., 1993) ascertained cases based on a door-to-door community screening and direct assessment in a defined urban area. However, as the method was different from other studies, and the number of cases small, it has little bearing on the question at hand.)

Among these four developing country studies reporting incidence, the Chandigarh study provides the most important evidence. It was part of the World Health Organization (WHO) Ten Country Study (Jablensky et al., 1992), in which both developed and developing country sites were included. In this landmark project, also referred to as the Determinants of Severe Mental Disorder Study (DOSMeD), the collection of comparable evidence in the same time period offers sound comparison of incidence rates across a variety of sociocultural settings. Furthermore, both an urban and a rural site were studied in Chandigarh.

The Ten Country Study

The Ten Country Study is often cited, in our view mistakenly, as providing the evidence for worldwide 'uniform' incidence and symptom expression of schizophrenia. Twelve centres in ten countries were represented: Denmark (Aarhus), India (Chandigarh urban, Chandigarh rural, Agra), Ireland (Dublin), USA (Honolulu, Rochester), England (Nottingham), Soviet Union (Moscow), Japan (Nagasaki), Czeckslovakia (Prague), Columbia (Cali), Nigeria (Ibadan). Cases were ascertained for 2 years, identifying first-contact patients with nonaffective psychosis in well-defined populations. Equivalent methods of ascertainment, assessment and diagnosis were implemented across sites. Eight sites had sufficiently complete case ascertainment to yield incidence rates. Urban and rural Chandigarh were the only developing country sites among the eight reporting incidence rates.

Two key findings were reported. The first was that the incidence of narrowly defined schizophrenia demonstrated no significant variation across sites. The observation of no significant variation for narrowly defined schizophrenia,

Table 2.1. Selected incidence studies (ICD-9 or CATEGO)

Site	Study Years	Author	Annual incidence rates per 1000		
			S+	SPO	ICD-9
Madras	87–88	Rajkumar et al. (1993)			0.35
Chandigarh Urban	78–80	Jablensky et al. (1992)	0.09	0.25	0.29[a]
Chandigarh Rural	78–80	Jablensky et al. (1992)	0.11	0.35	0.32[a]
Jamaica	1992	Hickling and Rodgers-Johnson (1995)	0.21	0.24	
Trinidad	1990	Bhugra et al. (1996)	0.16	0.22[b]	
Barbados	94–95	Mahy et al. (1999)	0.28	0.32[b]	
Moscow	79–81	Jablensky et al. (1992)	0.12	0.22	0.43[c]
Aarhus	78–80	Jablensky et al. (1992)	0.07	0.11	0.06[a]
Dublin	78–80	Jablensky et al. (1992)	0.09	0.14	0.21[a]
Honolulu	78–80	Jablensky et al. (1992)	0.09	0.09	0.13[a]
Nagasaki	79–81	Jablensky et al. (1992)	0.10	0.16	0.19[a]
Nottingham	78–80	Jablensky et al. (1992)	0.14	0.18	0.17[a]
Cantabria	89–91	Vazquez-Barquero et al. (1995)	0.13		0.19
Ireland	73–	Ninulaain et al. (1987)	0.17		
London	91–92	Goater et al. (1999)			0.22
London	91–93	Bhugra et al. (1997)		0.39[d]	
Salford	74–84	Bamrah et al. (1991)			0.19
Saskatchewan		D'Arcy et al. (1993)			0.10
Vancouver	82–85	Iancano and Beiser (1992)			0.08[e]

Notes:

CATEGO, computer algorithm diagnoses using Present State Exam; ICD, International Classification of Disease – ninth revision – Clinical Modification; S+, narrowly defined schizophrenia; SPO, broadly defined schizophrenia.

To facilitate comparison between developing and developed countries, only incidence study sites reporting CATEGO diagnoses or ICD-9 diagnoses are included in the table. For a more complete view of incidence studies see Eaton (1999).

[a] ICD-9 rates for the WHO Ten Country Study sites were calculated based on cases with 295 diagnoses reported in Jablensky et al. (1992; p. 29).

[b] Rates CATEGO SPO+.

[c] Moscow was a priori a developed country; this may be in error.

[d] Based on total population base and total cases over three reported ethnic groups in two health districts selected for ethnic diversity

[e] Based on mean rate between men and women given.

however, was based on CATEGO S+ diagnoses, which was the definition of 'narrow' schizophrenia in the Ten Country Study. CATEGO S+ criteria focus exclusively on first-rank, positive symptoms during the month before interview using the Present State Examination (PSE). The concordance between S+ and schizophrenia under modern diagnostic systems is not high (Mason et al., 1997). Because of these uncertainties about diagnosis, it is difficult to draw conclusions from S+ variation in the Ten Country Study. The second finding was that incidence of schizophrenia broadly defined demonstrated significant cross-country variation, with the highest rates being reported in Chandigarh, the only developing country sites.

Continuation studies of the initial WHO cohorts at both developed and developing country sites, and rediagnosis of cases using modern criteria, will contribute important information with respect to the generalizability of the S+ findings to schizophrenia currently conceived. *Preliminary* analyses of rediagnosed Chandigarh urban and rural site cases suggest that variation may be substantially greater than the S+ incidence findings would indicate. Cases were rediagnosed according to ICD-10 (World Health Organization, 1992) criteria, based on all information available at last follow-up. In the combined Chandigarh sites ($n=$ 209), lifetime diagnoses were assigned to 141 cases based on information available at 12–15 years of follow-up, to 15 based on information available at 5–11 years follow-up, and to 43 based on information available 0–4 years after intake; rediagnoses for 10 cases are currently unavailable. Based on known cases, urban and rural Chandigarh rates of lifetime ICD-10 F-20 schizophrenia in the original cohort are 1.85 (95% confidence interval (CI) 1.46–2.31) and 2.68 (95% CI 1.84–3.76) per 10000. These rates are intermediate between the rates of broadly defined schizophrenia (urban Chandigarh 3.5, rural Chandigarh 4.2 per 10000) and narrowly defined schizophrenia (urban Chandigarh 0.9, rural Chandigarh 1.1 per 10000) in the original report.

Interpretation of the Chandigarh incidence rates for ICD-10 schizophrenia is limited by the unavailability of similar incidence data from developed country sites in the Ten Country Study. However, somewhat comparable diagnoses are available for the Nottingham site. In a rediagnosis exercise, ICD-10 diagnoses were rendered based on information available at intake. The rate of ICD-10 F-20 schizophrenia was 1.41 per 10000 (95% CI 1.03–1.78) (Brewin et al., 1997). This rate is markedly lower than those reported above for the urban Chandigarh and rural Chandigarh sites. Therefore, comparison of the *preliminary* findings from Chandigarh and reports from Nottingham suggest that for ICD-10 schizophrenia there may be substantial variation across sites, as observed for broadly defined, not narrowly defined, schizophrenia in the original report.

Caribbean studies

The remaining incidence studies were conducted in Caribbean countries not plainly representative of developing countries. The level of socioeconomic development in the three Caribbean countries is relatively high for the developing world. Based on the United Nations Development Programme (1998), Barbados ranked 2nd, Trinidad 13th, and Jamaica 45th highest among developing nations. The health indicators and standards of living for these countries may be considered intermediate on the development continuum.

The three Caribbean studies (Hickling and Rodgers-Johnson, 1995; Bhugra et al., 1996; Mahy et al., 1999) emulated the design used in the WHO Ten Country Study: all patients making first contact with care agencies for a possible schizophrenic episode during a 1-year period were assessed for schizophrenia. The rates per 10000 person-years at risk for narrowly defined schizophrenia (CATEGO S+) were 2.1 (Jamaica), 1.6 (Trinidad) and 2.8 (Barbados). For schizophrenia using a broad CATEGO definition, the rates per 10000 were 2.4 (SPO schizophrenia, Jamaica), 2.2 (SPO+ schizophrenia,Trinidad) and 3.2 (SPO+ schizophrenia, Barbados). It should be noted that the rates for the narrow and broad diagnoses are quite similar, as there were few non-S+ cases reported by these sites. Relative to findings in the Ten Country Study, the point estimates for CATEGO S+ incidence rates in the Caribbean countries (range 1.6–2.8 per 10000) were higher than those reported at any Ten Country Study site (range 0.7–1.4 per 10000). For schizophrenia broadly defined using equivalent diagnostic classifications (SPO, SPO+) the Caribbean rates are higher than those reported by the WHO study developed country sites, except Moscow, and similar to those reported by developing country sites.

What does the total evidence suggest about variation in incidence of schizophrenia between developing and developed countries? Clearly there are insufficient data to support the claim that there is no difference in incidence between these two settings. However, the existing evidence is also insufficient for any inference of systematic variation across developing and developed countries. In sum, a strong case can be made for variation in incidence across place, but a patterned distribution based on country level of development is inconclusive.

Nonaffective acute remitting psychosis

It would be wrong, however, to conclude that no evidence has emerged from incidence studies relating to systematic variation in any nonaffective psychoses between developing and developed countries. Susser and collaborators found evidence for a distinct nonaffective psychotic disorder that mainly occurs in the developing world. Susser and Wanderling (1994) reported a marked variation in incidence of nonaffective acute remitting psychosis (NARP) between developed and developing country settings. The incidence of NARP was 10-fold greater in the developing than developed country settings in the Ten Country Study.

Susser and colleagues have argued that such results support the idea of a distinct disorder. Biological as well as cultural influences are suspected in the aetiology of these psychotic disorders (Collins et al., 1996, 1999). In one study, patients with NARP were more likely to have experienced fever in the 12 weeks preceding onset than controls (odds ratio 6.2).

Moreover, this class of remitting psychotic disorders constitutes a potential source of misclassified cases in studies of schizophrenia. In fact, all patients with NARP that Susser and Wanderling (1994) identified had been diagnosed, by their definition of NARP, with ICD-9 schizophrenia. The influence of NARP on incidence rates of schizophrenia, however, does not explain most of the difference between developed and developing countries in the incidence of schizophrenia broadly defined in the Ten Country Study, or the differential in incidence suspected based on the preliminary data on ICD-10 schizophrenia. Differences remained after removing those with NARP.

Some other differences between developing and developed countries remain unexplained. In particular, differences in the frequencies of psychotic individuals diagnosed as catatonic in the Ten Country Study (10% in developing countries and extremely rare in developed countries) have not been accounted for. Together with the finding of high rates of NARP in developing country settings, the evidence suggests possible aetiologic and disease diversity across the developing/developed divide.

Course and outcome

Scattered early reports that complete remission of schizophrenia was common in developing countries, in spite of the unavailability of treatment, suggested that course and outcome were more favourable in these settings (e.g. Lambo, 1960; Rin and Lin, 1962; German, 1972). The subsequent evolution of evidence did not disturb this initial impression (Murphy and Raman, 1971; Jablensky et al., 1992; Leff et al., 1992) (Table 2.2). A study on the island of Mauritius (Murphy and Raman, 1971), examining 12-year outcomes of all patients with a clinical diagnosis of schizophrenia on first admission to the local hospital, found that 64% had no symptoms and were independent. The authors also compared their results with a British study (Brown et al., 1966) and concluded that schizophrenic psychosis had a better overall prognosis in Mauritius than in Britain.

In this context, the WHO embarked upon an ambitious course of research to examine the issue of varied outcomes in different cultural settings. Two large multi-centre studies, the International Pilot Study of Schizophrenia (IPSS) and the Ten

Table 2.2. Selected studies in developing countries[a]

Author(s)	Location	Number	Duration of follow-up (years)	Followed	Mortality	Course[b]	Clinical outcome	Social functioning and work
Leff et al.[c] (1992)	IPSS: 8 countries; 3 developing countries	727	5	73% (531/727)	5% (52/1065)[d]		Symptoms (approximately)[e]	Social impairment
	Agra					42% best; 10% worst;	69% asymp; 24% psych;	13% severe; 87% mod/mild/none;
	Cali					11% best; 21% worst;	25% asymp; 37% psych;	17% severe; 83% mod/mild/none;
	Ibadan					33% best; 10% worst	68% asymp; 17% psych	19% severe; 81% mod/mild/none
Kulhara and Wig (1978)	Chandigarh	174	4.5–6	57% (100/174)	7% (13/174)	29% no disturbance; 32% chronic disturbance		58% normal role performance 50% normal social and clinical adjustment
Waxler (1979)	Sri Lanka	44	5	96% (42/44)	2% (1/44)	40% best; 29% worst	45% asymp; 69% not psychotic	
Lo and Lo (1977)	Hong Kong	133	10	62% (82/133)	3% (4/133)	21% rem; 12% worst	65% remission, or relapse with mild deterioration; 9% in hospital	43% independent normal functioning; 26% dependent
Thara et al. (1994)	Madras	90	10	84% (76/90)	10% (9/90)	14% best; 7% worst		60% employed
Leon (1989)	Cali	101	10	83% (84/101)	2% (2/101)	8% best; 13% continuous severe	51% complete/partial recovery; 25% overt psychosis/deterioration	50% no/min/mild impairment; 11% severe impairment
Murphy and Raman (1971)	Mauritius	90	12	98%	8% (7/90)	59% best; 21% worst	64% no symptoms and independent	
Dube et al. (1984)	Agra	140[d]	13–14	69% (96/140)[d]	12% (17/140)[d]	46% best	59% recovered 'normal'; 33% residual/active schizophrenia	59% normal global clinical/social outcome
Lee et al. (1998)	Hong Kong	100	15	70% (70/100)	11% (11/100)	22% best; 2% worst	53% recovered (last 2 years)	54% employed in last 2 years + 23% full-time housework; 67% never received disability

| Tsoi and Wong (1991) | Singapore | 330 | 15 | 88% (292/330) | 15% (48/330) | 32% recover | 55% not in treatment; 17% inpatient |
| Susser et al. (1998); Mojtabai et al. (2001) | Chandigarh urban and rural | 209 | 15 | 57% 118/209 | 12% 24/209 | | 32% working and not in treatment; 48% working |

Notes:

asmyp, asymptomatic; psych, psychotic; mod, moderate; min, minimal; rem, lasting remission; recov, recovered; SMR, standardized mortality ratio.

[a] Follow-up for 5 or more years; only data from last follow-up of the cohort is included unless otherwise indicated. The percentages for course and outcome pertain to those where a given outcome is known.

[b] Best, single episode complete recovery; worst, continuous, episode of inclusion continues throughout follow-up.

[c] Data on outcome for IPSS study sites in developed countries appear in Table 2.3.

[d] Data based on entire study sample; outcomes reported for schizophrenia.

[e] Estimates based on Figure 1, p. 136, Leff et al., 1992.

Table 2.3. Selected studies in developed countries[a]

Author(s)	Location	Number	Duration of follow-up (years)	Followed	Mortality	Course[b]	Clinical outcome	Social functioning and work
Leff et al. (1992)[c]	IPSS: 8 countries; 5 developed countries	727	5	73% (531/727)	5% (52/1065)[d]		Symptoms (approximately)[e]	Social impairment
	Aarhus					6% best; 40% worst	5% asymp; 63% psych	50% sev; 50% mild/mod/none
	London					5% best; 14% worst	12% asymp; 40% psych	27% sev; 73% mild/mod/none
	Moscow					6% best; 21% worst	2% asymp; 58% psych	23% sev; 77% mild/mod/none
	Prague					9% best; 23% worst	42% asymp; 41% psych	30% sev; 70% mild/mod/none
	Washington DC					17% best; 23% worst	6% asymp; 47% psych	25% sev; 75% mild/mod/none
Scottish Schizophrenia Research Group (1992)	Scotland	49	5	86% (42/49)	2% (1/49)	18% good	46% no symptoms	75% male unemployment
Shepherd et al. (1983)	Buckinghamshire	49	5	100% (49/49)	2% (1/49)	22% best; 43% poor	59% no first rank symptoms at 5-year f-u	30% mod/sev social impairment; 24% mod/sev work impairment
Mason et al. (1995, 1996); Harrison et al. (1994, 1996)	Nottingham	67	13	87% (58/67)	7% (5/67)	25% not readmitted; 33% continuous course	48% psychotic at 11–13 years 49% no/mild symptoms at 11–13 years	32% good social adjustment; 43% poor 37% employed
Wiersma et al. (1998)	The Netherlands	82[d]	15	77% (63/82)	11% (9/82)	18.3% good; 11% worst	27% complete remission	53% receiving disability/unemployment benefit at 2-year f-u
Helgason (1990)	Iceland	107	20	98% of living (82/84)	21% (23/107)		26% no/minor symptoms; 21% severe	45% socially isolated; 5% 'normal interaction' 17% fulltime employed

Notes:

asymp, asymptomatic; mod, moderate; sev, severe; f-u, follow-up. [a] Follow-up for 5 or more years; only data from last follow-up of cohort included unless otherwise indicated. The percentages for course and outcomes pertain to those where a given outcome is known. [b] Best, single episode complete recovery; worst, continuous, episode of inclusion continues throughout follow-up; good, no relapse, no schizophrenic symptoms at follow-up or first episode followed by complete or partial remission; poor, no return to normality. [c] Data on outcome for IPSS study sites in developing countries appear in Table 2.2. [d] Data based on entire study sample; outcomes reported for schizophrenia (Leff et al., 1992), and for functional psychosis (Wiersma et al., 1998). [e] Estimates based on Figure 1, p. 196, Leff et al. 1992.

Country Study described above, forged the methodological basis for studying outcome in transcultural settings. These studies still provide the best available evidence.

International Pilot Study of Schizophrenia

The IPSS, carried out simultaneously in nine countries (World Health Organization, 1973, 1979), had a prospective design and implemented standardized instruments for data collection and assessments. The countries included were Columbia (Cali), Denmark (Aarhus), India (Agra), England (London), Nigeria (Ibadan), USA (Washington DC), Czech Republic (Prague), Soviet Union (Moscow) and Taiwan (Taipei). Of the 1202 patients identified for study, 811 were diagnosed with schizophrenia; 75% of those with an initial diagnosis of schizophrenia were assessed at 2-year follow-up.

The IPSS strengthened the idea that the outcome of schizophrenia might be better in developing than in developed countries (Tables 2.2 and 2.3). The result is illustrated by the overall outcome. Overall outcome was rated in five categories based on combined criteria in three outcome domains: percentage of follow-up time spent in psychotic episode, presence or absence of social impairment, and type of remission after episodes. 'Good' represents the two best categories, and 'poor' the two worst categories of overall outcome. The three centres reporting the highest proportion of patients with 'good' overall outcome were in developing countries (Agra 66%, Cali 53%, and Ibadan 86%). The three centres reporting the highest proportion of patients with 'poor' overall outcome were in developed countries (Aarhus 48%, London 41%, and Washington 45%).

Eight of the nine centres went on to participate in a 5-year follow-up study (follow-up 74%), in which the outcome profile in developing country sites remained superior to that found in developed country sites (Leff et al., 1992). Approximately two-thirds of the patients at the Ibadan site and two-thirds of the patients at the Agra site were asymptomatic at the 5-year follow-up, and the pattern of course for these two sites was exceptional, in both the high proportion of patients with best course and the low proportion of patients with worst course ratings. Clinical course reports from Cali were more comparable to those from developed country sites.

Long-term outcomes (10 years or more) were reported separately by two developing country sites and one developed country site, extending the evidence. Leon (1989) was able to trace and assess 83% of the Cali IPSS patients with an initial diagnosis of schizophrenia 10 years after inclusion. Overall clinical outcome at 10 years was good (complete or partial recovery) in 51% of the patients. Dube et al. (1984) traced and examined 62 of the 140 IPSS patients in Agra 13–14 years after inclusion. Sustained remission was observed in 46% of those with an initial diagnosis of schizophrenia, and 59% were judged to be clinically 'normal' at assessment.

Carpenter and Strauss (1991) assessed 40% of the original Washington DC IPSS cohort at 11 years and found little change in the functioning of patients (in terms of social contacts, employment or symptoms) compared with functioning at 2 years.

The Ten Country Study

The IPSS was followed by another study coordinated by the WHO, the Ten Country Study described above (Sartorius et al., 1986; Jablensky et al., 1992). Data on outcome after 2 years were obtained for 78% ($n = 1078$) of the original sample. The outcome for patients diagnosed with broad schizophrenia was more favourable in developing countries than in developed countries, for example, on five of the six measures of 'best outcomes' examined.

Though limited, these reports support the view that patients fare better, on average, in the developing countries. Additional evidence from follow-up at the Chandigarh sites raises the possibility that there may be greater *variability* in outcomes in developing countries (Mojtabai et al., 2001). In Chandigarh, there was a group of subjects that did poorly in the first 2 years ($n = 15$); nearly half had died by the time of the 15-year follow-up. In two patients, malnutrition was a contributing cause of death. These findings are generally consistent with another study conducted in Brazil. Menezes and Mann (1996) carried out a 2-year follow-up of a prevalent sample of 120 patients with schizophrenia who had been consecutively admitted to psychiatric hospitals of a catchment area of São Paulo, Brazil and found an eightfold increased risk of dying compared with the general population (standardized mortality ratio 8.4), and a dramatically increased risk for suicide.

Several explanations of the fundamental differences in outcome between developed and developing countries in the Ten Country Study beg consideration. Artifact is one potential explanation. It is possible that the disease 'mix' in developing countries (higher incidence of non-S+ schizophrenia, higher proportion NARP) is at the foundation of the improved prognosis. However, improved or better course and outcomes apply to both acute and nonacute onset disease, and that broadly and narrowly defined (Jablensky et al., 1992). The 'mix' may be different, but it does not explain all of the difference in prognosis. Other explanations relating to background characteristics of the underlying samples and ascertainment bias have been considered (Jablensky et al., 1992; Hopper and Wanderling, 2000); however, none has been shown to account for the difference.

International Study of Schizophrenia

Further development of this finding has been taken on by the WHO International Study of Schizophrenia (ISoS). This is a collaborative project based on numerous cohorts including the original IPSS and Ten Country Study cohorts. Using the ISoS sample, Hopper and Wanderling (2000) replicated the developed versus developing differential both in the long term (>13 years follow-up), and under ICD-10 diagnostic criteria for schizophrenia. They demonstrated that various biases (ascertainment bias, bias in loss to follow-up, diagnostic issues including NARP and classification systems for developing/developed countries) could not account for the differences in outcome.

Possible explanations for differences in outcome

It appears, therefore, that some aspect of the economic or cultural circumstance in developing countries may provide a more therapeutic context for recovery. The most commonly proposed explanations fall into four categories: family relationships, informal economies, segregation of the mentally ill and community cohesion.

Family relationships

Family relationships may be more conducive to recovery in developing country settings. In India and some other developing countries, families are closely involved in treatment, support, recuperation and rehabilitation of individuals with schizophrenia (Susser et al., 1996). An individual is never removed from the family's care; social integration within the family setting is not disrupted. Furthermore, data support the view that family expressed emotion, a characteristic predicting relapse in developed country populations, may differ in developing country settings (Leff et al., 1987; Wig et al., 1987).

Informal economies

Students of developing countries often argue that, in subsistence economies, reintegration into work roles is the rule rather than the exception (Warner, 1985). Based on data from developed countries, reintegration into work roles would seem to be beneficial (Bell and Lysaker, 1997). In low-income countries, informal economies may provide more diverse opportunities for this reintegration to occur.

Segregation of the mentally ill

In developing countries, individuals with mental illness are less likely to be segregated in hospitals or other institutions. It has also been suggested that mental illness may be less stigmatized in developing countries, although there are no convincing data on this point.

Community cohesion

Communities may differ on dimensions of social integration and isolation, potentially creating contexts that are more or less therapeutic, affecting chances for recovery.

Societal basis

The bases for each of these speculations are societal phenomena. That developing countries better serve those with schizophrenia than developed countries stands in contrast with what is known about the benefit to individuals of modern therapies (e.g. medication, family interventions), treatments often unavailable in these settings. One possible explanation is that societal level processes and system features of treatment as determinants of disease outcomes are responsible.

Conclusion

The contrasting experiences of developed and developing countries with respect to schizophrenia may be interpreted as providing evidence for socioenvironmental influences in this disorder. The findings in incidence rates are inconclusive; the evidence for differences in outcome, however, is clear and convincing.

Two main findings regarding the incidence of schizophrenia emerged from the landmark Ten Country Study: first, the incidence of schizophrenia narrowly defined showed little variation across sites; and second, the incidence of schizophrenia broadly defined was significantly higher in developing than developed country sites. The underpinnings of the narrow definition have been questioned, but the alternative posed by the broad definition is probably overinclusive. While we await incidence rates based on rediagnosis using modern diagnostic systems, the question of variation in incidence rates remains unresolved.

Course and outcome appear to be more favourable in developing countries. In light of the scarcity of treatment options, this finding is remarkable. A point deserving further investigation is that there may be a greater risk of adverse outcomes, as suggested by mortality rates in two developing countries.

REFERENCES

Bamrah JS, Freeman HL, Goldberg DP (1991) Epidemiology of schizophrenia in Salford, 1974–84. Changes in an urban community over ten years. British Journal of Psychiatry 159, 802–810.

Bell MD, Lysaker PH (1997) Clinical benefits of paid work activity in schizophrenia: one year follow-up. Schizophrenia Bulletin 23, 317–328.

Bhugra D, Hilwig M, Hossein B et al. (1996) First-contact incidence rates of schizophrenia in Trinidad and one-year follow-up. British Journal of Psychiatry 169, 587–592.

Bhugra D, Leff J, Mallett R, Der G, Corridau B, Rudge S (1997) Incidence and outcome of schizophrenia in whites, African Caribbeans and Asians in London. Psychological Medicine 27, 791–798.

Bresnahan MA, Brown AS, Schaefer CA, Begg MD, Wyatt RJ, Susser ES (2000) Incidence and cumulative risk of treated schizophrenia in the Prenatal Determinants of Schizophrenia study. Schizophrenia Bulletin 26, 297–308.

Brewin J, Cantwell R, Dalkin T et al. (1997) Incidence of schizophrenia in Nottingham. A comparison of two cohorts, 1978–80 and 1992–94. British Journal of Psychiatry 171, 140–144.

Brown GH, Bone M, Dalison B, Wing JK (1966) Schizophrenia and Social Care. London: Oxford University Press.

Carpenter WT, Strauss JS (1991) The prediction of outcome in schizophrenia IV: Eleven-year follow-up of the Washington IPSS cohort. Journal of Nervous and Mental Disease 179, 517–525.

Collins PY, Wig NN, Day R et al. (1996) Psychosocial and biological aspects of acute brief psychoses in three developing country sites. Psychiatric Quarterly 67, 177–193.

Collins PY, Varma VK, Wig NN, Mojtabai R, Day R, Susser E (1999) Fever and acute brief psychosis in urban and rural settings in north India. British Journal of Pyschiatry 173, 520–524.

d'Arcy C, Rawson NSB, Lydick E, Epstein R (1993) The Epidemiology of Treated Schizophrenia Saskatchewan 1976–1990. Gronigen, the Netherlands: World Psychiatric Association, Section of Epidemiology and Community Psychiatry.

Dube KC, Kumar N, Dube S (1984) Long term course and outcome of the Agra cases in the International Pilot Study of Schizophrenia. Acta Psychiatrica Scandinavica 70, 170–179.

Eaton WW (1999) Evidence for universality and uniformity of schizophrenia around the world: assessment and implications. In Search for the Causes of Schizophrenia, Vol. IV: Balance of the Century, WF Gattaz and H Hafner, eds. Berlin: Springer-Verlag, pp. 21–33.

German N (1972) Aspects of clinical psychiatry in sub-Saharan Africa. British Journal of Psychiatry 121, 461–479.

Goater N, King M, Cole E et al. (1999) Ethnicity and outcome of psychosis. British Journal of Psychiatry 175, 34–42.

Harrison G, Mason P, Glazebrook C, Medley I, Croudace T, Docherty S (1994) Residence of incident cohort of psychotic patients after 13 years of follow up. British Medical Journal 308, 813–816.

Harrison G, Croudace T, Mason P, Glazebrook C, Medley I (1996) Predicting the long-term outcome of schizophrenia. Psychological Medicine 26, 697–705.

Helgason L (1990) Twenty years' follow-up of first psychiatric presentation for schizophrenia: what could have been prevented? Acta Psychiatrica Scandinavica 81, 231–235.

Hickling FW, Rodgers-Johnson P (1995) The incidence of first contact schizophrenia in Jamaica. British Journal of Psychiatry 167, 193–196.

Hopper K, Wanderling J (2000) Revisiting the developed versus developing country distinction in course and outcome in schizophrenia: Results from ISoS, the WHO colloaborative follow-up project. Schizophrenia Bulletin 26, 835–846.

Iancano WG, Beiser M (1992) Are males more likely than females to develop schizophrenia? American Journal of Psychiatry 149, 1070–1074.

Jablensky A, Sartorius N, Ernberg G et al. (1992) Schizophrenia: manifestations, incidence and course in different cultures. Psychological Medicine, Monograph Supplement 20. Cambridge: Cambridge University Press.

Kulhara P, Wig NN (1978) The chronicity of schizophrenia in North West India: results of a follow-up study. British Journal of Psychiatry 132, 186–190.

Lambo TA (1960) Further neuropsychiatric observations in Nigeria. British Medical Journal 2, 1696–1704.

Lee PWH, Lieh-Mak F, Wong MC, Fung ASM, Mak KY, Lam J (1998) The 15-year outcome of Chinese patients with schizophrenia in Hong Kong. Canadian Journal of Psychiatry 43, 706–713.

Leff J, Wig NN, Gosh A et al. (1987) Influence of relatives' expressed emotion on the course of schizophrenia in Chandigarh. British Journal of Psychiatry 151, 166–173.

Leff J, Sartorius N, Jablensky A, Korten A, Ernberg G (1992) The International Pilot Study of Schizophrenia: five year follow-up findings. Psychological Medicine 22, 131–145.

Leon CA (1989) Clinical course and outcome of schizophrenia in Cali, Columbia: a 10-year follow-up study. Journal of Nervous and Mental Disease 177, 593–606.

Lo WH, Lo T (1977) A ten-year follow-up study of Chinese schizophrenics in Hong Kong. British Journal of Psychiatry 131, 63–66.

Mahy G, Mallett R, Leff J, Bhugra D (1999) First-contact incidence rate of schizophrenia on Barbados. British Journal of Psychiatry 175, 28–33.

Mason P, Harrison G, Glazebrook C, Medley I, Dalkin T, Croudace T (1995) Characteristics of outcome in schizophrenia at 13 years. British Journal of Psychiatry 167, 596–603.

Mason P, Harrison G, Glazebrook C Medley, I Croudace T (1996) The course of schizophrenia over 13 years. A report from the International Study on Schizophrenia (ISoS) coordinated by the World Health Organization (1996) British Journal of Psychiatry 169, 580–586.

Mason P, Harrison G, Croudace T, Glazebrook C, Medley I (1997) The predictive validity of a diagnosis of schizophrenia. British Journal of Psychiatry 178, 321–327.

Menezes PR, Mann AH (1996) Mortality among patients with nonaffective functional psychoses in the city of São Paulo. Revista de Saúde Pública 30, 304–309.

Mojtabai R, Varma VK, Malhotra S et al. (2001) Mortality and long-term course in schizophrenia with a 2-year poor course: a study in a developing country. British Journal of Psychiatry 178, 71–75.

Murphy HBM, Raman AC (1971) The chronicity of schizophrenia in indigenous tropical peoples: results of a twelve-year follow-up survey. British Journal of Psychiatry 118, 489–497.

Ninulaain M, O'Hare A, Walsh D (1987) Incidence of schizophrenia in Ireland. Psychological Medicine 17, 943–948.

Rajkumar S, Padmavati R, Thara R, Sarada Menon M (1993) Incidence of schizophrenia in an urban community in Madras. Indian Journal of Psychiatry 35, 18–21.

Rin H, Lin TY (1962) Mental illness among Formosan Aborigines as compared with the Chinese in Taiwan. Journal of Mental Science 108, 134–146.

Sartorius N, Jablensky A, Korten A et al. (1986) Early manifestations and first-contact incidence of schizophrenia in different cultures. Psychological Medicine 16, 909–928.

Scottish Schizophrenia Research Group (1992) The Scottish first episode schizophrenia study VIII. Five-year follow-up: clinical and psychosocial findings. British Journal of Psychiatry 161, 496–500.

Shepherd M, Watt D, Falloon I, Smeeton N (1983) The natural history of schizophrenia: a five-year follow-up study of outcome and prediction in a representative sample of schizophrenics. Psychological Medicine, Monograph Supplement 15. Cambridge: Cambridge University Press.

Susser E, Wanderling J (1994) Epidemiology of nonaffective acute remitting psychosis vs schizophrenia. Archives General Psychiatry 51, 294–301.

Susser E, Collins P, Schanzer B, Varma VK, Gittelman M (1996) Can we learn from the care of persons with mental illness in developing countries? American Journal of Public Health 86, 926–928.

Susser E, Varma VK, Mattoo SK et al. (1998) Long-term course of acute brief psychosis in a developing country setting. British Journal of Psychiatry 173, 226–230.

Thara R, Henrietta M, Joseph, A, Rajkumar S, Eaton WW (1994) Ten-year course of schizophrenia – the Madras longitudinal study. Acta Psychiatrica Scandinavica 90, 329–336.

Tsoi WF, Wong KE (1991) A 15-year follow-up study of Chinese schizophrenic patients. Acta Psychiatrica Scandinavica 84, 1248–1253.

United Nations Development Programme (1998) Human Development Report. New York: United Nations.

Vazquez-Barquero JL, Cuesta Nunez MJ, de la Varga M et al. (1995) The Cantabria first episode schizophrenia study: a summary of general findings. Acta Psychiatrica Scandinavica 91, 156–162.

Warner R (1985) Recovery from Schizophrenia: Psychiatry and Political Economy. London: Routledge & Kegan Paul.

Waxler NE (1979) Is outcome for schizophrenia better in non-industrial societies? The case of Sri Lanka. Journal of Nervous and Mental Disease 167, 144–158.

Wig NN, Menon DK, Bedi H et al. (1987) Distribution of expressed emotion component in relatives of schizophrenic patients in Aarhus and Chandigarh. British Journal of Psychiatry 151, 160–165.

Wiersma D, Nienhuis FJ, Slooff CJ, Giel R (1998) Natural course of schizophrenic disorders: a 15-year follow-up of a Dutch incidence cohort. Schizophrenia Bulletin 24, 75–85.

World Health Organization (1973) The International Pilot Study of Schizophrenia. Vol. 1. Geneva: World Health Organization.

World Health Organization (1979) Schizophrenia: An International Follow-up Study. Chichester, UK: Wiley.

World Health Organization (1992) Manual of International Statistical Classification of Diseases, Injuries and Causes of Death, 10th edn. Geneva: World Health Organization.

3

Temporal variation in the incidence, course and outcome of schizophrenia

Michaeline Bresnahan[1], Jane Boydell[2], Robin Murray[2] and Ezra Susser[1]

[1]Division of Epidemiology, Columbia University, New York, USA
[2]Institute of Psychiatry, Kings College London, UK

In 1871, Maudsley presented a paper entitled 'Is Insanity on the Increase?' (Maudsley, 1872). Over 100 years later, Der published a paper entitled 'Is Schizophrenia disappearing?' (Der et al, 1990). Investigations of time trends in schizophrenia encompass centuries of disease reports and records, and generations of research. In this chapter, we will examine the evidence for secular trends in the incidence and outcome of schizophrenia.

Time trends are of sustained research interest because they address a basic question: Are things getting better or worse? A quantitative answer to this question is central to health services planning: it provides a means to anticipate the future, and a means to judge past efforts. The analysis of time trends has yet another purpose. Examining secular trends may also contribute to our understanding of the nature and the determinants of disease. In seeking to describe temporal variations in a population's disease experience, we may obtain the first glimpse of factors influencing the occurrence and shaping the outcome of disorders. An underlying shift in the human gene pool can only occur over a great deal of time; in contrast, changes in the social, biological and physical environment may occur over a shorter span of time. These environmental influences are potentially reflected in variation in rates of disease over years and decades. In this endeavour, we are limited by the types of information available to establish these trends, particularly in psychiatric disorders, and must appreciate the implications of these limitations as we wend our way through these time effects.

Time trends in incidence

The 19th century: the growth of asylums

In the historical epidemiology of schizophrenia, the fulcrum of interest resides in the 19th century. The pace and scope of change in the social environment was

34

unprecedented in human history, with dramatic increases in population and the industrialization of many western countries. A heated debate developed in both Europe and North America, not only among psychiatrists but also among the general public, over whether insanity was increasing. One view was that there was a genuine increase in incidence; indeed, some have subsequently hypothesized that schizophrenia is a modern disease ushered in by these social transformations (Torrey, 1980; Hare, 1983). There are, however, many alternative explanations for the rising asylum populations in both Europe and the USA, which suggest that there was no increase in the occurrence of mental disease.

That there was a perceived 'fearful increase' in the number of individuals in need of asylum care is not contested (Rosen, 1959). Proponents of the view that the increase represented something other than increasing incidence offer many explanations implicating changes in the visibility, definition and provision of treatment for mental illness. Some consider that rapid urbanization meant that the seriously mentally ill could no longer be contained in communities as they had been in previously largely rural society (Scull, 1984). Perhaps related to these social changes, the view of insanity and of 'what constituted committable madness' may also have been expanding over the period of increase. (Scull 1984, p. 434). Even the mere existence of an asylum system has been seen as a possible cause of the increase – creating the need for care by posing an alternative to family care, and creating incentives for use and expansion of the system (e.g. Maudsley, 1877).

Credible arguments have been made, however, that the increasing asylum population indicated a real increase in mental illness. Though the contribution of schizophrenia to the trend is a matter of conjecture, some modern commentators have argued that the increase in insanity reflected an increase in the incidence of schizophrenia. The absence or rarity of schizophrenia in medical and literary descriptions of madness prior to the 1800s is used to buttress this argument. The trend has been explained variously as resulting from a greater number of vulnerable individuals surviving to the age of illness (lower infant and child mortality rates), and the increasing risk associated with modernization. Urbanization may have carried specific risk related to social changes in family and community structures, the nature of work (Cooper and Sartorius, 1977) and the spread of infectious disease (Torrey, 1980).

Unfortunately, the only data available on the time trend from the 19th century are on treated patients, and are prevalence not incidence data. Although historical studies of the treated prevalence of insanity in the 19th century are intriguing, conflicting interpretations of the evidence have not been, and indeed may never be, resolved (Goldhammer and Marshall, 1953; Cooper and Sartorius, 1977; Torrey, 1980; Hare, 1983; Scull, 1984; Jeste et al., 1985; Bark, 1988; Shepherd, 1993).

The 20th century

For most of the 20th century, the assumption was that the incidence of schizophrenia was relatively unchanging. It was only towards the end of the 20th century that the assumption of constant incidence came under intense scientific scrutiny. The evidence suggests that, if anything, the rate of schizophrenia declined over this century.

Both the trend and the uncertainty of the data are evident in a study in Wales that 'bookends' a 100-year period by comparing hospital utilization rates in two periods, 1894–96 and 1996 (Healy et al., 2001). This study also attempts to address one of the most vexing limitations of prior historical work: diagnostic uncertainty. The research was based on hospitalized cases arising in an area in Wales with relatively stable population size, urbanicity and ethnic mix over the 100 years captured. Using archival records, the 1894–96 cases were rediagnosed under ICD-10 (World Health Organization, 1992) criteria. Based on the newly rendered chart diagnoses, it was found that the annual rate of first hospitalizations for schizophrenia was not much different in 1996 than during the period 1894–96 (in 1996 0.9 and in 1894–96 0.7 per 10000, age 15–55 years). Assuming that treatment was far less accessible in 1894–6 than in 1996 (a reasonable assumption even though there are no empirical data to demonstrate this), the result of this rate comparison supports the view that the incidence of schizophrenia was either stable or declining.

Examining time trends: age–period–cohort effects

While data are insufficient for definite conclusions about changes over the centuries, with the advent of psychiatric registries and diagnostic systems we can now examine time trends in more detail. For the analyses of these data, epidemiologists call on the methods discussed in Chapter 1. Briefly, changes in incidence rates over time are measured in three metrics: age, period and cohort. Each indicate different underlying processes. Changes in the rates of disease over age reflect the human life cycle. Changes in the rates of disease measured over calendar years (historical period) reflect period effects and are potential indicators of factors acting near or at the time of disease onset (e.g. changes in diagnostic criteria and diagnostic practices). Changes in rates of disease measured over birth years reflect cohort effects and are potential indicators of early experience (e.g. prenatal exposures) as well as cumulative experience of groups of individuals born at a certain time. Age, period and cohort effects tend to be entangled, so it is important to specify which you are focusing on in the analysis of trends.

Declining incidence: period effects?

In the last two decades of the 20th century, reports started appearing of a possible decrease in the incidence of schizophrenia in several developed countries (e.g. Scotland, England and Wales, New Zealand, Denmark), beginning in the 1960s and extending into the 1990s (Table 3.1). The decline was usually reported as a period trend, that is a trend in rates reported over calendar years rather than over age or birth years. Therefore, we will first consider the hypothesized decline as a period effect. Period effects are of great interest because they may reflect changes in the environment proximal to the onset of illness. These would include aetiological influences such as head trauma or social environment.

Most studies have shown a decline in schizophrenia as defined by ICD-8 or ICD-9 criteria (World Health Organization, 1967, 1978; Joyce, 1987; Eagles et al., 1988; Der et al., 1990; Geddes et al., 1993; Munk-Jørgensen, 1995; Osby et al., 2001; Waddington and Youssef, 1994). Comparison between studies is difficult, however, because different methodologies and different definitions of schizophrenia have been used. In addition, many of these studies obtained diagnoses from routine case registers of uncertain reliability.

Considerable attention has been paid to establishing the validity of this period trend, as there are a number of potential sources of artifact (Kendell et al., 1993). For example, changes in the underlying age structure of the population can give rise to misleading declines in incidence when there is a decline in the number of individuals in the population who are at high risk ages for illness; age standardization of rates remove the influence of such age effects. Period trends reflecting something other than changes in underlying incidence can also emerge from ascertainment varying with changing treatment systems or diagnostic practices.

The observed decline in incidence in recent decades corresponds to a time of great service change in developed countries. Treatment systems were increasingly emphasizing community-based care. A shift from inpatient to outpatient care might account for findings of decline in studies based solely on first admissions (Harrison et al., 1991). However, several studies of incidence of treatment contacts – outpatient, inpatient and daypatient – support the period decline in incidence (Eagles et al., 1988; de Alarcon et al., 1990, Munk-Jørgensen and Mortensen, 1992; Brewin et al., 1997). There has been no indication that the proportion of never-treated cases has increased over this period, ruling out a final effect of service change in accounting for the decline.

Another threat to the validity of the period decline is changing diagnostic practices. Diagnoses are susceptible to change over time as diagnostic fashions come and go. This could lead to the impression of rate change even though the underlying population is experiencing no such change in the true rates of disorder. There was a shift in diagnostic practices with the introduction of effective treatments for disorders other than schizophrenia (e.g. lithium; Parker et al., 1985) and, with the publication of DSM-III (American Psychiatric Association, 1980), towards a narrower diagnosis of schizophrenia. The movement towards narrower diagnostic criteria for schizophrenia has not yet been excluded as a viable explanation of the observed decline in rates.

Table 3.1. Temporal variation in the incidence of schizophrenia: recent studies

Study	Location	Diagnosis	Case source	Birth years	Case detection interval	Incidence (percentage change)[a]
Boydell et al. (2001)	South London, UK	OPCRIT RDC	Case register Maudsley Hospital: first out/inpatient treatment		1965–97	Increase, doubled
Osby et al. (2001)	Stockholm, Sweden	ICD-8, ICD-9	Inpatient register: first admission		1978–94	Schiz: decrease; Schiz + paranoid psychosis: no change
Preti and Miotto (2000)	Italy	ICD-9	ISTAT all hospitals: first admission		1984–94	Increase
Allardyce et al. (2000)	Scotland	OPCRIT ICD-10, DSM-IV, clinical diagnosis	ISD and register: first treatment contact		1979–98	OPCRIT ICD-10, DSM-IV: no change; Clinical diagnosis: decrease
Suvisaari et al. (1999a)	Finland	ICD-8 and ICD-9; code by DSM-II-R criteria	Registers: first admission	1954–65[b]	1970–91	Schiz: decrease (M: −32.9%; F: −29.3%); Paranoid psychosis: increase
Brewin et al. (1997)	Nottingham, UK	ICD-10; consensus diagnosis	First treatment contact		1978–94[c]	Schiz: decrease (M + F −38.3%)
Balestrieri et al. (1997)	South Verona, Italy	ICD-10	Register: first treatment contact	1947–74[d]	1979–95	Schiz: decrease (M + F −88.9%)
Jones et al. (1997)	Tasmania, Australia	ICD-9	MH Registry treatment	1945–60[d]	1965–90	No decrease (M); decrease (F)
Takei et al. (1996)	Scotland	ICD-9	CSA: first admission	1923–73[b]	1966–90	Decrease (M −55%; F −39%)
Oldehinkel and Giel (1995)	Groningen, the Netherlands	ICD-9	Case register: first treatment contact		1976–90	No trend observed
Geddes et al. (1993)	Scotland	ICD-9	First admission		1969–88	Decrease (M −42.8%; F −57.1%)
Kendell et al. (1993)	Edinburgh, Scotland	ICD-9 OPCRIT RDC, DSM-III-R, ICD-10	First admission		1971–89	Inconclusive
van Os et al. (1993)	France	INSERM Codes			1973–82	No trend observed (M +25%; F −18.1%)
de Salvia et al. (1993)	Portogruaro, Italy	ICD-9	Case register: first treatment contact		1982–89	No trend observed
Munk-Jørgensen and Mortensen (1992)	Denmark	ICD-8	Registry: first admission daypatient and inpatient		1971–87	Decrease (M + F −50%)
Harrison et al. (1991)	Nottingham, UK	ICD-8/9	Register: first treatment contact		1975–87	No significant change (M + F −10.5%)
Castle et al. (1991)	Camberwell, UK	ICD-9, RDC, DSM-III; structured diagnosis/case reviews	Registry: first treatment contact		1965–84	Increase (UK born: +43.2% (RDC))
Bamrah et al. (1991)	Salford, UK	ICD-9; structured diagnosis/case reviews	Registry: first treatment contact		1974–84	Increase (M + F +64.7%)
Hafner and Gattaz (1991)	Manheim, Germany	ICD-9, CATEGO S+			1965–80	Stable, no significant change

Study	Country/Region	Diagnostic criteria	Case definition	Interval	Result
Der et al. (1990)	UK	Administrative diagnosis	First admission	M: 1970–78 F: 1970–86	Decrease (M −40%; F −50%)
de Alarcon et al. (1990)	Oxford, UK	Administrative diagnosis	First treatment contact	1975–86	Decrease (M); inconclusive (F)
Folnegovic et al. (1990)	Croatia	ICD-7, ICD-8, ICD-9; administrative diagnosis	First admission	1965–84	No significant change
Eagles et al. (1988)	Aberdeen, Scotland	ICD-8, ICD-9	Case register: first treatment contact	1969–84	Decrease (M + F −54%)
Joyce (1987)	New Zealand	–	First admissions	1967–77	Decrease (M + F −9%)
Munk-Jorgensen (1986)	Denmark	ICD-8	Psychiatric register: first admission	1970–84	Decrease (M −37%)
Munk-Jorgensen and Jorgensen (1986)	Denmark	ICD-8	Psychiatric register: first admission	1970–84	Decrease (F −44%)
Eagles and Whalley (1985)	Scotland	Discharge diagnosis, ICD-8	First admission	1969–78	Decrease (M + F −39.9%)
Parker et al. (1985)	New South Wales, Australia	ICD-8/9	First admission	1967–77	Decrease (M + F −9%)

Notes:

[a] Percentage change as [rate last year–rate first year]/rate first year or the rate change provided by authors.

[b] Age-period cohort analysis included.

[c] Compared 1978–80 and 1992–94.

[d] Interval: trends were analysed over birth years.

OPCRIT, Operational Checklist for Psychotic Disease; RDC, Research Diagnostic Criteria; ICD, International Classification of Disease; DSM, Diagnostic and Statistical Manual of Mental Disorders; ISTAT, Italian National Institute for Statistics; CSA, Common Services Agency; M, male; F, female.

An illustration of the perils of diagnosis comes from Scotland, one of the countries that has shown the most consistently reported decline (Eagles et al., 1988; Geddes et al., 1993; Takei et al., 1996). Allardyce et al. (2000) have recently shown that an apparent decline in the incidence of schizophrenia in southwest Scotland from 1979 to 1998 (summary rate ratio linear trend 0.77 (95% confidence interval (CI) 0.68–0.88)), based on clinician diagnosis in administrative records, was in fact the result of a narrowing of the concept of schizophrenia that clinicians were using. There was no change in the incidence when consistent OPCRIT-derived (Operational Checklist for Psychotic Disorders, McGuffin et al., 1991) ICD-10 and DSM-IV (American Psychiatric Association, 1994) diagnoses were used. However, some studies incorporating ICD-10 criteria partially support the hypothesis of declining period incidence. A study of incidence in Nottingham, in which the ICD-10 diagnoses were made by consensus, reported an increase in psychosis as a whole, though a decrease in narrowly defined schizophrenia over a 16-year period (1978–1994; Brewin et al., 1997).

Finally, the evidence for contemporary trends is not uniform. While most studies show a period decline in schizophrenia, there have also been other reports of no decline (Oldehinkel et al., 1995; Folnegovic et al., 1990) and reports of increasing rates (van Os et al., 1993; Preti and Miotto, 2000; Boydell et al., 2001; Tsuchiya and Munk-Jørgensen, 2002). Boydell and colleagues investigated changes in OPCRIT-derived Research Diagnostic Criteria (RDC: Spitzer et al., 1990) schizophrenia (i.e. broadly defined) from 1965 to 1997 in South London. This study had the advantage that it covered all patients presenting with schizophrenia either on an outpatient or an inpatient basis from a geographically defined area. Psychiatric care was provided by services linked to the Maudsley hospital and the case registers and records were maintained to relatively high standards. RDC diagnoses were made by OPCRIT ratings of these records. The incidence of RDC schizophrenia approximately doubled over 30 years.

In summary, based on period data, evidence for declining incidence is not conclusive. Clearly, some portion of the reported decline is accounted for by artifact. It is notable that authors have not offered any explanations of period effects (i.e. suggesting processes proximal to the onset of disorder) other than sources of artifact. We must also consider the possibility that some portion of the reported declines in incidence may actually reflect cohort effects, capturing aetiological influences acting early in life. Strictly speaking, period analyses are not appropriate to examine cohort effects.

Declining incidence: birth cohort effects?

If the decline in incidence rates was observed over birth cohorts (i.e. mapping rates by year of birth), this would suggest that at least part of a secular decline is determined by processes occurring early in life. There are fewer studies seeking to establish trends in incidence of schizophrenia over birth cohorts than over historical period. One example is a study of incidence in South Verona, Italy. Using computer-based diagnoses on first treatment contact, Balestrieri and colleagues (1997) reported an overall decrease over birth years in ICD-10 paranoid and undifferentiated schizophrenia, with a consistent decline observed in males.

As in the previously described studies, however, the cohort and period effects are entangled. Discriminating between cohort and period effects (i.e. changes in incidence over birth years and changes in incidence over calendar years), in an attempt to disentangle the influence of aetiological factors acting early in life from factors acting closer to the time of disease onset, requires that they be considered simultaneously. Two studies have used age–period–cohort analysis to separate these effects. Takei et al. (1996) found most of the decrease in clinical diagnosis of schizophrenia in Scotland between 1966 and 1990 was accounted for by period effects (88%), but there was still a small cohort effect. Suvisaari et al. (1999a) found both period and cohort effects in a nationwide Finnish study of people born between 1954 and 1965 that demonstrated a significant decline in relatively early-onset, narrowly defined schizophrenia.

Factors contributing to observed birth cohort effects have received some attention, but findings are inconclusive (e.g. Eagles et al., 1995; Procopio and Marriot, 1998; Suvisaari et al., 1999b) and explanations speculative. Prenatal nutritional deficiency has been associated with risk of schizophrenia (Susser and Lin, 1992; Susser et al., 1996); therefore, generally improving nutrition could explain part of the decline. A more systematic assessment of influences on the nutritional status of populations may be illuminating (e.g. fortification of the food supply, dietary recommendations to pregnant women and uptake of prenatal vitamins, trends in breast feeding and neonatal nutrition). Maternal exposure to infectious disease during pregnancy, including polio and rubella, has been associated to varying degrees with schizophrenia (Susser et al., 1999; Suvisaari et al., 1999c; Brown et al., 2000). Effective immunization programmes have impacted on these prenatal exposures and correspond to the principal years involved in the decline. Obstetric complications have been associated with risk of schizophrenia (Ch. 5). The influence of improvements in obstetrics and neonatal care may be 'double-edged', causing both decreases in mortality among those who may have died without intervention and improved health of those who would survive without intervention. The balance of these influences in terms of the number of at-risk infants surviving is not clear and is probably changing over time.

Time trends in course and outcome

When William Farr turned his attention to assessing mortality in asylums during the 19th century, the findings were grim. He found annual mortality rates of patients in these institutions ranging from 11 to 27%; the latter was 'as high as the rate of mortality experienced by the British troops upon the western coast of Africa and by the population of London when the plague rendered its habitations desolate' (Susser and Adelstein, 1975, p. 429). At the end of the 19th century, the circumstances remained bleak, as borne out in the study by Healy et al. (2001). Excluding individuals diagnosed with dementias and organic disorders, the death rate of those admitted to the Denbigh Asylum in Wales during the period 1894–96 was 24%. Clearly, the mortality rate in the 20th century was lower than that in the 19th century. This decline was related to higher standard of living and lower mortality in the general population. It probably also reflected better accommodation of individuals with schizophrenia, although these individuals remained at much higher risk of death than the general population (Ch. 15).

During the 20th century, an apparent decline in the numbers of individuals with the most severe forms of schizophrenia (Bleuler, 1978; Jablensky et al., 1992; Jablensky, 1997) gave rise to speculation that schizophrenia is becoming more benign. Consequently, the companion to the hypothesis of declining incidence was the hypothesis of diminishing severity of schizophrenia (Hare, 1983; Zubin et al., 1983; Harrison and Mason, 1993). However, establishing time trends for a broader set of outcomes than mortality has proven difficult. Outcome is multidimensional (e.g. clinical or social outcomes), requires longitudinal assessment of patients and can be defined at various moments following the diagnosis of disease (e.g. short- and long-term outcomes). Lacking systematic data, several authors have addressed outcome trends in meta-analyses (Warner, 1985, 1995; Hegarty et al., 1994) and substantive reviews (e.g. Shepherd et al., 1989) of rather heterogeneous follow-up studies.

An ambitious meta-analysis of outcome studies constructed a foundation for analysing trends in outcome over a 100-year period (Hegarty et al., 1994). The analysis focused on studies in which there was a diagnosis of schizophrenia or dementia praecox with numerical outcome data for this diagnostic group, a mean length of follow-up of at least 1 year with less than a third of the study population lost to follow-up. All inclusion criteria were met by 320 studies, representing 51 800 subjects. In the final analysis, outcomes at the beginning and end of the century were roughly comparable ('improved': 1895–1955 35% and 1986–1992 36%).

In an analysis based on much of the same outcome research, Warner (1985) focused on economic influences on trends over roughly the same time interval. Warner examined 68 studies conducted exclusively in developed country settings. Studies were assessed to determine the proportion recovered. Graphing recovery rates for the North American and European studies combined against US and UK unemployment rates, Warner observed a close correspondence between more favourable outcomes and periods of low unemployment.

Some investigators have focused our attention on shorter periods of time and outcomes deriving from clinical contexts. Before and after designs have been used to examine the impact of neuroleptic medications (Wyatt, 1991; Wyatt and Henter, 1998). These studies suggest, for the most part, rather modest improvements in outcome over time related to medication effects. An interesting early example was a study of psychiatric hospitalizations in Norway (Ødegård, 1964). This study evaluated the impact of the introduction of antipsychotic medications into the treatment mix in 1954 on psychiatric outcomes. Based on data from a national register of all individuals with psychosis admitted to psychiatric hospitals, Ødegård compared the outcomes for patients first admitted to the hospital in 1936–40 (largely pre-war), 1948–52 (preneuroleptic medication) and 1955–59 (postneuroleptic medication). Two treatment outcomes were assessed: length of hospital stay, and discharge from hospital with no readmission in following 12 months. Based on the comparison of pre- and postneuroleptic period outcomes, he concluded that there was a slight improvement associated with the introduction of new medications. Because of the narrow time frame involved, other significant changes in treatment systems or practices were considered an unlikely explanation for the difference observed. The graphical data including the pre-war, preneuroleptic, and postneuroleptic cohorts of first admissions for functional psychosis illustrate, however, that a larger more decisive difference in discharge outcomes was observed between the first two time periods. The author attributed the earlier improvement to social changes and speculated that low unemployment during the post-war period may have played a role.

It is puzzling that the overall change is modest, despite the introduction of medications. Perhaps accounting for the unimpressive improvements in outcome, evidence indicates that most persons with schizophrenia do not receive recommended care, including appropriate medication (Lehman and Steinwachs, 1998). Competing factors may also be involved. These could include other dimensions of treatment systems, economic fluctuations, levels of support provided to the disabled, supplies of low-income housing and trends in substance use. The data used to detect trends in outcome, however, are unsystematic and do not yield insight into these and other factors. Given these limitations, the adequacy of the data for establishing trends in schizophrenia outcomes remains in question.

Today, at the start of the 21st century, trends in extreme negative outcomes are a matter of concern. The possibility of worsening trends in suicide among individuals with schizophrenia has been raised by Mortensen and Juel (1993) (Chs. 14 and 15). A recent study in Stockholm County reported increases in the relative risk for mortality associated with schizophrenia in the period 1976–95 (Osby et al., 2000). Finally, individuals with schizophrenia in some countries, notably the USA, have been devastated by homelessness, human immunodeficiency virus (HIV) and addiction disorders (Cournos and McKinnon, 1997; Susser et al., 1997; Herman et al., 1998).

Conclusions

The contemporary incidence of schizophrenia appears to be in decline, although the data are not conclusive. The decline seems mainly to reflect period effects, pointing to the potential important role of social environment, but it is entirely unclear what these social factors might be. Recent improvements deriving from economic advantage and related improvements in health (e.g. prenatal nutrition, maternal immunization and infection control) might be sufficient for a major socioeconomic impact to be plausible. The most compelling changes, however, are most relevant to the decline over birth cohorts rather than to period effects.

Changes in outcome are more difficult to judge. Based on meta-analyses of a large literature on schizophrenia outcomes, improvements in course or outcome from beginning to end of the 20th century are modest. This is surprising in light of the rather dramatic impact of modern medications on symptoms. Perhaps the explanation lies in countervailing influences of the modern social environment; conceivably these may be similar to influences accounting for worse outcome in developed countries in comparison with developing countries. Perhaps the explanation lies in the reality that most patients do not receive the recommended treatment or necessary care (Lehman, 2001).

REFERENCES

Allardyce J, Morrison G, McCreadie RG (2000) Schizophrenia is not disappearing in south-west Scotland. British Journal of Psychiatry 177, 38–41.

American Psychiatric Association (1980) Diagnosis and Statistical Manual of Mental Disorders, 3rd edn. Washington, DC: American Psychiatric Press.

American Psychiatric Association (1994) Diagnostic and Statistical Manual IV, 4th edn. Washington, DC: American Psychiatric Press.

Balestrieri M, Rucci P, Nicolaou S (1997) Gender-specific decline and seasonality of births in operationally defined schizophrenics in Italy. Schizophrenia Research 27, 73–81.

Bamrah JS, Freeman HL, Goldberg DP (1991) Epidemiology of schizophrenia in Salford, 1974–84. Changes in an urban community over ten years. British Journal of Psychiatry 159, 802–810.

Bark NM (1988) On the history of schizophrenia. Evidence of its existence before 1800. New York State Journal of Medicine July, 374–383.

Bleuler M (1978) The Schizophrenic Disorders: Long-Term Patient and Family Studies. New Haven: Yale University Press.

Boydell J, van Os J, Lambri M et al. (2001) Doubling in incidence of schizophrenia in south-east London from 1965–1997. British Journal of Psychiatry, in press.

Brewin J, Cantwell R, Dalkin T et al. (1997) Incidence of schizophrenia in Nottingham. A comparison of two cohorts, 1978–80 and 1992–94. British Journal of Psychiatry 171, 140–144.

Brown A, Cohen P, Greenwald S et al. (2000) Non-affective psychosis after prenatal exposure to rubella American Journal of Psychiatry 157, 438–443.

Castle D, Wessely S, Der, G, Murray RM (1991) The incidence of operationally defined schizophrenia in Camberwell, 1965–84. British Journal of Psychiatry 159, 790–794.

Cooper J, Sartorious, N (1977) Cultural and temporal variations in schizophrenia: speculation on the importance of industrialization. British Journal of Psychiatry 130, 50–55.

Cournos F, McKinnon K (1997) HIV seroprevalence among people with severe mental illness in the United States: a critical review. Clinical Psychological Review 17, 259–269.

de Alarcon J, Seagroatt V, Goldacre M (1990) Trends in schizophrenia (letter). Lancet 335, 852–853.

Der G, Gupta S, Murray RM (1990) Is schizophrenia disappearing? Lancet 335, 513–516.

de Salvia D, Barbato A, Pierandrea S, Zadro F (1993) Prevalence and incidence of schizophrenic disorders in Portogruaro: an Italian case register study. Journal of Nervous and Mental Disorders 181, 275–282.

Eagles JM, Whalley LJ (1985) Decline in the diagnosis of schizophrenia among first admissions to Scottish mental hospitals in 1969–78. British Journal of Psychiatry 146, 151–154.

Eagles JM, Hunter D, McCance C (1988) Decline in the diagnosis of schizophrenia among first contacts with psychiatric services in North-East Scotland, 1969–1984. British Journal of Psychiatry 152, 793–798.

Eagles JM, Hunter D, Geddes JR (1995) Gender-specific changes since 1900 in the season-of-birth effect in schizophrenia. British Journal of Psychiatry 167, 469–472.

Folnegovic Z, Folnegovic-Smalc V, Kulcar Z (1990) The incidence of schizophrenia in Croatia. British Journal of Psychiatry 156, 363–365.

Geddes JR, Black RJ, Whalley LJ, Eagles JM (1993) Persistence of the decline in the diagnosis of schizophrenia among first admissions to Scottish hospitals from 1969 to 1988. British Journal of Psychiatry 163, 620–626.

Goldhammer H, Marshall AW (1953) Psychosis and Civilization. New York: Free Press.

Häfner H, Gattaz WF (1991) Is schizophrenia disappearing? European Archives of Psychiatry and Clinical Neurology 240, 374–376.

Hare E (1983) Was insanity on the increase? British Journal of Psychiatry 142, 439–455.

Harrison G, Mason P (1993) Schizophrenia-falling incidence and better outcome? British Journal of Psychiatry 163, 535–541.

Harrison G, Cooper JE, Gancarczyk R (1991) Changes in the administrative incidence of schizophrenia. British Journal of Psychiatry 161, 811–816.

Healy D, Savage M, Michael P et al. (2001) Psychiatric bed utilization: 1896 and 1996 compared. Psychological Medicine 31, 779–790.

Hegarty JD, Baldessarini RJ, Tohen M, Waternaux C, Oepen G (1994) One hundred years of schizophrenia: a meta-analysis of the outcome literature. American Journal of Psychiatry 151, 1409–1416.

Herman DB, Susser ES, Jandorf L, Lavelle J, Bromet EJ (1998) Homelessness among individuals with psychotic disorders hospitalized for the first time: findings from the Suffolk County Mental Health Project. American Journal of Psychiatry 155, 109–113.

Jablensky A (1997) The 100-year epidemiology of schizophrenia. Schizophrenia Research 28, 111–125.

Jablensky A, Sartorius N, Ernberg G et al. (1992) Schizophrenia: manifestations, incidence and course in different cultures. Psychological Medicine, Monograph Supplement 20. Cambridge, UK: Cambridge University Press.

Jeste DV, del Carmen R, Lohr JB, Wyatt RJ (1985) Did schizophrenia exist before the eighteenth century? Comprehensive Psychiatry 26, 493–503.

Jones IH, Kirkby KC, Hay DA, Daniels BA, Longmore LM (1997) Decline in diagnoses of schizophrenia in Tasmania during the period 1965–1990. Acta Psychiatrica Scandinavica 95, 13–18.

Joyce PR (1987) Changing trends in first admissions and readmissions for mania and schizophrenia in New Zealand, 1974 to 1984. Australian and New Zealand Journal of Psychiatry 21, 82–86.

Kendell RE, Malcolm DE, Adams W (1993) The problem of detecting changes in the incidence of schizophrenia. British Journal of Psychiatry 162, 212–218.

Lehman A (2001) Keeping practice current. Psychiatric Services 52, 1132.

Lehman A, Steinwachs D (1998) Patterns of usual care for schizophrenia: initial results from the Schizophrenia Patient Outcomes Research Team (PORT) client survey. Schizophrenia Bulletin 24, 11–20.

Maudsley H (1872) Is insanity on the increase? British Medical Journal i, 36–39.

Maudsley H (1877) The alleged increase of insanity. Journal of Mental Science 23, 45–54.

McGuffin P, Farmer A, Harvey I (1991) A polydiagnostic application of operational criteria in studies of psychotic illness. Archives of General Psychiatry 48, 764–770.

Mortensen PB, Juel K (1993) Mortality and causes of death in first admitted schizophrenic patients. British Journal of Psychiatry 163, 183–189.

Munk-Jørgensen P (1986) Decreasing first-admission rates of schizophrenia among males in Denmark from 1970 to 1984. Acta Psychiatrica Scandinavica 73, 645–650.

Munk-Jørgensen P (1995) Decreasing rates of incident schizophrenia cases in psychiatric service: a review of the literature. European Psychiatry 10, 129–141.

Munk-Jørgensen P, Jorgensen P (1986) Decreasing rates of first admission diagnoses of schizophrenia among females in Denmark 1970–84. Acta Psychiatrica Scandinavica 74, 379–383.

Munk-Jørgensen P, Mortensen PB (1992) Incidence and other aspects of the epidemiology of schizophrenia in Denmark, 1971–1987. British Journal of Psychiatry 161, 489–495.

Ødegård O (1964) Pattern of discharge from Norwegian psychiatric hospitals before and after the introduction of psychotropic drugs. American Journal of Psychiatry 120, 772–778.

Oldehinkel AJ, Giel R (1995) Time trends in the care-based incidence of schizophrenia. British Journal of Psychiatry 167, 77–782.

Osby U, Correia N, Brandt L, Ekbom A, Sparen P (2000) Time trends in schizophrenia mortality in Stockholm County, Sweden: cohort study. British Medical Journal 321, 483–484.

Osby U, Hammar N, Brandt L et al. (2001) Time trends in first admissions for schizophrenia and paranoid psychosis in Stockholm County, Sweden. Schizophrenia Research 47, 247–254.

Parker G, O'Donnell M, Walter S (1985) Changes in the diagnoses of the functional psychoses associated with the introduction of lithium. British Journal of Psychiatry 146, 377–382.

Preti A, Miotto P (2000) Increase in first admissions for schizophrenia and other major psychoses in Italy. Psychiatry Research 94, 139–152.

Procopio M, Marriot PK (1998) Is the decline in diagnoses of schizophrenia caused by the disappearance of a seasonal aetiological agent? An epidemiological study in England and Wales. Psychological Medicine 28, 367–373.

Rosen G (1959) Social stress and mental disease from the eighteenth century to the present, some origins of social psychiatry. Millbank Memorial Fund Quarterly 37, 5–32.

Scull A (1984) Discussion: was insanity increasing? A response to Edward Hare. British Journal of Psychiatry 144, 432–436.

Shepherd M (1993) Historical epidemiology and the functional psychoses. Psychological Medicine 23, 301–304.

Shepherd M, Watt D, Falloon I, Smeeton N (1989) The natural history of schizophrenia: a five-year follow-up study of outcome and prediction in a representative sample of schizophrenics. Psychological Medicine, Monograph Supplement 15. Cambridge, UK: Cambridge University Press.

Spitzer RL, Williams JBW, Gibbon M (1990) User's Guide for the Structured Clinical Interview for DSM-III-R (SCID). Washington, DC: American Psychiatric Association.

Stephens JH (1978) Long-term prognosis and followup in schizophrenia. Schizophrenia Bulletin 4, 25–45.

Susser M, Adelstein A (1975) Vital Statistics: A Memorial Volume of Selections from the Reports and Writings of William Farr. Metuchen, NJ: Scarecrow Press for the New York Academy of Medicine.

Susser E, Lin SP (1992) Schizophrenia after prenatal exposure to the Dutch Hunger Winter of 1944–1945. Archives of General Psychiatry 49, 983–988.

Susser E, Neugebauer R, Hoek HW, Brown AS (1996) Schizophrenia after prenatal famine: Further evidence. Archives of General Psychiatry 53, 25–31.

Susser E, Colson P, Jandorf L et al. (1997) HIV infection among young adults with psychotic disorders. American Journal of Psychiatry 154, 864–866.

Susser E, Brown AS, Gorman JM (1999) Prenatal Exposures in Schizophrenia. Washington, DC: American Psychiatric Press.

Suvisaari JM, Haukka JK, Tanskanen AJ, Lonnqvist JK (1999a) Decline in the incidence of schizophrenia in Finnish cohorts born from 1954 to 1965. Archives of General Psychiatry 56, 733–740.

Suvisaari JM, Haukka JK, Tanskanen AJ, Lonnqvist JK (1999b) Decreasing seasonal variation of births in schizophrenia. In: Incidence and Risk Factors of Schizophrenia in Finland. Helsinki: Publications of the National Public Health Institute.

Suvisaari J, Haukka J, Tanskanen A, Hovi T, Lonnqvist J (1999c) Association between prenatal exposure to poliovirus infection and adult schizophrenia. American Journal of Psychiatry 156, 1100–1102.

Takei N, Lewis G, Sham PC, Murray RM (1996) Age-period-cohort analysis of the incidence of schizophrenia in Scotland. Psychological Medicine 26, 963–973.

Torrey EF (1980) Schizophrenia and Civilization. New York: Jason Aronson.

Tsuchiya KJ, Munk-Jørgensen P (2002) First-admission rates of schizophrenia in Denmark, 1980–1997: have they been increasing? Schizophrenia Research 54, 187–191.

van Os J, Galdos P, Lewis G, Bourgeois M, Mann A (1993) Schizophrenia sans frontieres:

concepts of schizophrenia among French and British psychiatrists. British Medical Journal 307, 489–492.

Waddington JL, Youssef HA (1994) Evidence for a gender-specific decline in the rate of schizophrenia in rural Ireland over a 50-year period. British Journal of Psychiatry 164, 171–176.

Warner R (1985) Recovery from Schizophrenia: Psychiatry and Political Economy. New York: Routeledge.

Warner R (1995) Schizophrenia: a 100-year retrospective [letter]. American Journal of Psychiatry 152, 1693.

World Health Organization (1967) Manual of International Statistical Classification of Diseases, Injuries and Causes of Death, 8th edn. Geneva: World Health Organization.

World Health Organization (1978) Manual of International Statistical Classification of Diseases, Injuries and Causes of Death, 9th edn. Geneva: World Health Organization.

World Health Organization (1992) Manual of International Statistical Classification of Diseases, Injuries and Causes of Death, 10th edn. Geneva: World Health Organization.

Wyatt RJ (1991) Neuroleptics and the natural course of schizophrenia. Schizophrenia Bulletin 17, 325–351.

Wyatt RJ, Henter ID (1998) The effects of early and sustained intervention on the long-term morbidity of schizophrenia. Journal of Psychiatric Research 32, 169–177.

Zubin J, Magaziner J, Steinhauer SR (1983) The metamorphosis of schizophrenia: from chronicity to disability. Psychological Medicine 13, 551–571.

4

Urbanization, migration and risk of schizophrenia

Jane Boydell and Robin Murray

Institute of Psychiatry, King's College London, UK

Influence of urban life

Historical context

A number of early studies (reviewed by Freeman, 1994) have shown that the rates of schizophrenia are increased in inner city areas in Western societies. One of the first papers to demonstrate this clearly was the classic monograph of Faris and Dunham (1939), who showed that first admission rates of schizophrenia were particularly high in certain areas of inner city Chicago and then decreased again towards the periphery of the city. There were considerable differences within the inner city area itself: rates were higher in the disorganized 'hobohemia' area than in the more cohesive working class and ethnic minority areas. The authors suggested that characteristics of certain neighbourhoods, such as social isolation and lack of cohesion, may be responsible for the increased rates of schizophrenia. Interestingly, in contrast to schizophrenia, the incidence of manic depression was not higher in the inner city, a finding that has recently been replicated by Mortensen et al. (1999).

Sadly, the refinements of Faris and Dunham's study and their discussion of possible causes of the increased rates of schizophrenia were largely ignored for many years. During the latter half of the 20th century, the generally accepted view was that the high rates of schizophrenia in the inner city could be accounted for by the tendency of people with schizophrenia, or with incipient schizophrenia, to move into the more urbanized and deprived areas. This was known as the 'social drift' hypothesis. A variant on this theme implied that the more able move out to better areas in the suburbs, as a city develops, leaving a residual population in the centre with a high risk of psychiatric disorders. This was known as the 'social residue' theory. The idea that causal agents are associated with urbanization (the 'breeder' hypothesis) was largely dismissed.

In an ingenious study looking back at the 19th century, Torrey et al. (1997a) used the comprehensive 1880 census of the 'insane' in the USA to examine the association between urbanicity and severe mental illness. 'Insanity' in 1880 included people who would be considered to have a psychotic illness today but, of course, also many others. Torrey and coworkers calculated prevalence rates for different degrees of urbanicity: urban was defined as including the 30 largest cities; semi-urban was 50% or more people living in towns of >4000; semi-rural was 25–50% living in towns of ⩾4000; rural was 1–25% living in towns of >4000; and completely rural was no-one living in a town of >4000. Odds ratios (OR) were calculated using completely rural as a baseline and showed a strong linear trend (OR: urban 1.66, semi-urban 1.46, semi-rural 1.44, rural 1.37). This study is important, despite its limitations, because a gradient was found between areas that would all be considered rural today.

Recent studies

Most recent studies on urbanization as a risk factor for schizophrenia have come from Northern Europe, where good-quality national records have made large-scale epidemiological studies possible. In the first of these, Lewis et al. (1992) investigated the association between place of upbringing and incidence of schizophrenia using data from a cohort of over 49 000 male Swedish conscripts, linking it to the Swedish National Psychiatric Register. There was a strong significant linear trend (chi-squared 9.9; $p = 0.002$), with the highest rate of clinically diagnosed ICD-8 (World Health Organization, 1967) schizophrenia in those who had mostly lived in cities (Stockholm, Goteborg, Malmo) while they were growing up (crude OR 1.65). There were intermediate rates in large towns (>50 000; crude OR 1.39) and small towns (<50 000; crude OR 1.28) with the lowest rates found in country areas, which were taken as baseline. A similar, though weaker, trend was found for other psychoses. Adjusting for family finances, parental divorce and family psychiatric history (relative 'on medication for nervous trouble') had little effect. Adjusting for cannabis use and any psychiatric disorder at conscription (as these may have been part of a prodrome) reduced but did not eliminate the associations. The authors suggested that causal environmental factors are implicated as the association remained after adjusting for family history. However, this study could not distinguish between place of birth, place of upbringing and place of residence at the onset of psychosis.

Subsequently, Marcelis et al. (1998) used the Dutch National Psychiatric Register and the Dutch Birth Register to explore further whether urban birth is specifically associated with schizophrenia. Urban birth was linearly associated with later psychosis and there were quantitative differences between diagnostic categories in the strength of the association. The incidence rate ratio (IRR) linear trend was 1.39 for broadly defined schizophrenia, 1.18 for affective psychosis and 1.27 for other psychoses. The strongest association was for narrowly defined schizophrenia and urban exposure (incidence rate ratio/linear trend 1.44; 95% confidence interval

(CI)/1.39–1.5). This study also found an interaction with gender in that the effect of urbanicity on all psychosis was greater for men than for women. The effect of urban birth was greatest for individuals from the most recent birth cohorts and with early-onset disease even after correcting for length of follow-up.

In a separate study in the Netherlands, Peen and Decker (1997) also found a significant positive correlation between admission rates for clinically diagnosed ICD-9 (World Health Organization, 1978) schizophrenia and degree of urbanization. This correlation was not accounted for by differences in the availability of psychiatric services, as the average length of hospital admission and average number of readmissions did not differ between urban and rural areas.

In the largest study to date, Mortensen et al. (1999) investigated the effect of place and season of birth on risk of admission with ICD-8 schizophrenia in a large Danish population-based cohort of 1.75 million. The relative risk associated with birth in Copenhagen compared with birth in rural areas was 2.40 (95% CI 2.13–2.7). There was a clear dose–response relationship for urbanicity, in that the larger the town of birth, the greater the risk. A family history of schizophrenia did not explain or affect the results. Mortensen and colleagues calculated that the population attributable risk for urban birth was 34.6%, compared with 9% for having a mother with schizophrenia. Therefore, the effect of urban birth was much larger than the effect of having a relative affected with schizophrenia (though having an affected parent does not equate with genetic predisposition). Like the original study of Faris and Dunham (1939), Mortensen and his colleagues (1999) found the incidence of manic depression to be fairly evenly distributed across rural and urban areas.

Dauncey and colleagues (1993) examined where patients had lived 5 years before their first admission in Nottingham, UK but were unable to find evidence for systematic geographic drift. Furthermore, it is unlikely that the drift occurred in the previous parental generation, as the magnitude of this movement would need to have been extremely high to explain the findings. For example, in the Danish study, Mortensen and colleagues (1999) calculated that nearly 50 000 children born in the capital and its suburbs needed to have a parent who transmitted a genetic risk equal to that transmitted by a parent with diagnosed schizophrenia to account for the urban excess. Furthermore, a family history of schizophrenia did not explain or affect the urban–rural difference. This is also relevant for the social residue theory (that those at greater risk are left behind in an area as it becomes less desirable). The evidence for an early effect is strong but there may also be an effect of urbanization around the time of onset for non-early-onset schizophrenia, and there is recent evidence of a cumulative effect of urban exposure throughout childhood.

Most of the studies investigating urbanicity and psychosis have used admission data to measure incidence and have relied on national case registers of clinical diagnoses. This enables wide coverage but leaves the possibility that bias (owing to referral, admission, and diagnostic practices for instance) may have affected the results. In an attempt to address this, Allardyce et al. (2001) examined case note data on all incident cases (both admitted and not admitted) of psychosis from two areas in the UK: a largely rural part of southwest Scotland and urban south London. Case records of all individuals who developed their first psychosis were rated, whether or not they were admitted, to obtain computer-generated diagnoses of schizophrenia according to Research Diagnostic Criteria (RDC; Spitzer et al., 1990), thereby avoiding potential bias introduced by different admission policies and diagnostic traditions. The incidence was 61% higher in the urban than in the rural area (standardized incidence ratio 1.61; 95% CI 1.42–1.81), and once again the urban excess was more marked in males than females.

Timing of exposure: urban birth, upbringing or residence

As urban birth is strongly correlated with both urban upbringing and residence at the time of onset of psychosis, it is not clear whether the urban risk factor is operating at the time of gestation and birth, at around the time of onset, or throughout the period in between. This question was investigated by Marcelis et al. (1999) in the Netherlands among a cohort of all people born between 1972 and 1978, using a national psychiatric database of first admissions that included information on place of birth and of residence. Individuals were followed up through the register until the oldest were 23. Urban exposure was defined as living in the 'Randstad', three provinces where the population density is 1000 persons/km^2, in contrast to all other provinces, where the population density is 300 persons/km^2. Using population and internal migration data, they characterized the birth cohort as exposed born/exposed resident (EBER), exposed born/nonexposed resident (EBNR), nonexposed born/exposed resident (NBER) and nonexposed born/nonexposed resident. The relative risk for narrowly defined schizophrenia was 2.05 (95% CI 1.18–3.57) for EBNR and 1.96 (95% CI 1.55–2.46) for EBER, implying that there is no additional risk for urban residence at the time of onset, above that of urban birth. However, this study could not distinguish between urban birth and urban upbringing and only applied to relatively early-onset schizophrenia.

Few studies have been able to separate out the effects of place of birth and place of upbringing. Astrup and Ødegård (1961) found a stronger effect of city upbringing amongst those who had moved to the city. However, Pedersen and Mortensen (2001), using a comprehensive national registration system that accurately recorded every change of residence, have shown that schizophrenia risk increased with the number of years (between 0 and 20 years of age) that an individual lived in an urbanized area and with increasing degree of urbanization. Relative risk for those who had spent their entire childhood in the capital was 2.75 (95% CI 2.31–3.28) compared with 1 for those who had always lived in the most rural areas. Further details of this study are awaited but it suggests aetiological factors of a pervasive and long-term nature are operating in urbanized areas.

Possible explanations for the risk-increasing effect of cities

Social class

It has been suggested that social class might confound the urban/rural difference. Hare (1955) studied all male admissions in a UK city over 5 years and found a marked excess of schizophrenia amongst people from social class 4 and 5. Castle et al. (1993) carried out a case-control study in south London and found that people with schizophrenia were more likely to have been born in the socially deprived areas and to have fathers with manual occupations. Ohta et al. (1992) did not find a significant urban/rural difference in Nagasaki and attributed this to there being few social class differences between areas. It is unlikely that the entire urban effect can be attributed to social class as some of the positive findings have come from countries where there is a higher standard of living in cities than in the rural areas. Furthermore, in the Swedish conscript study of Lewis et al. (1992), the urban effect remained after adjusting for 'family finances'. It is entirely possible, however, that the aetiological agent(s) might be related to both urbanization and low social class, for example aspects of nutrition.

Obstetric complications

Obstetric complications are considered to be a risk factor for schizophrenia (Ch. 5). Since pre- and perinatal complications are more common among the urban working classes, Eaton et al. (2000) tested the hypothesis that the urban–rural difference may be mediated by obstetric complications in a Danish case-control study. Birth in Copenhagen was a strong risk factor for schizophrenia, as discussed earlier. Prospectively measured obstetric complications had a moderate relationship to early-onset schizophrenia but the relationship of urban birth to schizophrenia was unaffected by adjusting for obstetric complications. Recent data from the Netherlands has raised the question of whether or not malnutrition during pregnancy (Susser et al., 1996, 1998; Hoek et al., 1998) increases risk of schizophrenia, though this finding has yet to be replicated. Again, it is conceivable that mothers in poor inner city areas have poorer nutrition, but there is no empirical evidence that this explains the urban effect.

Infectious disease

Increased maternal exposure to infectious disease at the time of fetal brain development is a possible risk factor for schizophrenia (Ch. 5) and another possible mechanism to explain the increased incidence of schizophrenia in cities, since many infections are transmitted more readily in crowded urban environments. Brown et al. (2000) suggested that maternal exposure to rubella is associated with increased risk of schizophrenia. Polio and measles may also be relevant. Mothers who had children who developed schizophrenia were more likely to have had toxoplasmosis during pregnancy, as evidenced by IgM antibodies (an indicator of recent infection) (Torrey et al., 2001).

Drug abuse

The relationship between drug use and psychosis is complex (Ch. 16), but if we accept that drug abuse can increase the incidence of schizophrenia, then this could confound the association between urbanization and schizophrenia. However, the early studies were carried out before recreational drug use was so prevalent. Furthermore, this issue was also addressed in the Swedish conscript study by Lewis et al. (1992), and the effect of urban upbringing remained after adjusting for cannabis use.

Psychosocial stress

Three prospective studies have found an association between life events and onset of psychosis (Ventura et al., 1989; Malla et al., 1990; Bebbington et al., 1993). Once again, it is possible that adverse life events may be more common in the inner city, but there is no direct evidence that this explains the increased urban risk of schizophrenia. Indeed, given that the effect size for life events is greater in affective psychosis than schizophrenia, this hypothesis would have predicted an increased urban incidence of manic-depression, which, as we noted earlier, has not been found.

Social isolation

Hare (1956) reported that social isolation, as measured by the proportion of single person households in a geographical area, is associated with increased rates of schizophrenia The findings were not accounted for by movement into the area of people with, or developing, schizophrenia. There has been a recent resurgence of interest in these ideas. Thornicroft et al. (1993) noted that clustering of individuals with schizophrenia in deprived areas occurs only in urban areas and suggested that social isolation is an important mediator of this. However, it is difficult to distinguish between cause and effect in this context. Related to these ideas is the theory that disruption of social networks decreases an individual's capacity to cope with psychosocial stress and increases the risk of schizophrenia. Van Os et al. (2000) found evidence for person–environment interaction in the Netherlands. People who were single had a slightly higher risk of developing psychosis if they lived in a neighbourhood with fewer single people than if they lived in a neighbourhood with many other single people. The authors suggested that single status might give rise to perceived (or actual) social isolation if most other people are living with a partner. The question of whether social isolation may increase risk of schizophrenia (or whether a close relationship may be protective) is also raised by Jablensky et al. (1997), who showed that marriage had a protective effect and that this was not simply a consequence of better-adjusted males being able to marry.

Summary

There is substantial, but not universal, evidence that urban birth and/or upbringing are associated with an increased risk of psychosis – at least in Western societies as there is little evidence regarding developing countries. The effect appears to be increasing and to be stronger for narrowly defined schizophrenia, early-onset schizophrenia and males. Although we cannot totally discount the effects of the 'social drift' hypothesis, it cannot account for the results of recent studies that implicate urban birth, implying a return to the 'breeder' hypothesis.

An important question is whether the causal aetiological factors associated with urban birth have a general effect on the population at large or only on those who develop schizophrenia. To address this, van Os et al. (2001) examined psychiatric symptoms in a large Dutch study of the general population ($n = 7500$). Psychotic-like symptoms (isolated delusions or hallucinations) were found in 17.5% of the community sample, largely in people who had never presented to psychiatric services. Furthermore, the prevalence of such symptoms increased with increasing urbanization (i.e. just like schizophrenia).

Possible causal factors associated with urbanization include those resulting from the high concentration of people in an area (population density) or living unit (overcrowding), and those resulting from the deprivation that is so commonly seen with urbanization. Many factors that influence fetal and early child development and are relevant to the neurodevelopmental model of schizophrenia (Murray et al., 1992; Murray and Fearon, 1999; Ch. 5) such as infectious disease, obstetric complications, poor nutrition and pollution, are more prevalent in cities. Increased head injury, drug abuse and psychosocial stress, especially from noise and isolation, are also possible agents

Influence of season of birth on the incidence of schizophrenia

There is a small but significantly increased risk for schizophrenia and other psychoses among individuals born in late winter and early spring (Bradbury and Miller, 1985). More than 250 studies were reviewed by Torrey et al. (1997b), who concluded that the results were remarkably consistent in showing a 5–8% winter excess.

It was once fashionable to attribute this to an 'age-incidence' effect, i.e. more of the people born early in the year will have developed schizophrenia simply because they are a number of months older than those born later in the year (Lewis, 1989).

However, this notion cannot be sustained since the excess in the southern hemisphere, though weaker than in the northern hemisphere, occurs in their spring, which is in the second half of the calendar year. McGrath et al. (1995) carried out an ingenious test of the seasonal effect by examining the dates of birth of schizophrenic patients in Queensland and contrasted those born in Australia with those who were born in Europe. The latter group showed an excess of births early in the year (i.e. the European spring) while the former group showed the excess later (in the Australian spring). Furthermore, recent studies that have calculated person-years have still shown an effect. Other methodological problems such as inaccuracy of data, duplication of subjects, choice of controls, taking account of migration, choice of period of analysis, sample size, and use of appropriate statistics have been taken into consideration and the finding still holds (Adams and Kendell, 1999). The large methodologically robust Danish study described above (Mortensen et al., 1999) showed a season of birth effect with a peak rise in early March (relative risk 1.1; 95% CI 1.06–1.18).

Possible causes of the season of birth effect

The cause or causes of the season of birth effect are not yet clear despite decades of speculation and investigation. One theoretical possibility concerns the procreational habits of parents of people with schizophrenia. However the birth dates of siblings of individuals with schizophrenia show no seasonal variation (Torrey, 1989), although one study suggested that the siblings of people with manic depression may show some seasonal variation (Hare, 1976). Increased pregnancy and birth complications in winter, nutritional deficiencies and season variations of trace elements have all been implicated but not definitively proven. Effects of higher temperature, light and weather have been suggested but not substantiated (Torrey et al., 1997b). Few studies have investigated the deficit of schizophrenia in those born in summer months, although this might be just as informative.

Maternal exposure to influenza

Investigators have theorized that the spring excess of births of individuals with schizophrenia could be secondary to prenatal exposure to viruses such as those causing influenza, which are more prevalent during winter. Suvisaari et al. (2000) addressed this issue in a large nationwide sample of all Finnish patients with schizophrenia born between 1950 and 1969. They found that seasonal variation was particularly marked in patients born between 1955 and 1959 but decreased in those born from 1960 onwards. The authors suggested that poliomyelitis or influenza epidemics could account for their findings. A full discussion of maternal influenza as a risk factor for schizophrenia can be found in Chapter 5.

Season of birth and the urban effect

Since many infections are passed on more readily in crowded areas, researchers have enquired whether the season of birth effect is greater in urban than rural settings, and early studies reported positive results (O'Callaghan et al., 1995). Takei et al. (1995) tested the hypothesis that winter birth and urban birth potentiate each other in a sample of first-admission patients with schizophrenia born 1936–1963 in England and Wales. They calculated that city birth was only associated with an increased risk of schizophrenia in those born in autumn (OR 1.19; 95% CI 1.057–1.347) and winter (OR: 1.21 95% CI 1.079–1.364) but not summer or spring. Verdoux et al. (1997) found a greater season of birth effect in densely populated areas in France (20% excess for >136 inhabitants/km^2). However, the Danish study discussed above did not find any interaction between urbanicity and season of birth (Mortensen et al., 1999) or urbanicity and exposure to influenza (Westergaard et al., 1999). Similarly, the large population-based studies described above from Finland (Suvisaari et al., 2000) and the Netherlands (Marcelis et al., 1998) did not find a significant interaction between season and place of birth. Overall, it seems that the urban effect can operate independently of season of birth. The season of birth effect is not only seen in highly populated areas but there is some evidence, mainly from UK, Ireland and France, that the two can interact. It could be that household overcrowding rather than population density is the important determinant.

Differences between people with schizophrenia according to their season of birth

Considerable endeavour has been directed towards identifying differences between summer- and winter-born patients with schizophrenia (Torrey et al., 1997b). Some studies have reported lower skin conductance (Ohlund et al., 1990, 1991; Katsanis et al., 1992) and increased computed tomographic scan abnormalities in the winter born (Sacchetti et al., 1992; d'Amato et al., 1994). Studies of seasonality in obstetric complications and schizophrenia have yielded mixed results (Jones et al., 1991; Cantor-Graae, 1994): Bary and Bary (1964) suggested that the winter birth effect was only seen in lower socioeconomic groups, but this has not been confirmed (Ødegård, 1974). Large studies have not shown increased seasonality in men (Dalen, 1975; Torrey and Torrey, 1980). An interaction between season of birth and genetic risk has been sought, the majority of studies showing that those with no family history are more likely to have been winter born; however, studies in the other direction have also been reported (Torrey et al., 1997b).

In short, there do not seem to be any consistent correlations between winter birth with symptom patterns or subtypes, and no consistent neuropsychological differences have been found. It is perhaps not surprising that this line of research has been relatively unproductive, since the fact that the season of birth effect is small suggests that the majority of summer- and winter-born people with schizophrenia are subject to similar aetiological factors. This means that most studies have insufficient power to detect what will only be small differences.

Migration, ethnic minority status and incidence of schizophrenia

Historical context

As early as 1932, Ødegärd (1932) showed that Norwegian migrants to the USA had an increased risk of psychosis. One early interpretation was that this resulted from selective migration, in that those at risk, less connected with their families, are more likely to leave their homeland. An alternative interpretation was that the alienation and suspicion engendered in the migrant by their unfamiliar surroundings led to psychosis. Thus, Ødegärd (1932) wrote:

Everywhere you are surrounded by people with strange and unfamiliar ways . . . They do not seem to be as friendly as the people at home and many of them do their best to profit by your lack of experience. Even if you have not had any disagreeable experiences yourself, your imagination is stirred by all the stories you have heard about how crooked and dangerous they may be. You notice that your own appearance, clothing and language points you out to everyone as a greenhorn.

In the 1940s and 1950s, a number of studies from the USA (particularly New York) and Canada demonstrated high rates of admission for schizophrenia amongst migrants. Interestingly, not all migrant groups showed the same pattern. Jewish migrants did not show any excess of psychosis and UK-born migrants to the USA had lower rates than the native USA-born individuals, although the second generation (children of UK-born migrants) had higher rates than both the native born and their own parents (Malzberg, 1969).

Interest in this topic has grown with new evidence that the incidence of psychosis is high amongst migrant groups and their children (Thomas et al., 1993; King et al., 1994). Mortensen et al. (1999) found that children born in Greenland to Danish mothers had a relative risk of 3.71 for schizophrenia. The most striking findings have come from the UK, where numerous studies have reported an increased incidence of psychosis among African-Caribbean people (Harrison et al., 1988; Castle et al., 1991; van Os et al., 1996a). Increased rates have also been found in the UK amongst people of African origin (van Os et al., 1996a). King et al. (1994) found higher rates of schizophrenia amongst Asians in the UK. Although this was not confirmed by Bhugra et al. (1997), neither of these studies had sufficient power to be definitive. Increased rates have also been found in Carribean and some other migrant groups living in the Netherlands (Selten and Sijben, 1994; Selten et al., 2001).

Methodological problems

There are serious methodological problems associated with migration and minority group research, which will be outlined below.

Category fallacy

The possibility of 'category fallacy', that the categories of mental illness used in one culture cannot be applied to another, is still raised. However, even when migration between very similar cultures is considered, there is still evidence of an increased risk. Bruxner et al. (1997) found higher rates of hospital admission with psychosis among British, Irish and southern European migrants to Western Australia and the risk persisted many years after migration.

Misdiagnosis

A related question is whether psychiatrists in the host country may wrongly diagnose schizophrenia in migrants because of prejudice or a lack of understanding of their cultural norms. However, one study (Hickling et al. 1999), which invited a black Caribbean psychiatrist to rediagnose African-Caribbean patients at a south London hospital, found that a similar proportion were subsequently diagnosed as having schizophrenia (although there was disagreement as to whether individual patients had schizophrenia). A related theory is that migrants might be more likely to come into contact with services, through lack of family support or because primary and secondary care doctors might be more likely to refer or admit a patient from a different background to themselves. These various theories are reviewed by Sharpley et al. (2001).

Estimating the denominator

A major methodological problem with migration research is the accurate estimation of the denominator. Mortensen et al. (1997) suggested that transient visitors contribute to the excess of psychosis found in migrant studies. However, northern European countries such as the Netherlands and Denmark seem to have the most accurate and comprehensive data and still report the effect. Furthermore, even studies that have taken these pitfalls into account have still found increased rates of psychosis in several migrant and minority groups (van Os et al., 1996a) as have case-control studies that avoided the need for denominator data (Wessely et al., 1991).

Separating the effects of migration and ethnicity

Migration and ethnic minority status are related but not synonymous. They may
influence rates of schizophrenia by different mechanisms, but so far most studies
have not attempted to separate the two. This separation may be relevant to understanding the higher rates that some have reported in second- rather than first-
generation African-Caribbean immigrants in the UK (Harrison et al., 1988). As
third-generation children in Europe enter the 'at-risk' age group, it should be possible to separate out the effects of being a migrant from those of being a member
of an ethnic minority.

A different illness?

There has been considerable debate as to whether migrants with psychosis have the
same illness as their host population. Hutchinson et al. (1999a) compared
symptom profiles in 96 white patients and 64 African-Caribbean patients hospitalized in south London who met the criteria for broadly defined schizophrenia
(RDC). They identified six symptom dimensions from factor analysis of Present
State Examination (PSE) symptoms: mania, depression, first-rank delusions, other
delusions, hallucinations and mixed mania/catatonia. African-Caribbean patients
were slightly over-represented on the mixed mania/catatonia dimension (which
included incoherent speech and inappropriate affect) but this did not reach significance. Other studies have shown high levels of affective, particularly manic, symptoms presenting concurrently with the more classical schizophrenic ones (van Os
et al., 1996b).

There have also been claims that migrants to Western countries from developing
countries who develop schizophrenia have a different outcome than white patients
with such a diagnosis (Mackenzie et al., 1995; Callan, 1996). A 4-year follow-up
study of consecutive admissions with recent-onset psychosis in south London compared course and outcome of psychotic illness between 53 African-Caribbeans and
60 British-born Whites (McKenzie et al., 1995). African-Caribbeans were more
often admitted involuntarily and more often imprisoned over the follow-up period.
However, with regard to clinical outcome, the Caribbeans were less likely to have
had a continuous unremitting illness course (adjusted OR 3). These results suggest
that the high incidence of schizophrenia observed in UK African-Caribbeans is
coupled with a less-deteriorated illness course. More recent studies comparing
outcome among African-Caribbean and white British patients with psychosis have
reported decreased likelihood of a continuous illness course in African-Caribbean
patients. However, the differences between the African-Caribbean and white
patients were not large (Harrison, 1999; McKenzie et al., 2001).

Possible causes of the migration effect

Genes or environment

Genetic predisposition cannot be the sole explanation for the increased rates of psychosis in the African-Caribbeans in the UK, since the increased risk is not shared by the population of origin in the Caribbean (Bhugra et al., 1997; Mahy et al., 1999). However, Hutchinson et al. (1996) found that the morbid risk for schizophrenia among siblings of second-generation (African-Caribbeans born in the UK) psychotic probands was approximately seven times higher than that for their white counterparts, although morbid risks for schizophrenia were similar for parents and siblings of white and first-generation African-Caribbean patients. This study replicates the work of Sugarman and Crauford (1994) and suggests the operation of gene–environment interaction. The question, therefore, arises as to the nature of this environmental factor, which appears to be present in the UK but not the Caribbean countries.

Neurodevelopmental impairment

Increased exposure, or susceptibility, to neurodevelopmental insult such as obstetric complications (Glover et al., 1989; Harrison, 1990; Hutchinson et al., 1997) have been largely excluded as possible explanations. The possibility of prenatal exposure to infection has been raised, as migrant mothers may not have developed immunity to influenza or other viruses and, therefore, their fetuses may have been more likely to have been affected by prenatal exposure to viral infections. However, Selten et al. (1998) examined the numbers of migrants in the Nertherlands with schizophrenia from Surinam and the Dutch Antilles who were born after the 1957 influenza epidemic. They found that individuals who were in the second trimester at the peak of the epidemic were at no greater risk of schizophrenia.

Drug abuse

The role of drug abuse as an aetiological factor in migrant populations is controversial. McGuire et al. (1995) found no difference in drug abuse between their White and African-Caribbean patients in south London. Selten et al. (1997) found that consumption of cannabis was lower amongst Caribbean migrants to the Netherlands than amongst the native population but the incidence rates of schizophrenia were higher in the former.

Social causation

The combination of more affective symptoms and a less-deteriorated course has led to the theory that factors in the social environment might cause psychosis in those migrants predisposed but who might not otherwise develop the disease (McKenzie et al., 1995). Racism (overt and institutionalized), social isolation and reduced social networks may contribute (Hutchinson et al., 1999b). Boydell et al. (2001) have recently found that incidence rates of broadly defined schizophrenia increased in ethnic minorities as the proportion of ethnic minorities in the locality fell, suggesting that social experience contributes to the development of the disorder. Janssen et al. (2002) measured subjective experience of discrimination and subsequent development of psychotic illness years later. Experience of discrimination strongly predicted the development of a psychotic illness (OR 2.8; CI 1.9–4.2). Ethnic minority status was no longer significant when experience of discrimination was controlled for. Some people may be more susceptible to the deleterious effects of such events than others because they are less able to derive support from those around them (Sharpley et al., 2001). Mallett et al. (1998) demonstrated that one of the main distinguishing features of first-onset patients of Caribbean origin with psychosis in London was that they lived alone and additionally were separated from their mother at an early age, while Bhugra et al. (1997) found that unemployment was particularly high amongst people of Caribbean origin first presenting with schizophrenia. Interest has recently focused on the cognitive processing of external events and whether this increases the risk of psychosis. Attributional style (particularly making external attributions) could be a pathway through which discrimination and social adversity could lead to psychosis (Sharpley et al., 2001).

Urbanization

Increased rates of schizophrenia amongst migrants and ethnic minorities might be attributed (at least in part) to the urban effect discussed earlier, as most migrants live in cities and often in the most deprived areas. This might explain why second-generation African-Caribbeans seem to have higher rates than their parents (Hutchinson et al., 1999a,b). Malzberg (1969) found that controlling for urbanicity reduced but did not explain the excess of psychosis amongst migrants to the USA.

Summary

When high rates of psychosis were identified in migrant groups, it was thought that a single risk factor would be found to explain the excess. Maternal exposure and low resistance to viral agents during gestation were considered but have largely been excluded. The evidence of increased rates across many disparate groups argues against specific biological or genetic factors and suggests that social and psychological aetiological factors are operating. It is likely that the same environmental factors are acting on the minority as on the majority group, but the former are more exposed or less protected against them.

REFERENCES

Adams W, Kendell RE (1999) Annual variation in birth rate of people who subsequently develop schizophrenia. British Journal of Psychiatry 175, 522–527.

Allardyce J, Boydell J, van Os J et al. (2001) A comparison of the incidence of schizophrenia in rural Dumfries and Galloway and urban Camberwell. British Journal of Psychiatry 179, 335–339.

Astrup C, Ødegård O (1961) Internal migration and mental illness in Norway. Psychiatric Quarterly 34, 116–130.

Bary H, Bary H (1964) Season of birth: an epidemiological study in psychiatry. Archives of General Psychiatry 11, 385–391.

Bebbington P, Wilkins S, Jones P et al. (1993) Life events and psychosis. Initial results from the Camberwell Collaborative Psychosis Study. British Journal of Psychiatry 162, 72–79.

Bhugra D, Leff J, Mallett R et al. (1997) Incidence and outcome of schizophrenia in Whites, African Caribbeans and Asians in London. Psychological Medicine 27, 791–798.

Boydell J, vanOs J, McKenzie K et al. (2001) The incidence of schizophrenia in ethnic minorities is highest in London neighbourhoods which are mainly white. British Medical Journal 7325, 1336–1338.

Bradbury TN, Miller GA (1985) Season of birth in schizophrenia: a review of the evidence, methodology and etiology. Psychological Bulletin 98, 569–594.

Brown A, Cohen P, Greenwald S et al. (2000) Non-affective psychosis after prenatal exposure to rubella. American Journal of Psychiatry 157, 438–443.

Bruxner G, Burvill P, Fazio S, Febbo S (1997) Aspects of psychiatric admissions of migrants to hospitals in Perth, Western Australia. Australian and New Zealand Journal of Psychiatry 31, 532–542.

Callan AF (1996) Schizophrenia in Afro-Caribbean immigrants. Journal of the Royal Society of Medicine 89, 253–256.

Cantor-Graae E, McNeil T, Sjostrom K et al. (1994) Obstetric complications and their relationship to other aetiological risk factors in schizophrenia. A case-control study. Journal of Nervous and Mental Disorders 182, 645–650.

Castle D, Wessley S, Der G, Murray R (1991) The incidence of operationally defined schizophrenia in Camberwell, 1965–1984. British Journal of Psychiatry 171, 140–144.

Castle D, Scott K, Wessely S et al. (1993) Does social deprivation during gestation and early life predispose to later schizophrenia? Social Psychiatry and Psychiatric Epidemiology 28, 1–4.

Dalen P (1975) Season of Birth: A study of Schizophrenia and other Mental Disorders. New York: American Elsevier.

d'Amato T, Rochet T, Dalery J, Chauchat JH, Martin JP, Marie-Cardine M (1994) Seasonality of birth and ventricular enlargement in chronic schizophrenia. Psychiatry Research. 55, 65–73.

Dauncey K, Giggs J, Baker K, Harrison G (1993) Schizophrenia in Nottingham: lifelong residential mobility of a cohort. British Journal of Psychiatry 163, 613–619.

Eaton W, Mortensen P, Frydenberg M (2000) Obstetric factors, urbanization and psychosis. Schizophrenia Research 43, 117–1233.

Faris R, Dunham H (1939) Mental Disorders in Urban Areas. Chicago: University of Chicago Press.

Freeman H (1994) Schizophrenia and city residence. British Journal of Psychiatry 164(Suppl. 23), 39–50.

Glover G (1989) Why is there a high rate of schizophrenia in British Caribbeans? British Journal of Hospital Medicine 42, 48–51.

Hare E (1955) Mental illness and social class in Bristol. British Journal of Preventative and Social Medicine 9, 191–195.

Hare E (1956) Mental illness and social conditions in Bristol. Journal of Mental Science 102, 349–357.

Hare E (1976) The season of birth of psychiatric patients. British Journal of Psychiatry 129, 49–54.

Harrison G (1990) Searching for the causes of schizophrenia: the role of migrant studies. Schizophrenia Bulletin 16, 663–671.

Harrison, G (1999) Outcome of psychosis in people of African-Caribbean family origin. British Journal of Psychiatry 175, 43–49.

Harrison G, Owens D, Holten A et al. (1988) A prospective study of severe mental disorder in Afro-Caribbean patients. Psychological Medicine 18, 643–657.

Hickling W, McKenzie K, Mullen R et al. (1999) A Jamaican psychiatrist evaluates diagnoses at a London hospital. British Journal of Psychiatry 175, 283–285.

Hoek HW, Brown AS, Susser E (1998) The Dutch famine and schizophrenia spectrum disorders. Social Psychiatry and Psychiatric Epidemiology 33, 373–379.

Hutchinson G, Takei N, Fahy TA et al. (1996) Morbid risk of schizophrenia in first-degree relatives of white and African-Caribbean patients with psychosis. British Journal of Psychiatry 169, 776–780.

Hutchinson G, Takei N, Bhugra T et al. (1997) Increased rate of psychosis among African-Caribbeans in Britain is not due to an excess of pregnancy and birth complications. British Journal of Psychiatry 171, 145–147.

Hutchinson G, Takei N, Sham P, Harvey I, Murray RM (1999a) Factor analysis of symptoms in schizophrenia: differences between White and Caribbean patients in Camberwell [in process citation]. Psychological Medicine 29, 607–612.

Hutchinson G, Mallett R, Fletcher H (1999b) Are the increased rates of psychosis reported for the population of Caribbean origin in Britain an urban effect? International Review of Psychiatry 11, 122–128.

Jablensky A, Cole SW (1997) Is the earlier age at onset of schizophrenia in males a confounded finding? Results from a cross-cultural investigation. British Journal of Psychiatry 170, 234–240.

Janssen I, Hanssen M, Bak M et al. (2002) Evidence that ethnic group effects on psychosis risk are confounded by experience of discrimination. Schizophrenia Research 53(Suppl.), 34.

Jones P, Goodman R, Owen M, Lewis S, Murray R (1991) Neurodevelopment and the chronological curiosities of schizophrenia. In: Developmental Neuropathology of Schizophrenia, Mednick SA, ed. New York: Pleneum Press, pp. 191–201.

Katsanis J, Ficken J, Iacono W, Beiser M (1992) Season of birth and electrodermal activity in functional psychoses. Biological Psychiatry 31, 841–855.

King M, Coker E, Leavey G et al. (1994) Incidence of psychotic illness in London: a comparison of ethnic groups. British Medical Journal 309, 1115–1119.

Lewis G, David A, Andreasson S et al. (1992) Schizophrenia and city life. Lancet 340, 137–140.

Lewis MS (1989) Age-incidence and schizophrenia. Part 1 The season of birth controversy. Schizophrenia Bulletin 15, 59–73.

Mahy G, Mallett R, Leff J, Bhugra D (1999) First-contact incidence rate of schizophrenia in Barbados. British Journal of Psychiatry 175, 28–33.

Malla A, Cortese L, Shaw TS et al. (1990) Life events and relapse in schizophrenia: a one year prospective study. Social Psychiatry and Psychiatric Epidemiology 25, 221–224.

Mallett R, Hutchinson G, Leff J (1998) Social conditions and schizophrenia in African-Caribbeans: Edward Hare revisited. In: Proceedings of the Royal College of Psychiatrists Winter Meeting, No. 39.

Malzberg B (1969) Are immigrants psychologically disturbed? In: Changing Perspectives in Mental Illness, Plog S, Edgerton R, eds. New York: Holt, Rinehart and Winston, pp. 395 -421.

Marcelis M, Navarro-Mateu F, Murray R, Selten JP, van Os J (1998) Urbanization and psychosis: a study of 1942–1978 birth cohorts in the Netherlands. Psychological Medicine 28, 871–879.

Marcelis M, Takei N, van Os J (1999) Urbanization and risk for schizophrenia: does the effect operate before or around the time of illness onset? Psychological Medicine 29, 1197–1203.

McGrath J, Welham J, Pemberton M (1995) Month of birth, hemisphere of birth and schizophrenia. British Journal of Psychiatry 167, 783–785.

McGuire P, Jones P, Harvey M (1995) Morbid risk of schizophrenia in relatives of patients with cannabis-associated psychosis. Schizophrenia Research 15, 277–281.

McKenzie K, van Os J, Fahy T et al. (1995) Psychosis with good prognosis in Afro-Caribbean people now living in the United Kingdom [see comments]. British Medical Journal 311, 1325–1328.

McKenzie K, Samele C, van Horn E, Tattan T, van Os J, Murray RM (2001) A comparison of the outcome and treatment of psychosis in people of Caribbean origin living in the UK and British Whites. British Journal of Psychiatry 178, 160–165.

Mortensen PB, Cantor-Graae E, McNeil TF (1997) Institution increased rates of schizophrenia among immigrants: some methodological concerns raised by Danish findings [see comments]. Psychological Medicine 27, 813–820 [see comment in Psychological Medicine (1998) 28, 496–497].

Mortensen P, Pedersen C, Westergaard T et al. (1999) Effects of family history and place and season of birth on the risk of schizophrenia. New England Journal of Medicine 340, 603–608 [correspondence New England Journal of Medicine (1999) 341, 370–372].

Murray R, Fearon P (1999) The developmental 'risk factor' model of schizophrenia. Journal of Psychiatric Research 33, 497–499.

Murray RM, O'Callaghan E, Castle DJ et al. (1992) A neurodevelopmental approach to the classification of schizophrenia. Schizophrenia Bulletin 18, 319–332.

O'Callaghan E, Cotter D, Colgan K et al. (1995) Confinement of winter birth excess in schizophrenia to the urban born and its gender specificity. British Journal of Psychiatry 66, 51–54.

Ødegård O (1932) Emigration and insanity: a study of mental disease among Norwegian born population in Minnesota. Acta Psychiatrica Neurologica Scandinavica Suppl. 4.

Ødegård O (1974) Season of birth in the general population and in patients with mental disorder in Norway. British Journal of Psychiatry 125, 397–405.

Ohlund L, Ohman A, Alm T et al. (1990) Season of birth and electrodermal unresponsiveness in male schizophrenics. Biological Psychiatry 27, 328–340.

Ohlund L, Ohman A, Ost L (1991) Electrodermal orienting response, maternal age and season of birth in schizophrenia. Psychiatry Research 36, 223–232.

Ohta Y, Nakane Y, Nishihara J, Takemoto T (1992) Ecological structure and incidence rates of schizophrenia in Nagasaki City. Acta Psychiatrica Scandinavica 86, 113–120.

Pedersen CB, Mortensen PB (2001) Urbanization and schizophrenia; evidence of a cumulative negative effect of urban residence during upbringing. Schizophrenia Research Suppl. 41, 65–66.

Peen J, Dekker J (1997) Admission rates for schizophrenia in the Netherlands: an urban/rural comparison. Acta Psychiatrica Scandinavica 96, 301–305.

Sacchetti E, Calzeroni A, Vita A et al. (1992) The brain damage hypothesis of the seasonality of births in schizophrenia and major affective disorders: evidence from computerised tomography. British Journal of Psychiatry 160, 390–397.

Selten JP, Sijben N (1994) First admission rate for schizophrenia in immigrants to the Netherlands: the Dutch National Register. Social Psychiatry and Psychiatric Epidemiology 29, 71–72.

Selten JP, Slaets JP, Kahn RS (1997) Schizophrenia in Surinamese and Dutch Antillean immigrants to the Netherlands: evidence of an increased incidence [see comments]. Psychological Medicine 27, 807–811 [comment in Psychological Medicine (1998) 28, 496].

Selten JP, Slaets J, Kahn R (1998) Prenatal exposure to influenza and schizophrenia in Surinamese and Dutch Antillean immigrants to the Netherlands. Schizophrenia Research 30, 101–103.

Selten JP, Veen N, Feller W, Blom JD et al. (2001) Incidence of psychotic disorders in immigrant groups to the Netherlands. British Journal of Psychiatry 178, 1–7.

Sharpley M, Hutchinson G, McKenzie K, Murray RM (2001) Understanding the excess of psychosis among the African-Caribbean population in England. Review of current hypotheses. British Journal of Psychiatry 178(Suppl. 40), 60–68.

Spitzer RL, Williams JBW, Gibbon M (1990) User's Guide for the Structured Clinical Interview for DSM-III-R (SCID). Washington, DC: American Psychiatric Press.

Sugarman P, Crauford D (1994) Schizophrenia in the Afro-Caribbean community. British Journal of Psychiatry 164, 474–480.

Susser E, Neugebauer R, Hoek H et al. (1996) Schizophrenia after prenatal famine: further evidence. Archives of General Psychiatry 53, 25–31.

Susser E, Hoek H, Brown A (1998) Neurodevelopmental disorders after prenatal famine. American Journal of Epidemiology 147, 213–216.

Suvisaari JM, Haukka JK, Tanskanen AJ, Lonnqvist JK (2000) Decreasing seasonal variation of births in schizophrenia. Psychological Medicine 30, 315–324.

Takei N, Sham P, O'Callaghan E et al. (1995) Schizophrenia increased risk associated with winter and city birth. Journal of Epidemiology and Community Health 49, 106–107.

Thomas CS, Stone K, Osborn M et al. (1993) Psychiatric morbidity and compulsory admission among UK born Europeans, Afro-Caribbeans and Asians in central Manchester. British Journal of Psychiatry 163, 91–99.

Thornicroft G, Bisoffi G, de Salva D, Tansella M (1993) Urban–rural differences in the associations between social deprivation and psychiatric service utilization in schizophrenia and all diagnoses: a case-register study in northern Italy. Psychological Medicine 23, 487–496.

Torrey EF (1989) The epidemiology of schizophrenia: questions needing answers. In: Schizophrenia: Scientific Progress, Schulz S, Tamminga C, eds. New York: Oxford University Press.

Torrey EF, Torrey B (1980) Sex differences in the seasonality of schizophrenic births [letter]. British Journal of Psychiatry 137, 101–102.

Torrey EF, Bowler A, Clark K (1997a) Urban birth and residence as risk factors for psychoses: an analysis of 1880 data. Schizophrenia Research 25, 169–176.

Torrey EF, Miller J, Rawlings R, Yolken R (1997b) Seasonality of births in schizophrenia and bipolar disorder: a review of the literature. Schizophrenia Research 28, 1–38.

Torrey EF, Weis S, Yolken RH (2001) An epizootic etiology of schizophrenia: is it time to put the cat out? Schizophrenia Research 49, 49.

van Os J, Castle DJ, Takei N, Der G, Murray RM (1996a) Psychotic illness in ethnic minorities: clarification from the 1991 census. Psychological Medicine 26, 203–208.

van Os J, Takei N, Castle DJ et al. (1996b) The incidence of mania: time trends in relation to gender and ethnicity. Social Psychiatry and Psychiatric Epidemiology 31, 129–136.

van Os J, Driessen G, Gunther N et al. (2000) Neighbourhood variation in incidence of schizophrenia. Evidence for person–environment interaction. British Journal of Psychiatry 176, 243–248.

van Os J, Hanssen M, Bijl RV, Vollebergh W (2001) Prevalence of psychotic disorder and community level of psychotic symptoms: an urban–rural comparison. Archives of General Psychiatry 58, 663–668.

Ventura J, Nuechterlein KH, Lukoff D, Hardesty JP (1989) A prospective study of stressful life events and schizophrenic relapse. Journal of Abnormal Psychology 98, 407–411.

Verdoux H, Takei N, Cassou R et al. (1997) Seasonality of birth in schizophrenia: the effect of regional population density. Schizophrenia Research 23, 175–180.

Wessely S, Castle D, Der R et al. (1991) Schizophrenia and Afro-Caribbeans: a case-control study. British Journal of Psychiatry 159, 795–801.

Westergaard T, Mortensen P, Pedersen C et al. (1999) Exposure to prenatal and childhood infections and the risk of schizophrenia. Archives of General Psychiatry 56, 993–998.

World Health Organization (1967) Manual of International Statistical Classification of Diseases, Injuries and Causes of Death, 8th edn. Geneva: World Health Organization.

World Health Organization (1978) Manual of International Statistical Classification of Diseases, Injuries and Causes of Death, 9th edn. Geneva: World Health Organization.

Part II

The developmental epidemiology of schizophrenia

Introduction

The term developmental epidemiology was originally confined to the study of the distribution and risks of childhood disorders (Costello and Angold, 1995) but has extended to include the study of early antecedents and risk factors for adult-onset illness and chronic diseases (Buka and Lipsitt, 1994). It is also known as 'life-course epidemiology' (Kuh and Ben-Schlomo, 1997). Developmental epidemiology studies causation in the context of development and investigates causal chain mechanisms and person–environment interaction.

From its first descriptions, schizophrenic psychosis had a longitudinal dimension. Thomas Clouston (1892) recognized a syndrome of 'developmental insanity' in which developmental physical abnormalities were associated with early-onset psychotic phenomena, particularly in men. While defining the schizophrenia syndrome more clearly, both Kraepelin (1896) and Bleuler (1911) noted that people who developed the psychotic syndrome were often different from their peers before psychosis began, but these observations were incorporated into the psychodynamic formulations prevalent at the time.

During the 1980s, a 'neurodevelopmental hypothesis' of schizophrenia became prominent (Murray & Lewis, 1987; Weinberger, 1987). This hypothesis broadly proposed that interaction between early pathology or insult and normal processes of structural and functional brain development yielded a nervous system prone to psychosis. Jones (1999) has pointed out that the neurodevelopmental hypothesis of schizophrenia 'is not really a hypothesis at all, rather a general position or thesis . . . that has directed research towards early life in terms of causation'.

Central to a developmental model of schizophrenia is the identification of pre- and perinatal risk factors and the demonstration of childhood manifestations of deviance long before the frank onset of the illness. Cannon and colleagues in Chapter 5 examine the evidence for pre- and perinatal risk factors for schizophrenia, including such diverse risk factors as winter/spring birth, urban birth, prenatal infection, prenatal stress, prenatal malnutrition and birth complications. The authors conclude that there is now secure evidence for the existence of pre- and perinatal risk factors for schizophrenia and warn that there is little to be gained from continuing to replicate these findings. Research should instead focus on collaboration with other disciplines to elucidate the mechanisms behind these intriguing associations.

The existence of a developmental theory of schizophrenia implies that the presence of developmental abnormalities should be detectable during childhood and adolescence. In Chapter 6, Cannon and colleagues seek to clarify the nature of these childhood developmental abnormalities by drawing on two robust sources of evidence: general population birth cohort studies and genetic high-risk studies. Despite their very different designs, the studies indicate that children who later go on to develop schizophrenia show early motor, language, cognitive, emotional and sociobehavioural developmental abnormalities compared with their peers or siblings. There is some evidence for a dose–response relationship and the most likely unifying mechanism is a genetic one. More refined and detailed study of these developmental trajectory disorders will be a challenge for the future.

The next two chapters chart the development of schizophrenia through the prodromal stage and the first episode. In Chapter 7, Häfner outlines the various stages of the prodrome and the problems in defining when onset actually occurs. In Chapter 8, Clarke and O'Callaghan acknowledge these problems but point out the value of studying the illness from its first episode. Using this strategy, we can get information about risk factors, brain structure and functional abnormalities in schizophrenia without bias from treatment or chronicity.

Although the peak age of onset for schizophrenia is in the late teens and early twenties, the disorder can also have its onset in childhood or in old age. In Chapter 9, Orr and Castle provide an overview of the characteristics of early- and late-onset schizophrenia and conclude that 'detailed comparative studies of these groups of patients can enhance our understanding of schizophrenia at any age'.

REFERENCES

Bleuler E (1911) Dementia praecox oder Gruppe der Schizophrenien. Leipzig: Deutick.

Buka SL, Lipsitt AP (1994) Towards a developmental epidemiology. In: Developmental Follow-up: Concepts, Domains and Methods, Freidman SL, Haywood HC, eds. New York: Academic Press, pp. 331–350.

Clouston TS (1892) Clinical Lectures on Mental Diseases, 3rd edn. London: Churchill.

Costello EJ, Angold A (1995) Developmental epidemiology. In: Developmental Psychopathology Vol. 1, Cicchetti D, Cohen DJ, eds. New York: Wiley, pp. 23–56.

Jones PB (1999) Longitudinal approaches to the search for the causes of schizophrenia: past, present and future. In: Search for the Causes of Schizophrenia Vol. IV, Balance of the Century, Gattaz WF, Häfner H, eds. Darmstadt: Steinkopf and Berlin, Springer, pp. 91–119

Kraepelin E (1896) Dementia praecox. In: Psychiatrie, 5th edn. Leipzig: Barth, pp. 426–441.

Kuh D, Ben-Schlomo Y (1997) A Life Course Approach to Chronic Disease Epidemiology. Oxford: Oxford University Press.

Murray RM, Lewis SW (1987) Is schizophrenia a neurodevelopmental disorder? British Medical Journal 295, 681–682.

Weinberger DR (1987) Implications of normal brain development for the pathogenesis of schizophrenia. Archives of General Psychiatry 44, 660–669.

5

Prenatal and perinatal risk factors for schizophrenia

Mary Cannon[1], Robert Kendell[2], Ezra Susser[3] and Peter Jones[4]

[1]Institute of Psychiatry, Kings College London, UK
[2]Department of Psychiatry, University of Edinburgh, UK
[3]Division of Epidemiology, Columbia University, New York, USA
[4]Division of Psychiatry, University of Cambridge, UK

Historical context

A neurodevelopmental model of schizophrenia

The existence of pre- and perinatal risk factors for schizophrenia as outlined in this chapter is central to the notion of schizophrenia as a neurodevelopmental disorder. The 'neurodevelopmental hypothesis' of schizophrenia proposes a subtle deviance in early brain development, the full adverse consequences of which are not manifest until adolescence or early adulthood. The hypothesis came to prominence in the late 1980s (Murray and Lewis, 1987; Weinberger, 1987), though similar models had been proposed by other researchers decades, even centuries, earlier (Clouston, 1891, 1892; Southard, 1915; Pasamanick et al., 1956).

The 1980s version of the neurodevelopmental hypothesis originated from a number of strands of evidence available at that time, including retrospective studies revealing a pattern of abnormalities in neurological and behavioural characteristics during childhood (Watt, 1978; Aylward et al., 1984), histopathological studies indicating developmental abnormalities in the hippocampus (Kovelman and Scheibel, 1984; Jakob and Beckman, 1986) and neuroimaging studies showing cerebral ventricular enlargement (Johnstone et al., 1976; Weinberger et al., 1979), even at the time of the first episode (Turner et al., 1986). Not all of this evidence has withstood the test of time, particularly the original histopathological findings. However, new, convincing information to support the neurodevelopmental hypothesis has emerged from epidemiological investigations, longitudinal studies of high-risk offspring, imaging studies and recent, robust neuropathological investigations (for review see Marenco and Weinberger, 2000; McDonald et al., 2000).

The neurodevelopmental hypothesis is now viewed as an aetiological model that directs research towards early life (Jones, 1999). These early risk factors for schizophrenia represent some of the most challenging and interesting targets of schizophrenia epidemiology.

Prenatal risk factors for schizophrenia

Time and place of birth

There is consistent evidence for a 5–8% winter/spring excess of births for both schizophrenia and mania/bipolar disorder (Hare et al., 1974; Bradbury and Miller, 1985). It appears to be a robust finding, at least in the northern hemisphere (Hare, 1975; Kendell and Adams, 1991; Mortensen et al., 1999), although the effect seems to be absent, or at least much weaker, in the southern hemisphere (McGrath and Welham, 1999). The cause of the 'season of birth' effect is not known. An environmental factor that fluctuates with the season and has its effects around the time of birth is the presumptive explanation and seasonal infections are the most popular candidate (Torrey et al., 1997). Detailed reviews of this literature are provided by Cotter et al. (1995) and Torrey et al. (1997) and the topic is discussed further in Chapter 4.

The risk of developing schizophrenia has consistently been found to be increased among those born in cities compared with those born in rural areas (Torrey and Bowler, 1990; Lewis et al., 1992; Takei et al., 1995; Marcelis et al., 1998; Mortensen et al., 1999), but effect sizes are small, ranging between 1.5 and 2.5. Many earlier studies presented good evidence that the excess of schizophrenia found in the central areas of large cities was largely a result of migration into these areas of adolescents and young adults a few months or years before they developed overt schizophrenia (Gerard and Houston, 1953; Hare, 1956). Therefore, attempts have been made to tease apart the effects of urban birth and urban living. Marcelis et al. (1999) found that the greatest risk was for those born in urban areas with no additional effect of later urban residence. Urban dwellers who were not born in the city were not at increased risk of schizophrenia. These results indicate that the urban risk factor or factors associated with an increase in risk of schizophrenia appear to act in early life rather than around the time of illness onset. Linear trends for risk of schizophrenia with increasing population density of area of birth have been noted (Marcelis et al. 1998; Mortensen et al., 1999). However, like winter/spring birth, urban birth is a proxy variable that could encompass a large number of possible risk factors, including prenatal and childhood infections, the prevalence of which tends to increase with increasing population density. This topic is discussed in detail in Chapter 4.

Prenatal infection as a risk factor for schizophrenia

Prenatal influenza

Much of the evidence regarding the role of prenatal infections has come from ecological or population-association studies. In 1988, Mednick and colleagues demonstrated that the offspring of women who were in the second trimester of pregnancy during the 1957–58 influenza A_2 pandemic in Helsinki were about twice as likely to be hospitalized with a diagnosis of schizophrenia as those not exposed during pregnancy or exposed earlier or later in pregnancy. There have been many attempts to replicate this intriguing finding in different populations using an ecological design (Kendell and Kemp, 1989; Mednick et al., 1990; Kendell and Adams, 1991; O'Callaghan et al., 1991; Torrey et al., 1992; Erlenmeyer-Kimling et al., 1994; McGrath et al., 1994; Kunugi et al., 1995; Izumoto et al., 1999). The effect sizes demonstrated in these studies are small – somewhere between 1.5 and 2.0 (Cannon and Jones, 1996) – and not all ecological studies have replicated the association (Torrey et al., 1988; Kendell and Kemp, 1989; Selten and Slaets, 1994; Susser et al., 1994; Selten et al. 1999; Westergaard et al., 1999), but this is not inconsistent with a small effect on the threshold of detectability. The balance of evidence suggests that maternal influenza in the 1957 epidemic was associated with a slightly raised incidence of schizophrenia if it occurred in the second trimester of pregnancy, particularly the fifth or sixth month (for review, see McGrath et al., 1995; Wright et al., 1999). In most studies where the sexes are examined separately, the positive association was found mainly or exclusively in females (Kendell and Kemp, 1989; Mednick et al., 1990; O'Callaghan et al., 1991; Adams et al., 1993; McGrath et al., 1994; Takei et al., 1994, 1996; Izumoto et al., 1999) but no satisfactory explanation has yet been offered for this. Likewise, the association with prenatal influenza does not adequately account for the 'season-of-birth effect' reviewed in the previous section (Torrey et al., 1991).

Studies of longer-term trends in the association between the timing of influenza epidemics and the birth dates of people with schizophrenia have yielded generally positive results in most (Barr et al., 1990; Sham et al., 1992; Adams et al., 1993; Takei et al. 1994) but not all (Torrey et al., 1988; Selten and Slaets, 1994; Morgan et al., 1997) studies. Those studies based on whole countries or large regions (such as Western Australia) will, in general, be less powerful than those based solely in urban areas where infection is concentrated (Kendell and Kemp, 1989), and studies based on highly mobile populations, such as occur in the USA (Torrey et al., 1988), will be weak because the ecological design assumes that most people are still living in the state or region in which they were born when they develop schizophrenia two or three decades later.

The ecological design has many limitations. There may be unknown confounding with other factors, such as maternal fever or medication, that could explain the association. Another major limitation of the design is the so-called 'ecological fallacy': we cannot be certain that the individuals in the population who were exposed to influenza in utero are the same individuals who are diagnosed with schizophrenia as adults.

The application of cohort and case-control methodology to this question then followed. Two case-control studies replicated the association between second trimester exposure to influenza and later schizophrenia but relied on maternal recall for information about the exposure (Stöber et al., 1992; Wright et al., 1995). Two cohort studies have failed to support the influenza–schizophrenia association (Crow and Done, 1992; Cannon et al., 1996). The British 1958 birth cohort study (National Child Development Study (NCDS)) collected information on all children born in one week in March 1958. In the first study, mothers were asked after they had given birth whether they had suffered influenza (the 1957 A_2 pandemic) during pregnancy. There was no association between reported maternal influenza and schizophrenia in the offspring (Crow et al., 1991; Crow and Done, 1992). Cannon and colleagues (1996) followed a group in Dublin who had been exposed to the same 1957 pandemic. Valid information on exposure had been collected for an earlier report by Coffey and Jessop (1959, 1963). There was no evidence of an excess of schizophrenia in the exposed group during adult life, although a secondary analysis suggested a link with affective disorder.

The negative results of these cohort studies must, of necessity, be viewed in the light of their limited power to detect an effect (Adams and Kendell, 1996) and the evidence that self-report of influenza infection is not an accurate indication of serological infection (Elder et al., 1996). Certainly the prevalence of recall of pregnancy infection in the NCDS (Crow and Done, 1992) was much lower than would have been expected given the severity of the influenza pandemic only a few months previously.

Other prenatal infections

Interest in prenatal infection as a risk factor for schizophrenia is not restricted to influenza. Influenza lends itself to study because of the frequent occurrence of well-defined epidemics. Brown et al. (2000a) showed that second trimester exposure to a wide variety of respiratory infections (including influenza, pneumonia, tuberculosis and acute bronchitis among others) was associated with a significantly increased risk of schizophrenia spectrum disorders in the Prenatal Determinants of Schizophrenia Study (adjusted relative risk 2.13). These results indicate that several infections, both bacterial and viral, may increase the risk of schizophrenia presumably through some common pathogenic mechanism. An ecological study from Finland by Suvisaari and colleagues (1999) found an association between second trimester exposure to poliovirus infection and later schizophrenia. Jones and colleagues (1999) have followed a large group of individuals whose mothers were identified during pregnancy as suffering from identified viral infections (Fine et al., 1985) and have found evidence relating neurotrophic virus exposure with a range of adverse central nervous system (CNS) outcomes, including mental retardation, epilepsy and psychosis.

Prenatal rubella

Brown and colleagues (2000b) investigated a cohort of individuals who were serologically documented to have sustained in utero exposure to rubella and found that the rubella-exposed subjects, most of whom were exposed in the first trimester, had a substantially higher risk (relative risk 5.2) of developing nonaffective psychoses than those who were not exposed, independent of hearing status. The cohort methodology with proof of individual exposure status is robust and the effect size for the association between prenatal rubella and schizophrenia is much larger than that reported for prenatal influenza. These findings suggest that nonaffective psychosis may be a remote neuropsychiatric consequence of prenatal rubella.

Neonatal and early childhood infection

The time window during which early exposure to infection may exert an effect appears to extend into childhood. The North Finland 1966 birth cohort contains all live births (12058 in total) to women in northern Finland (Oulu and Lapland provinces) during 1966 (Rantakallio, 1969). Rantakallio and colleagues (1997) identified through record linkage all cohort members who had been hospitalized during childhood for a CNS infection (mainly encephalitis and meningitis). They then identified those members of the cohort who had been hospitalized for psychiatric illness. Of 145 in the group with serologically diagnosed childhood CNS infections who had survived to age 16 years, four (2.8%) developed schizophrenia, compared with 0.7% of the unexposed majority. This fourfold relative risk may even underestimate the true risk because of the restriction to severe exposure. The relative incidence of schizophrenia was particularly high among a group of 16 individuals who contracted neonatal coxsackievirus B meningitis during an epidemic in one maternity unit.

There is biological plausibility for this high relative risk to be interpreted in terms of causality, the CNS was known to have been affected, and similar findings emerged in this sample for mental retardation and childhood epilepsy (Rantakallio and von Wendt, 1986). An estimate of the population attributable fraction (the amount by which the population burden of schizophrenia would be reduced if the effect of the exposure, if causal, were removed) is around 4%. As with any causal inference, one must consider the possibility of reverse causality. The CNS may already have been abnormal in the individuals who developed infection and schizophrenia, and these abnormalities may have made them liable to CNS infection. Unknown genetic or epigenetic factors may be necessary components of the causal pathway.

Prenatal infection: possible mechanisms and future directions

What are the possible aetiological mechanisms underlying the association between prenatal exposure to infection and later schizophrenia? Brown et al. (2000a) offer a number of possibilities: hyperthermia, medication, and the maternal inflammatory response to infection (proinflammatory cytokines and chemokines) (Nelson et al., 1998). Immune mechanisms have also been suggested (Fatemi et al., 1999;

Wright et al., 1999). The role of genetic vulnerability remains unclear (Murray et al., 1992).

These are all interesting possibilities. The availability of stored prenatal serum from birth cohorts in the USA, who are now in the period of risk for schizophrenia may help to answer some of these questions and test these hypotheses more precisely (Susser et al., 2000). A new generation of studies on the prenatal infection and schizophrenia story is beginning. Using stored prenatal serum samples from the Providence cohort of the National Collaborative Perinatal Project, Buka et al. (2001) has reported a strong association between maternal antibodies to herpes simplex virus type 2 gG2 glycoprotein and later psychosis (odds ratio (OR) 5.8; confidence interval (CI) 1.7–19.3). The investigators also found an association between adult psychosis and maternal levels of certain cytokines, but these were preliminary results. The future of this field of enquiry lies in the combination of molecular biological techniques to define exposure (Yolken and Torrey, 1995), molecular genetics to define susceptibility and the opportunistic use of population-based samples.

Other putative prenatal epigenetic risks

Prenatal famine

A series of ecological studies of exposure to prenatal famine (Susser and Lin, 1992, 1994; Susser et al., 1996) have demonstrated dose–response relationships between maternal nutritional deprivation during the Nazi blockade of the Netherlands in the winter of 1944–45 and risk of later schizophrenia in the offspring. The initial finding to emerge from these studies was that birth cohorts exposed to the famine in early but not late gestation had a twofold increase in risk for schizophrenia (Susser and Lin, 1992; Susser et al., 1996). A subsequent study using military conscription data demonstrated that prenatal famine during early gestation was associated with a twofold elevation in risk for schizoid or schizotypal personality disorders (Hoek et al., 1996). The authors postulate that severe nutritional deprivation is the aetiological mechanism involved (Butler et al., 1999; Hoek et al., 1999) and this possibility has received indirect support from a finding that a short interval between siblings is associated with an increased risk of schizophrenia (Westergaard et al., 1999). Again, there is biological plausibility for this putative cause; congenital CNS defects in this population were related to famine exposure in a similar fashion (Stein et al., 1975). Confounding and interaction with genetic effects are issues that the investigators are tackling by studying the individuals and by more detailed studies of nutritional status in birth cohorts (Hoek et al., 1999).

Rhesus incompatibility

Rhesus (Rh) incompatibility, characterized by a Rh-negative mother pregnant with a Rh-positive fetus, has been associated with an elevated risk for schizophrenia.

Hollister et al. (1996) used data on males from the Danish Perinatal Cohort and found an elevated risk for schizophrenia among offspring of Rh-incompatible pregnancies compared with Rh-compatible pregnancies. Rhesus incompatibility can give rise to haemolytic disease of the newborn, which results, among other things, in childhood neuromotor abnormalities and behavioural disorders such as emotional instability. It is possible that schizophrenia is yet another possible consequence of rhesus haemolytic disease (Hollister and Brown, 1999). Rhesus haemolytic disease occurs most commonly in mothers who have already delivered a Rh-positive child, thus triggering the production of the antibody against the Rh(D) antigen. As hypothesized, the risk for schizophrenia among males in the Danish Perinatal Cohort Study was increased over threefold in second and later-born offspring from Rh-incompatible pregnancies, but there was no increased risk for first-born offspring (Hollister et al., 1996).

Prenatal stress

Psychosocial stress may play a role in the precipitation of the adult schizophrenia syndrome (Brown and Birley, 1968; Steinberg and Durrell, 1968). Stress may also act early in life, even in the prenatal period, and play a role in predisposition (Kinney, 2001). A classic paper by Huttunen and Niskanen (1978) show a greatly increased risk of schizophrenia (OR 6.2) among individuals whose fathers died before the child's birth compared with those whose fathers died in the first year after birth. This appears to provide evidence for the involvement of prenatal stress in the aetiology of schizophrenia.

The possibility of an association between prenatal exposure to stress and schizophrenia has been investigated in a series of ingenious ecological studies based around discrete, highly stressful events. Van Os and Selten (1998) demonstrated a small increased risk of schizophrenia among individuals in the Netherlands who were in utero during the Nazi invasion in May 1940. Selten et al. (1999) found a nonsignificant increased risk of psychosis (RR 1.8; 95% CI 0.9–3.5) among those exposed during gestation to the 1953 Dutch Flood Disaster. Kinney et al. (1999) report a similar effect for prenatal exposure to a tornado in Worcester, Massachusetts.

More subtle forms of prenatal stress may also have an effect. In the 1966 North Finland birth cohort, both maternal depression in late pregnancy (Jones et al., 1998) and 'un-wantedness' of a pregnancy by the mother (Myhrman et al., 1996) were independently associated with a modest increase in the risk of schizophrenia in the offspring. The reasons for the pregnancy being unwanted were unknown, as was the attitude of the mother once the child was born. Many potential confounders such as maternal age, physical conditions and socioeconomic status were taken into account, but a diluted genetic effect cannot be excluded. Mednick and Schulsinger (1968) reported from the Copenhagen High Risk Study that 69% of the mothers of the high-risk children who suffered severe early psychiatric breakdown were under severe stress (e.g. jailing of a husband) at the time of the pregnancy compared with 29% of the mothers of the 'well' high-risk children. This finding suggests an interaction between genetic vulnerability to psychosis and prenatal exposure to stress.

There is a considerable animal literature concerning the effects of prenatal stress on brain development and behaviour of the offspring (for review, see Suomi 1997). The effect is thought to be mediated by glucocorticoid effects on the fetal hypothalamo–pituitary–adrenal axis. Glucocorticoids increase susceptibility to hypoxic-ischaemic injury both in rats and in cultured fetal hippocampal neurons (Sapolsky and Pulsinelli, 1985; Tombaugh et al., 1992), and maternal anxiety during pregnancy is associated with increased uterine artery resistance (Teixeira et al., 1999). Therefore, the effects of prenatal stress could mediate the association with some of the other obstetric complications noted in schizophrenia and discussed below.

Perinatal risk factors for schizophrenia: obstetric complications

Case-control studies

There is a large literature on the possible role of obstetric complications (OCs) in schizophrenia (for reviews, see McNeil, 1988, 1995; Cannon, 1997; McNeil et al., 2000). Before 1997, most of the studies showing an association were of case-control design using maternal recall for assessment of the exposure. They also had small sample sizes and were prone to various forms of bias. Geddes and Lawrie (1995) carried out a meta-analysis of the results from 16 case-control studies and two cohort studies published by that time, and reached three main conclusions: (i) a pooled OR of 2.0 (95% CI 1.6–2.4) suggested that OCs did have a small effect on increasing risk for schizophrenia (ii) there was evidence for selection and publication bias; and (iii) there was significant heterogeneity between the results from the case-control studies and the two birth cohort studies.

Geddes and colleagues followed up this work by carrying out an individual patient data meta-analysis of 12 case-control studies that had used the same rating scale (Lewis and Murray scale) to measure the exposure (Geddes et al., 1999). Significant associations (with effects sizes of 1.5–3.0) were found between schizophrenia and premature rupture of membranes, gestational age shorter than 37 weeks and use of resuscitation or incubator, and there was an almost significant association with birthweight <2500 g. Studies using birth record data found a significant association with pre-eclampsia while the studies based on maternal recall found a significant association with forceps delivery, indicating that agreement between birth records and maternal recall varies for different categories of birth complication.

Population-based studies

Because of methodological problems associated with the classic case-control design, particularly when measuring such early exposures, cohort and population-based study designs have now been exploited to investigate the relationship between OCs and later schizophrenia. This 'phase' of the OC and schizophrenia literature began in earnest in about 1997 and continues to date. Details of the designs and results of these population-based studies are given in Table 5.1. They all have the following characteristics: large and psychiatrically well-defined schizophrenic samples drawn from population-based registers; use of standardized, prospectively collected obstetric information from birth records or registers; general population control subjects with OC information from the same source and context; and control of demographic confounding factors through either matching or statistical adjustment. It can be seen from the results of the studies listed in Table 5.1 that these methodological advances have not confirmed the earlier findings. Moreover, although the designs of these studies are broadly similar, their results are quite diverse and no consensus has yet been reached. What are the reasons for this?

Methodological issues

The studies are drawn from different populations, in terms of geography, cohort and period effects and age of onset. Measurement of obstetric exposures is highly dependent on the quality of the birth record information available. Obstetric practices and the nomenclature and meaning of different complications vary between countries and over time. For example, 'uterine inertia' is a Scandinavian concept not mentioned in birth records from the UK or USA. Another problem is that many complications are not recorded in sufficient detail to give useful aetiological information: bleeding during pregnancy is mentioned in many studies but there is usually no information on timing or amount of bleeding. Equally, it is often unclear whether caesarian section was an elective or emergency procedure. The problems inherent in this field of study can be illustrated by examining two large studies based on broadly the same dataset and with similar methodology, but which find different, even contradictory, associations between various obstetric exposures and schizophrenia (Dalman et al., 1999; Hultman et al., 1999). As discussed previously with regard to prenatal infection, even small methodological differences can have a major influence on study results when one is dealing with small relative risks on the threshold of detectability.

There are so many discrete exposures wrapped up in the term 'obstetric complication' that it is essentially meaningless to consider them as one risk factor (Zornberg et al., 2000a). If the field is to progress, it must define and clarify the exposures under scrutiny. There are many distinct associations to be considered in terms of chance, bias or confounding before beginning to judge how any association should be interpreted as causal or not. A broad definition of OCs should no longer be used as it will not increase our understanding of the field. Greater definition of the exposure (such as prenatal measurement of maternal antibodies) or use of quantitative measures (such as birthweight, head circumference) are likely to show larger and more consistent effects.

Statistical power issues

Unfortunately, when one gets to the level of individual OCs as risk factors for schizophrenia, one rapidly runs into difficulties with statistical power, particularly if the obstetric factors have small effect sizes. The meta-analysis of Geddes et al. (1999) with 700 cases and 835 controls had 90% power to detect an OR of 2.0 at a population prevalence of 5%, but only 44% power to detect an OR of 1.5. As shown in Table 5.1, many of the cohort studies did not have sufficient statistical power to detect an odds ratio of 2.0 for an obstetric exposure with a population prevalence of 10%. These figures are actually conservative. Many OCs occur at a population prevalence of less than 10% and reported effect sizes are often less than 2.0. At best, the power of the largest studies to detect OR values of 1.5 was less than 70%.

The issue of interactive effects is even more problematic. Pregnancy, birth and neonatal complications do not act independently of each other. Pregnancy factors that have been associated with schizophrenia, such as rhesus incompatibility and prenatal stress (see previous section) can increase the risk for hypoxic-ischaemic damage during delivery. Current studies have negligible statistical power to detect such interactive effects.

Some studies try to overcome these problems by examining only one exposure based on a prior hypothesis, and this has proved relatively fruitful, showing significant effects for the putative risk-increasing mechanism of hypoxic–ischaemic damage (Buka et al., 1993; Cannon et al., 2000; Rosso et al., 2000; Zornberg et al., 2000b). The main problem with this approach is that no two sets of researchers have used exactly the same combinations of exposures. This makes direct comparisons between the studies or synthesis of the results difficult, and it prevents pooling of data between studies.

Timing of exposure

As with infections, the period of risk during which hypoxic brain damage may lead to later schizophrenia appears to extend beyond birth. In the North Finland 1966 cohort, a group of CNS insults that had hypoxia as a common mechanism was identified and termed 'perinatal brain damage' (PBD) (Rantakallio et al., 1987). This exposure has been used to investigate possible causes of mental handicap and childhood epilepsy. Given this link with other developmental CNS disorders, there was an a priori hypothesis for an association with schizophrenia. Of 125 survivors

Table 5.1. Summary of studies of obstetric complications and schizophrenia with epidemiological design

Study	Country	Design (cohort or case-control)	No. cases (% female)	No. controls	Match criteria	Diagnosis	Birth years	Age range cases (years)
Done et al. (1991)	UK	Cohort: NCDS	35 (39)	16812	N/A	PSE S+	1958	16–28
Buka et al. (1993)	US	Cohort: NCPP (Providence centre)	8 (32)	685	N/A	DSM-III	1960–66	18–27 (mean 23)
Sacker et al. (1995)	UK	Cohort: NCDS	35 (39)	16812	N/A	PSE S+	1958	16–28
Jones et al. (1998)	Finland	Cohort: 1966 North Finland Birth Cohort	76 (32.9)	1074	N/A	DSM-III-R	1966	27–28
Hultman et al. (1999)	Sweden	Case-control	167 (34.9)	835	Sex, dob, hosp	ICD-9	1973–79	15–21
Dalman et al. (1999)	Sweden	Cohort	238 (41.6)	507278	N/A	ICD-9	1973–77	15–22
Kendell (1) et al. (2000)	Scotland	Case-control	296 (21.3)	296	Sex, dob, hosp, mat age, parity, seg	ICD-9, ICD-10	1971–74	22–26
Kendell (2) et al. (2000)	Scotland	Case-control	156 (24.4)	156	Sex, dob, hosp, mat age, parity, seg	ICD-9, ICD-10	1975–78	18–21
Byrne et al. (2000)	Ireland	Case-control	431 (40.6)	431	Sex, dob, hosp, mat age, parity, seg	ICD-9	N/S	N/A
Cannon et al. (2000)	US	Cohort: NCPP (Philadephia centre)	72 (35.3)	7941 normal; 63 siblings	N/A	DSM-IV	1959–66	19–36
Rosso et al. (2000)	Finland	Case-control	80 (52)	56 controls; 61 siblings	Sex, age, seg	ICD-8	1955	36
Zornberg et al. (2000b)	US	Cohort: NCPP (Providence centre)	12 (32)	681	N/A	DSM-IV	1960–66	18–27 (mean 23)
Dalman et al. (2001)	Sweden	Case-control	524(34)	1043	Sex, hosp, dob, parish	ICD-8 ICD-9	N/S	Mean 29.5

Notes:
NCPP, National Collaborative Perinatal Project; NCDS, National Child and Development Study; PSE, Present State Examination; DSM, Diagnostic and Statistical Manual [of Mental Disorders]; ICD, International Classification of Disease; N/A, not applicable; N/S, not specified; dob, date of birth; hosp, hospital; mat, maternal; seg, socioeconomic group; OC, obstetric complications;

Power[a]	Source of cases	Source of obstetric information	Findings
40	Mental Health Enquiry 1974–86	Midwife report	No overall association between risk factors for perinatal death and later schizophrenia. Low maternal weight and medications given to baby were associated with narrowly defined schizophrenia
10	Follow-up tracing and lay interviewer	NCPP records	Nonsignificant increased risk of psychosis in those exposed to chronic fetal hypoxia (OR 2.6)
40	Mental Health Enquiry 1974–86	Midwife report	Re-analysis of Done et al. (1991). The following variables were associated with increased risk of narrowly defined schizophrenia: low maternal weight, maternal psychological problems, smoking in pregnancy, poor antenatal attendance, rhesus negative, parity >2, previous births <2500 g, bleeding in pregnancy, untrained person delivering, baby's weight <2500 g, other drugs given to baby
50	National Hospital Discharge Register to 1993	Midwife report	Low birthweight (OR 2.4; 1–5.6); combination of low birthweight and prematurity (OR 3.5; 1.3–9.6) and perinatal brain damage (OR 6.9; 2.9–16.3) were associated with schizophrenia
80	National Hospital Discharge Register 1987–(?)1994	Birth register: obstetrician	Schizophrenia was associated with multiparity (OR 2.0); bleeding during pregnancy (OR 3.5); winter birth (OR 1.4); small for gestational age (males only OR 3.2); parity >4 (males only OR 3.6)
95	National Hospital Discharge Register 1987–95	Birth register: obstetrician	Increased risk of pre-eclampsia (OR 2.5); vacuum extraction (OR 1.7); malformations (OR 2.4), parity 1 (OR 1.3); bleeding during pregnancy (OR 2.0); threatened premature delivery (OR 2.3); gestational age <32 weeks (OR 2.7); prolonged delivery (OR 1.6); uterine inertia (OR 2.4; ponderal; index <20 (OR 3.4); respiratory illness (OR 1.5); birthweight <2500 g (males only OR 2.2); birthweight <1500 g (females only OR 6.0); small for gestational age (males only OR 1.9); pre-eclampsia remained significant after adjusting for all other complications
78	National Hospital Admission Register to 1996	Birth register: obstetrician or midwife	No association found between any OC and schizophrenia
50	National Hospital Admission Register to 1996	Birth register: obstetrician or midwife	Emergency caesarian section (OR 3.7; CI 1.02–13.1) and labour >12 hours were associated with subsequent schizophrenia
92	Dublin Psychiatric Case Register 1972–92	Labour ward records	No overall differences in rates of OC. Caesarian section and narrow maternal pelvis commoner among cases; males with early-onset schizophrenia had greater frequency and severity of OCs than controls
55	The Penn Longitudinal Database	NCPP records	Hypoxia-related complications >3 increased the risk of schizophrenia (OR 3.84) and particularly early-onset schizophrenia (OR 7.3)
25	Finnish Hospital Discharge Register	Birth records: midwife	Risk of early-onset schizophrenia increases (OR 2.16; CI 1.3–3.5) per hypoxia-related OC
15	Rediagnosis of interview information from Buka et al. (1993)	NCPP records	Re-analysis of Buka et al. (1993). Composite variable entitled 'hypoxic-ischaemia-related fetal/neonatal complications' associated with schizophrenia (OR 4.56; CI 2.42–8.6)
99	Stockholm county inpatient register 1971–94	Birth records: midwife	Signs of asphyxia at birth were associated with increased risk for schizophrenia (OR 4.4; CI 1.9–10.3) after adjusting for other complications and confounders

OR, odds ratio; CI, confidence interval.

[a] Power to detect an odds ratio of 2.0 with 95% confidence for an exposure with a prevalence of 10% among controls.

of PBD, six (4.8%) developed schizophrenia in adult life: a sevenfold relative risk (Jones et al., 1998). The estimate of the proportion of schizophrenia in the general population that may be attributable to this mechanism was 5–8% in this study.

Specificity

The specificity of these obstetric exposures for schizophrenia is not established (Tarrant and Jones, 1999). It is possible that other mental disorders, such as affective disorders, have similar obstetric risk factors, but these have not been investigated to the same extent. We do not advocate repeating the whole cycle of investigation again for other disorders but recommend including them as additional groups in the investigation of mechanisms. Another approach would be to follow up a cohort of individuals who have suffered certain pre- and perinatal complications and assess a range of outcomes during development – a return to the approach advocated by Pasamanick and colleagues many decades ago (1956).

Meta-analysis of findings from population-based studies

The standardized fashion of reporting results and the methodological similarities of the population-based studies lend themselves to a meta-analytic approach. Meta-analysis provides a method for integrating quantitative data from multiple studies by using a weighted average of the results in which larger studies have more influence than smaller studies. It improves the estimates of effect size, increases the statistical power and helps to make sense out of studies with conflicting conclusions (Fleiss, 1993; Egger et al., 1997).

Cannon et al. (2002) carried out a meta-analytic synthesis of the prospective 'population-based' studies that had published data on individual OCs and found that three groups of complications were significantly associated with schizophrenia: (i) complications of pregnancy (bleeding, diabetes, rhesus incompatibility, preeclampsia); (ii) complications of delivery (uterine atony, asphyxia, emergency caesarian section); and (iii) abnormal fetal growth and development (low birthweight, congenital malformations, reduced head circumference). Pooled estimates of effect sizes were generally small (OR values < 2). Interactive effects and independence of obstetric risk factor could not be examined using this design. A meta-analysis of individual patient data on these population-based studies, such as that carried out by Geddes et al. (1999) on case-control studies, may help to elucidate such issues.

Conclusions and speculations on the study of pre- and perinatal risk factors for schizophrenia

Investigation of the role of pre- and perinatal risk factors in the genesis of schizophrenia provides a good example of the development of epidemiological thought and methodology since the 1960s, beginning with ecological studies, then progressing through case-control studies to general population cohorts and enriched samples where specific exposures are identified. What conclusions can be drawn from the large literature reviewed in this chapter?

It seems that many pre- and perinatal risk factors are somehow involved in increasing the risk for schizophrenia in later life. Those with the best evidence to date are prenatal (probably second trimester) exposure to influenza and other respiratory infections, prenatal rubella, hypoxia-related OCs and low birthweight or intrauterine growth retardation. Evidence is less secure for prenatal stress or prenatal malnutrition, principally because of the difficulties in obtaining suitable samples in which to examine these exposures.

Gene–environment interaction

The effect sizes for these prenatal and perinatal risk factors are small, with OR values or relative risks of around 2 (Table 5.2). Similarly, the results of genetic studies in the 1990s suggest that multiple genes with small effect sizes are involved in causation of schizophrenia (Chs. 10 and 11). Taken together, these and other findings indicate that we are likely to be dealing with interactive effects of prenatal and genetic factors. The presence of interactive effects has implications for statistical power, model-building and study design (for further discussion of these issues, see Ch. 12).

Schizophrenia has been posited as a neurodevelopmental disease with a strong genetic component (Jones and Murray, 1991; Tsuang, 2000). Genes control the development of the brain and nervous system but the environment modifies it. Insults such as second trimester infection or hypoxia during delivery may interact with the genotype to increase the risk of schizophrenia. The story probably does not end at birth, as brain maturation continues through the first two decades of life and is influenced by experience.

Programming

In thinking about causation, we will increasingly have to take into account the dynamic interplay between genes and environment in utero. While development is genetically programmed, the programme is continually modified in utero, as the expression of genes is determined in part – as when genes are turned on or off – by their molecular environment (Kandel, 1998). Furthermore, both epidemiological and animal studies increasingly support the view that the in utero environment has another, more profound, impact on the developmental programme (Barker, 1992; Liu et al., 2000). Depending upon the amount and the kind of nutrients that are available in utero, the fetus appears to select among alternative paths of development that entail different homeostatic setpoints. This may have evolved as a means to anticipate and thereby increase survival in widely variable postnatal environments. Thus, normal variation in the fetal environment may have important implications for offspring risk of schizophrenia because it modifies the developmental programme. We

Table 5.2. Estimate of approximate effect sizes for pre- and perinatal risk factors for schizophrenia

Pre- or perinatal risk factor	Approximate effect size (relative risk or odds ratio)
Place or time of birth	
Winter birth	1.15
Urban birth	1.5–2.4
Infection	
Prenatal influenza	2.0
Prenatal respiratory infection (T2)	2.1
Prenatal rubella	5.2
Prenatal poliovirus (T2)	1.05
Neonatal and childhood CNS infection	4.0
Malnutrition	
Prenatal famine (T1)	2.0
Prenatal stress	
Bereavement of spouse	6.2
Flood (T2)	1.8
War (T2)	
'Unwantedness'	2.4
Maternal depression (T3)	1.8
Obstetric complications	
General	2.0
Rhesus incompatibility	2.8
Hypoxia-related	2.1–4.4
Perinatal brain damage	7.0
Low birthweight (<2500 g)	1.6
Pre-eclampsia	2.5

Notes:
T1, T2, T3, trimesters 1–3, respectively.

do not yet know the relative importance for schizophrenia risk of specific fetal insults, such as infection, and of normal fetal variation such as in fetal nutrient supply.

The interplay between genes and environment may precede even the conception of the offspring at risk for schizophrenia. Recent findings confirm earlier reports that increasing paternal age is associated with an increased risk of schizophrenia (Hare and Moran, 1979; Malaspina et al., 2001). The most parsimonious interpretation attributes the effect to mutations in the male sperm line prior to conception. These mutations, in turn, are to a large extent environmentally determined, by both the cumulative life experience (age) and specific environmental exposures (e.g. toxins) of the biological father.

Techniques for investigating genetic and environmental risk factors are beginning to converge, with case-control and cohort designs being used for genetic association studies (Ch. 11). Molecular genetic studies are including measures of environment, and cohort studies are collecting both DNA samples and information on early and later environmental risk factors. In the first decade of the 21st century we may see the first reports of studies examining precisely measured genetic and environmental causes of schizophrenia in the same population.

Confounding and proxy variables

The precise nature of these early risk factors for schizophrenia is often unclear, which makes interpretation of the aetiological mechanism involved very difficult. In the case of season of birth or urban birth, one is dealing with a 'proxy' variable that encompasses many even smaller unknown risk factors, possibly interacting with each other to produce an effect. The association with prenatal infection could be confounded by fever or medication. The association with hypoxia-related birth complications could be confounded by earlier prenatal factors or sociodemographic factors. Current approaches do not easily allow us to explore these issues further, other than just to report an association, and these problems can never be resolved within the framework of a uni-level, risk factor model. As a result, investigations of pre- and perinatal risk factors for schizophrenia have become 'stuck' at this point, reporting risk factors of vanishingly small effect over and over again – an example of circular epidemiology (Kuller, 1999). In epidemiological research in general, it has been postulated that the vogue for risk factor epidemiology is reaching the limits of its usefulness (Taubes, 1995; Susser, 1998; Fearon et al., 2001) and that other approaches which incorporate, but are not restricted by, the traditional individual risk factor approach should also be utilized (Susser and Susser, 1996; Schwartz et al., 1999).

Future directions

Some related approaches for future research into early life exposures and schizophrenia have emerged during the 1990s and are already being put into practice. These include new conceptual approaches to causality and collaborative approaches.

New conceptual approaches to causality
Longitudinal or life-course approach

First, risk factors have traditionally been modelled as static characteristics of the individual, but disease causation can be a dynamic process that involves a time dimension and an interplay of causal interactions (Kreiger, 1994). Introducing the element of development over time is necessary, and causation should be considered in terms of a pathway over a life course, rather than in terms of a certain set of risk factors at a certain point in time. Developmental, or life-course, epidemiology is concerned with early-life risk factors for adult diseases. This far-reaching, longitudinal approach is transforming our understanding of a number of chronic physical disorders (Barker and Osmond, 1986; Barker et al., 1989, 1990; Barker, 1992; Kuh and Ben-Shlomo, 1997) and is likely to do the same for schizophrenia (Keshavan and Murray, 1997). The life-course model incorporates such elements as cumulative insults over the life course, critical periods of susceptibility throughout life, and interaction between early and late factors (Kuh and Ben-Schlomo, 1997). For schizophrenia, this process has been conceptualized by some as a 'self-perpetuating cascade of abnormal function' (Jones et al., 1994; also see Tarrant and Jones, 1999; Waddington et al., 1999; Bramon et al., 2001).

Multilevel approach

Second, a new paradigm should allow for causes to be considered at multiple levels of organisation: a multilevel eco-epidemiology (Susser and Susser, 1996). The prevailing methods are well suited for finding factors that influence the risk of disease within individuals but not for finding causes best characterized at higher levels of organization, such as societal context, or at lower levels of organization, such as genes and molecules. This means that in an investigation of schizophrenia we may need to consider characteristics of the society, such as level of development (Ch. 2), characteristics of individuals, including development over time (Ch. 6), and genetic and molecular factors (Chs. 11 and 12). Not only does the environment vary over time but genes are expressed at varying times and to varying extents. Statistical and epidemiological methods that can encompass dynamic and multilevel processes will need to be developed and refined. As an example of future directions, these principles are being applied to the study of causes of schizophrenia in the Prenatal Determinants of Schizophrenia Study (PDS) (Susser et al., 2000).

Collaborative ventures

The collection or opportunistic use of increasingly large cohorts will be necessary; researchers will need to think in terms of tens or hundreds of thousands of subjects. The need for these large cohorts will arise once strong associations are established from molecular genetic studies; they will allow us to model epigenetic effects involving small pre- and perinatal risk factors and combinations of genes. This will be a major challenge for traditional cohort designs. Whether necessary samples and investigations can be funded will be a matter for society as much as for scientists (Jones, 1999). Collaboration and cross-fertilization will be needed with researchers in other disciplines, such as neuroimaging, genetics, statistics, molecular and developmental biology, and also with other chronic disease epidemiologists investigating the early origins of adult health, for instance in the area of cardiovascular disease or diabetes (Leon and Ben-Schlomo, 1999; McKeigue, 1999). The same cohorts and methods can often be useful to researchers in different fields. It is increasingly evident that mental and physical health are linked in many ways throughout life, and research on early adult exposures should consider outcomes in both domains (Susser et al., 1999).

We now have the chance to enter a 'new age of epidemiology for schizophrenia' (Susser et al., 2000). The combination of new paradigms and larger cohorts, with the tools of modern epidemiology and biomedical science, has the potential greatly to advance our understanding of the causal pathways to schizophrenia.

Acknowledgements

This work was made possible by the support of the Wellcome Trust (MC), the EJLB Foundation (MC), the Theodore and Vada Stanley Foundation (ESS, PBJ), NARSAD (ESS) and NIMH (ESS).

REFERENCES

Adams W, Kendell RE (1996) Influenza and schizophrenia [letter]. British Journal of Psychiatry 169, 791–792.

Adams W, Kendell RE, Hare EH (1993) Epidemiological evidence that maternal influenza contributes to the aetiology of schizophrenia: an analysis of Scottish, English and Danish data. British Journal of Psychiatry 163, 522–534.

Aylward E, Walker E, Bettes B (1984) Intelligence in schizophrenia: meta-analysis of the research. Schizophrenia Bulletin 10, 430–459.

Barker DJP (1992) Fetal and Infant Origins of Adult Disease. London: British Medical Journal.

Barker DJP, Osmond C (1986) Childhood respiratory infection and chronic bronchitis in England and Wales. British Medical Journal 293, 1271–1275.

Barker DJP, Winter PD, Osmond C, Margetts B, Simmonds SJ (1989) Weight in infancy and death from ischaemic heart disease. Lancet ii, 577–580.

Barker DJP, Bull AR, Osmond C, Simmonds SJ (1990) Fetal and placental size and risk of hypertension in adult life. British Medical Journal 301, 259–262.

Barr CE, Mednick SA, Munk-Jørgensen P (1990) Exposure to influenza epidemics during gestation and adult schizophrenia: a 40 year study. Archives of General Psychiatry, 47, 869–874.

Bradbury TN, Miller GA (1985) Season of birth in schizophrenia: a review of evidence, methodology, and etiology. Psychological Bulletin 98, 569–594.

Bramon E, Kelly J, van Os J, Murray RM (2001) The cascade of increasingly deviant development that culminates in the onset of schizophrenia. NeuroScience News 4, 5–19.

Brown AS, Cohen P, Greenwald S, Susser E (2000a) Nonaffective psychosis after prenatal exposure to rubella. American Journal of Psychiatry 157, 438–443.

Brown AS, Schaefer CA, Wyatt RJ et al. (2000b) Maternal exposure to respiratory infections and adult schizophrenia spectrum disorders: a prospective birth cohort study. Schizophrenia Bulletin, 26, 287–296.

Brown GW, Birley JLT (1968) Crises and life changes and the onset of schizophrenia. Journal of Health and Social Behaviour 9, 203–214.

Buka SL, Tsuang MT, Lipsitt LP (1993) Pregnancy/delivery complications and psychiatric diagnosis. A prospective study. Archives of General Psychiatry 50, 151–156.

Buka SL, Tsuang MT, Torrey EF, Klebanof MA, Bernstein D, Yolken RH (2001) Maternal infections and subsequent psychosis among offspring. Archives of General Psychiatry 58, 1032–1037.

Butler PD, Printz D, Klugewicz D, Brown AS, Susser ES (1999) Plausibility of early nutritional deficiency as a risk factor for schizophrenia. In: Prenatal Exposures in Schizophrenia, Susser ES, Brown AS, Gorman JM, eds, Washington, DC: American Psychiatric Press, pp. 163–193.

Byrne M, Browne R, Mulryan N et al. (2000) Labour and delivery complications and schizophrenia. Case-control study using contemporaneous labour ward records. British Journal of Psychiatry 176, 531–536

Cannon M, Jones P (1996) Schizophrenia: neuroepidemiology of schizophrenia. Journal of Neurology, Neurosurgery and Psychiatry 61, 604–613.

Cannon M, Cotter D, Coffey VP et al. (1996) Prenatal exposure to the 1957 influenza epidemic and adult schizophrenia: a follow-up study. British Journal of Psychiatry 168, 368–371.

Cannon M, Jones PB, Murray RM (2002) Obstetric complications and schizophrenia. An historical review and meta-analysis. American Journal of Psychiatry in press.

Cannon TD (1997) On the nature and mechanisms of obstetric influences in schizophrenia: a review and synthesis. International Review of Psychiatry 9, 387–397.

Cannon TD, Rosso IM, Hollister JM, Bearden CE, Sanchez, Hadley T (2000) A prospective cohort study of genetic and perinatal influences in the etiology of schizophrenia. Schizophrenia Bulletin 26, 351–366.

Clouston TS (1891) The Neuroses of Development. Edinburgh: Oliver and Boyd.

Clouston TS (1892) Clinical Lectures on Mental Diseases, 3rd edition. London: Churchill.

Coffey VP, Jessop WJE (1959) Maternal influenza and congenital deformities: a prospective study. Lancet ii, 935–938.

Coffey VP, Jessop WJE (1963) Maternal influenza and congenital deformities. A follow-up study. Lancet i, 748–751.

Cotter D, Larkin C, Waddington JL, O'Callaghan E (1995) Season of birth in schizophrenia: clue or cul-de-sac. In: The Neurodevelopmental Basis of Schizophrenia, Waddington JL, Buckley PB, eds. Texas: R.G. Landes, pp. 17–33.

Crow TJ, Done J (1992) Prenatal exposure to influenza does not cause schizophrenia. British Journal of Psychiatry 161, 390–393.

Crow TJ, Done DJ, Johnstone EC (1991) Schizophrenia and influenza. Lancet 338, 116–117.

Dalman C, Allebeck P, Culberg J, Grunewald C, Köster M (1999) Obstetric complications and the risk of schizophrenia: a longitudinal study of a national birth cohort. Archives of General Psychiatry 56, 234–240.

Dalman C, Thomas HV, David AS, Gentz J, Lewis G, Allebeck P (2001) Signs of asphyxia at birth increase the risk of schizophrenia: a population based case-control study. British Journal of Psychiatry 179, 403–408.

Done J, Johnstone EC, Frith CD, Golding J, Shepard PM, Crow TJ (1991) Complications of pregnancy and delivery in relation to psychosis in adult life: data from the British Perinatal Mortality Survey. British Medical Journal 302, 1576–1580.

Egger M, Davey Smith G, Phillips AN (1997) Meta-analysis: principles and procedures. British Medical Journal 315, 1533–1537.

Elder AG, O'Donnell B, McCruden AB, Symington IS, Carman WF (1996) Incidence and recall of influenza in a cohort of Glasgow healthcare workers during the 1993/1994 epidemic: results of serum testing and questionnaire. British Medical Journal 313, 1241–1242.

Erlenmeyer-Kimling L, Folnegovic Z, Hrabic-Zerjavic V, Borcic B, Folnegovic-Smalc V (1994) Schizophrenia and prenatal exposure to the 1957 influenza epidemic in Croatis. American Journal of Psychiatry 151, 1496–1498.

Fatemi SH, Emamian ES, Kist D et al. (1999) Defective corticogenesis and reduction in Reelin immunoreactivity in cortex and hippocampus of prenatally infected neonatal mice. Molecular Psychiatry 4, 145–154.

Fearon P, Cannon M, Murray RM (2001) A critique of the idea and science of risk factor research in schizophrenia. Journal of International Mental Health 30, 82–90.

Fine PEM, Adelstein AM, Snowman J, Clarkson JA, Evans SM (1985) Long term effects of exposure to viral infections in utero. British Medical Journal 290, 509–511.

Fleiss JL (1993) The statistical basis of meta-analysis. Statistical Methods in Medical Research 2, 121–145.

Geddes JR, Lawrie SM (1995) Obstetric events in schizophrenia: a meta-analysis. British Journal of Psychiatry 167, 786–793.

Geddes JR, Verdoux H, Takei N et al. (1999) Schizophrenia and complications of pregnancy and labor: an individual-patient data meta-analysis. Schizophrenia Bulletin 25, 413–423.

Gerard DL, Houston LG (1953) Family setting and the social ecology of schizophrenia. Psychiatric Quarterly 27, 90–101.

Hare EH (1956) Mental illness and social conditions in Bristol. Journal of Mental Science 102, 349–357.

Hare EH (1975) Season of birth in schizophrenia and neurosis. American Journal of Psychiatry 132, 1168–1171.

Hare EH, Moran PA (1979) Raised paternal age in psychiatric patients: evidence for the constitutional hypothesis. British Journal of Psychiatry 134, 169–177.

Hare EH, Price JS, Slater ETO (1974) Mental disorder and season of birth: a national sample compared with the general population. British Journal of Psychiatry 124, 81–86.

Hoek HW, Susser E, Buck KA, Lumey LH, Lin SP, Gorman JM (1996) Schizoid personality disorder after prenatal exposure to famine. American Journal of Psychiatry 153, 1637–1639.

Hoek HW, Brown AS, Susser ES (1999) The Dutch famine studies: prenatal nutritional deficiency and schizophrenia. In: Prenatal Exposures in Schizophrenia, Susser ES, Brown AS, Gorman JM, eds. Washington DC: American Psychiatric Press, pp. 135–161.

Hollister JM, Brown AS (1999) Rhesus incompatibility and schizophrenia. In: Prenatal Exposures in Schizophrenia, Susser ES, Brown AS, Gorman JM, eds. Washington, DC: American Psychiatric Press, pp. 197–214.

Hollister JM, Laing P, Mednick SA (1996) Rhesus incompatibility as a risk factor for schizophrenia in male adults. Archives of General Psychiatry 53, 19–24.

Hultman CM, Sparen P, Takei N, Murray RM, Cnattingius S (1999) Prenatal and perinatal risk factors for schizophrenia, affective psychosis and reactive psychosis of early onset: case-control study. British Medical Journal 318, 421–426

Huttunen M, Niskanen P (1978) Prenatal loss of father and psychiatric disorders. Archives of General Psychiatry 35, 427–431.

Izumoto Y, Inoue S, Yasuda N (1999) Schizophrenia and the influenza epidemics of 1957 in Japan. Biological Psychiatry 46, 119–124.

Jakob H, Beckmann H (1986) Prenatal developmental disturbances in the limbic allocortex in schizophrenics. Journal of Neural Transmission 65, 303–326.

Johnstone EC, Crow TJ, Frith CD, Husband J, Kreel L (1976) Cerebral ventricular size and cognitive impairment in chronic schizophrenia. Lancet ii, 944–946.

Jones P, Murray R (1991) The genetics of schizophrenia is the genetics of neurodevelopment. British Journal of Psychiatry 158, 615–623.

Jones P, Rodgers B, Murray R, Marmot M (1994) Childhood developmental risk factors for schizophrenia in the British 1946 birth cohort. Lancet 344, 1398–1402.

Jones PB (1999) Longitudinal approaches to the search for the causes of schizophrenia: past, present and future. In: Search for the Causes of Schizophrenia Vol. IV, Balance of the Century, Gattaz WF, Häfner H, eds. Darmstadt: Steinkopf and Berlin: Springer, pp. 91–119.

Jones PB, Rantakallio P, Hartikainen AL et al. (1998) Schizophrenia as a long-term outcome of pregnancy, delivery and perinatal complications: A 28-year follow-up of the 1966 North Finland general population birth cohort. American Journal of Psychiatry 155, 355–364.

Jones PB, Pang D, Piriach S, Fine PEM (1999) Prenatal viral infection and subsequent mental illness: a long-term cohort study of 6152 subjects. Schizophrenia Research 36, 45.

Kandel ER (1998) A new intellectual framework for psychiatry. American Journal of Psychiatry 155, 457–469.

Kendell RE, Adams W (1991) Unexplained fluctuations in the risk for schizophrenia by month and year of birth. British Journal of Psychiatry 158, 758–763.

Kendell RE, Kemp JW (1989) Maternal influenza in the aetiology of schizophrenia. Archives of General Psychiatry 46, 878–882.

Kendell RE, McInneny K, Jusczak E, Bain M (2000) Obstetric complications and schizophrenia: two case-control studies based on structured obstetric records. British Journal of Psychiatry 174, 516–522.

Keshavan MS, Murray RM (eds.) (1997) Neurodevelopmental Models of Psychopathology. New York: Cambridge University Press.

Kinney DK (2001) Prenatal stress and risk for schizophrenia. International Journal of Mental Health 29, 62–71.

Kinney DK, Hyman W, Greetham C, Tramer S (1999) Increased relative risk for schizophrenia and prenatal exposure to a severe tornado. Schizophrenia Research 36, 45–46.

Kovelman JA, Scheibel AB (1984) A neurohistological correlate of schizophrenia. Biological Psychiatry 19, 1601–1621.

Kreiger N (1994) Epidemiology and the web of causation: has anyone seen the spider? Social Science and Medicine 39, 887–903.

Kuh D, Ben-Shlomo Y (eds.) (1997) A Life-Course Approach to Chronic Disease Epidemiology. Oxford: Oxford University Press.

Kuller LH (1999) Circular epidemiology. American Journal of Epidemiology 150, 897–903.

Kunugi H, Nanko S, Takei N, Saito K, Hayashi N, Kazamatsuri H (1995) Schizophrenia following in utero exposure to the 1957 influenza epidemics in Japan. American Journal of Psychiatry 152, 450–452.

Leon D, Ben-Schlomo Y (1999) Preadult influences on cardiovascular disease and cancer. In: A Life Course Approach to Chronic Disease Epidemiology, Kuh D, Ben-Schlomo Y, eds. Oxford, UK: Oxford University Press, pp. 45–77.

Lewis G, David A, Andreasson S, Allebeck P (1992) Schizophrenia and city life. Lancet 340, 137–140.

Liu D, Diorio J, Day JC, Francis DD, Meaney MJ (2000) Maternal care, hippocampal synaptogenesis and cognitive development in rats. Nature Neuroscience 3, 799–806.

Malaspina D, Harlap S, Fennig S et al. (2001) Advancing paternal age and the risk of schizophrenia. Archives of General Psychiatry 58, 313–412.

Marcelis M, Navarro-Mateu F, Murray R, Selten JP, van Os J (1998) Urbanization and psychosis: a study of 1942–1978 birth cohorts in the Netherlands. Psychological Medicine 28, 871–879.

Marcelis M, Takei N, van Os J (1999) Urbanization and risk for schizophrenia: does the effect operate before or around the time of illness onset? Psychological Medicine 29, 1197–1203.

Marenco S, Weinberger DR (2000) The neurodevelopmental hypothesis of schizophrenia: following a trail of evidence from cradle to grave. Developmental and Psychopathology 12, 501–527.

McDonald C, Fearon P, Murray RM (2000) Neurodevelopmental hypothesis of schizophrenia 12 years on: data and doubts. In: Childhood Onset of Adult Psychopathology, Rapaport JL, ed. Washington, DC: American Psychiatric Press, pp. 193–222.

McGrath JJ, Welham JL (1999) Season of birth and schizophrenia: a systematic review and meta-analysis of data from the southern hemisphere. Schizophrenia Research 35, 237–242.

McGrath JJ, Pemberton MR, Welham JL, Murray RM (1994) Schizophrenia and the influenza epidemics of 1954, 1957 and 1959: a southern hemisphere study. Schizophrenia Research 14, 1–8.

McGrath JJ, Castle D, Murray RM (1995) How can we judge whether or not prenatal exposure to influenza causes schizophrenia. In: Neural Development and Schizophrenia. Theory and Research, Mednick SA, Hollister JM, eds. New York: Plenum Press.

McKeigue P (1999) Diabetes and insulin action. In: A Life Course Approach to Chronic Disease Epidemiology, Kuh D, Ben-Shlomo Y, eds. Oxford, UK: Oxford University Press, pp. 78–101.

McNeil TF (1988) Obstetric factors and perinatal injuries. In: Handbook of Schizophrenia Vol. 3: Nosology, Epidemiology and Genetics, Tsuang MT, Simpson JC, eds. Amsterdam: Elsevier Science, pp. 319–344.

McNeil TF (1995) Perinatal risk factors and schizophrenia: selective review and methodological concerns. Epidemiologic Reviews 17, 107–112.

McNeil T, Cantor-Graae E, Ishmail B (2000) Obstetric complications and congenital malformations in schizophrenia. Brain Research Reviews 31, 166–178.

Mednick SA, Schulsinger F (1968) Some premorbid characteristics related to breakdown in children with schizophrenic mothers. Journal of Psychiatric Research 6(Suppl. 1), 267.

Mednick SA, Machon RA, Huttunen MO, Bonett D (1988) Adult schizophrenia following prenatal exposure to an influenza epidemic. Archives of General Psychiatry 45, 189–192.

Mednick SA, Machon RA, Huttunen MO (1990) An update on the Helsinki influenza project [letter to editor]. Archives of General Psychiatry 47, 292.

Morgan V, Castle D, Page A et al. (1997) Influenza epidemics and incidence of schizophrenia, affective disorders and mental retardation in Western Australia: no evidence of a major effect. Schizophrenia Research 26, 25–39.

Mortensen PB, Pedersen CB, Westergaard T et al. (1999) Effects of family history and place and season of birth on the risk of schizophrenia. New England Journal of Medicine 340, 603–608.

Murray RM, Lewis SW (1987) Is schizophrenia a neurodevelopmental disorder? British Medical Journal 295, 681–682.

Murray RM, Jones PB, O'Callaghan E, Takei N, Sham PC (1992) Genes, viruses and neurodevelopmental schizophrenia. Journal of Psychiatric Research 26, 225–235.

Myhrman A, Rantakallio P, Isohanni M, Jones PB, Partanen U (1996) Does unwantedness of a pregnancy predict schizophrenia? British Journal of Psychiatry 169, 637–640.

Nelson KB, Dambrosia JM, Grether JK, Philips TM (1998) Neonatal cytokines and coagulation factors in children with cerebral palsy. Annals of Neurology 44, 665–675.

O'Callaghan E, Sham P, Takei N, Glover G, Murray RM (1991) Schizophrenia after prenatal exposure to 1957 A$_2$ influenza epidemic. Lancet 337, 1248–1250.

Pasamanick B, Rodgers ME, Lilienfield AM (1956) Pregnancy experience and behaviour disorder in children. American Journal of Psychiatry 112, 613–618.

Rantakallio P (1969) Groups at risk in low birth weight infants and perinatal mortality. Acta Paediatrica Scandinavica 193(Suppl.), 1–71.

Rantakallio P, von Wendt L (1986) A prospective comparative study of the etiology of cerebral palsy and epilepsy in a one-year birth cohort from Northern Finland. Acta Paediatrica Scandinavica 75, 586–592.

Rantakallio P, von Wendt L, Koivu M (1987) Prognosis of perinatal brain damage: a prospective study of a one year birth cohort of 12 000 children. Early Human Development 15, 75–84.

Rantakallio P, Jones P, Moring J, von Wendt L (1997) Association between central nervous system infections during childhood and adult onset schizophrenia and other psychoses: A 28-year follow- up. International Journal of Epidemiology 26, 837–843.

Rosso IM, Cannon TD, Huttunen T, Huttunen MO, Lönnqvist J, Gasperoni TL (2000) Obstetric risk factors for early-onset schizophrenia in a Finnish birth cohort. American Journal of Psychiatry 157, 801–807.

Sacker A, Done DJ, Crow TJ, Golding J (1995) Antecedents of schizophrenia and affective illness: obstetric complications. British Journal of Psychiatry 166, 734–741.

Sapolsky RM, Pulsinelli WA (1985) Glucocorticoids potentiate ischaemic injury to neurons: therapeutic implications. Science 229, 1397–1400.

Schwartz S, Susser E, Susser M (1999) A future for epidemiology. Annual Review of Public Health 20, 15–33.

Selten JPCJ, Slaets JPJ (1994) Evidence against maternal infection as a risk factor for schizophrenia. British Journal of Psychiatry 164, 674–676.

Selten J-P, van der Graaf Y, van Duursen R, Gispen-de Wied CC, Kahn RS (1999) Psychotic illness after prenatal exposure to the 1953 Dutch flood disaster. Schizophrenia Research 35, 243–245.

Sham PC, O'Callaghan E, Takei N, Murray GK, Hare EH, Murray RM (1992) Schizophrenia following pre-natal exposure to influenza epidemics between 1939 and 1960. British Journal of Psychiatry 160, 461–466.

Southard EE (1915) On the topographic distribution of cortex lesions and anomalies in dementia praecox with some account of their functional significance. American Journal of Insanity 71, 603–671.

Stein Z, Susser M, Saenger G, Marolla F (1975) Famine and Human Development: The Dutch Hunger Winter of 1944–45. New York: Oxford University Press.

Steinberg HR, Durrell J (1968) A stressful situation as a precipitant of schizophrenic symptoms, an epidemiologic study. British Journal of Psychiatry 114, 1097–1105.

Stöber G, Franzek E, Beckmann J (1992) The role of maternal infectious diseases during pregnancy in the aetiology of schizophrenia in offspring. European Psychiatry 7, 147–152.

Suomi SJ (1997) Long-term effects of different early rearing experiences on social, emotional, and physiological development in nonhuman primates. In: Neurodevelopment and Adult Psychopathology, Ch. 8, Keshavan MS, Murray RM, eds. Cambridge, UK: Cambridge University Press, pp. 104–116.

Susser E, Lin SP (1992) Schizophrenia after prenatal exposure to the Dutch hunger winter of 1944–1945. Archives of General Psychiatry 49, 983–988.

Susser E, Lin SP (1994) Schizophrenia after prenatal exposure to the Dutch hunger winter of 1944–1945. Archives of General Psychiatry 51, 333–334.

Susser ES, Lin SP, Brown AS, Lumey LH, Erienmeyer-Kimling L (1994) No relation between risk of schizophrenia and prenatal exposure to influenza in Holland. American Journal of Psychiatry 151, 922–924.

Susser E, Neugebauer R, Hoek HW et al. (1996) Schizophrenia after prenatal famine. Archives of General Psychiatry 53, 25–31.

Susser E, Brown A, Matte TD (1999) Prenatal factors and adult mental and physical health. Canadian Journal of Psychiatry 44, 326–334.

Susser E, Schaefer C, Brown A, Begg M, Wyatt RJ (2000) The design of the Prenatal Determinants of Schizophrenia Study (PDS). Schizophrenia Bulletin 26, 257–273.

Susser M (1998) Does risk factor epidemiology put epidemiology at risk? Peering into the future. Journal of Epidemiology and Community Health 52, 608–611.

Susser M, Susser E (1996) Choosing a future for epidemiology: II From black boxes to Chinese boxes and eco-epidemiology. American Journal of Public Health 86: 674–677.

Suvisaari J, Haukka J, Tanskanen A, Hovi T, Lönnqvist J (1999) Association between prenatal exposure to poliovirus infection and adult schizophrenia. American Journal of Psychiatry 156, 1100–1102.

Takei N, Sham P, O'Callaghan E, Murray GK, Glover G, Murray RM (1994) Prenatal exposure to influenza and the development of schizophrenia: is the effect confined to females? American Journal of Psychiatry 151, 117–119.

Takei N, Sham P, O'Callaghan E, Glover G, Murray RM (1995) Schizophrenia: increased risk associated with winter and city birth – a case-control study in 12 regions within England and Wales. Journal of Epidemiological and Community Health 49, 106–107.

Takei N, Mortensen PB, Klaening U, Murray RM, Sham PC, O'Callaghan E (1996) Relationship between in-utero exposure to influenza epidemics and risk of schizophrenia in Denmark. Biological Psychiatry 40, 817–824.

Tarrant J, Jones PB (1999) Precursors to schizophrenia: do biological markers for schizophrenia have specificity? Canadian Journal of Psychiatry 44, 335–349.

Taubes G (1995) Epidemiology faces its limits. Science 269, 164–169.

Teixeira JMA, Fisk NM, Glover V (1999) Association between maternal anxiety in pregnancy and increased uterine artery resistance index: cohort based study. British Medical Journal 318, 153–157.

Tombaugh G, Yang S, Swanson R, Sapolsky R (1992) Glucocortocoids exacerbate hypoxic and hypglycaemic hippocampal injury in vitro: biochemical correlates and a role for astrocytes. Journal of Neurochemistry 59, 137–146.

Torrey EF, Bowler A (1990) Geographical distribution of insanity in America: evidence for an urban factor. Schizophrenia Bulletin 16, 591–604.

Torrey EF, Rawlings R, Waldman IN (1988) Schizophrenic births and viral diseases in two states. Schizophrenia Research 1, 73–77.

Torrey EF, Bowler AE, Rawlings R (1991) An influenza epidemic and the seasonality of schizophrenic births. In: Psychiatry and Biological Factors, Kurstak E, ed. New York: Plenum Press, pp. 109–116.

Torrey EF, Bowler AE, Rawlings R (1992) Schizophrenia and the 1957 influenza epidemic. Schizophrenia Research 6, 100–107.

Torrey EF, Miller J, Rawlings R, Yolken RH (1997) Seasonality of birth in schizophrenia and bipolar disorder: a review. Schizophrenia Research 28, 1–38.

Tsuang M (2000) Schizophrenia: genes and environment. Biological Psychiatry 47, 210–220.

Turner SW, Toone BK, Brett-Jones JR (1986) Computerised tomographic scan changes in early schizophrenia. Psychological Medicine 16, 219–225.

Van Os J, Selten J-P (1998) Prenatal exposure to maternal stress and later schizophrenia: The may 1940 invasion of the Netherlands. British Journal of Psychiatry 172, 324–326.

Waddington JL, O'Callaghan E, Joussef H et al. (1999) Schizophrenia: evidence for a 'cascade' process with neurodevelopmental origins. In: Prenatal Exposures in Schizophrenia, Susser ES, Brown AS, Gorman JM, eds. Washington, DC: American Psychiatric Press, pp. 3–34.

Watt NF (1978) Patterns of childhood social development in adult schizophrenics. Archives of General Psychiatry, 35, 160–165.

Weinberger DR (1987) Implications of normal brain development for the pathogenesis of schizophrenia. Archives of General Psychiatry 44, 660–669.

Weinberger DR, Torrey EF, Neophytides AN, Wyatt RJ (1979) Lateral ventricular enlargement in chronic schizophrenia. Archives of General Psychiatry 36, 735–739.

Westergaard T, Mortensen PB, Pedersen CB, Wohlfahrt J, Melbye M (1999) Exposure to prenatal and childhood infections and the risk of schizophrenia. Archives of General Psychiatry 56, 993–998.

Wright P, Rifkin L, Takei N, Murray R (1995) Maternal influenza, obstetric complications and schizophrenia. American Journal of Psychiatry 152, 1714–1720.

Wright P, Takei N, Murray RM, Sham PC (1999) Seasonality, prenatal influenza exposure and schizophrenia. In: Prenatal Exposures in Schizophrenia, Susser ES, Brown AS, Gorman JM, eds. Washington, DC: American Psychiatric Press, pp. 89–112.

Yolken RH, Torrey EF (1995) Viruses, schizophrenia and bipolar disorder. Clinical Microbiology Reviews 8, 131–145.

Zornberg G, Buka SL, Tsuang MT (2000a) The problem of obstetrical complications and schizophrenia. Schizophrenia Bulletin 26, 249–256.

Zornberg GL, Buka SL, Tsuang MT (2000b) Hypoxic-ischaemia-related fetal/neonatal complications and risk of schizophrenia and other nonaffective psychoses: a 19 year longitudinal study. American Journal of Psychiatry 157, 196–202.

6

Childhood development and later schizophrenia: evidence from genetic high-risk and birth cohort studies

Mary Cannon[1], C. Jane Tarrant[2], Matti O. Huttunen[3] and Peter Jones[4]

[1]Institute of Psychiatry, King's College London, UK
[2]Department of Psychiatry, University of Nottingham, UK
[3]Department of Mental Health and Alcohol Research, National Public Health Institute, Helsinki, Finland
[4]Division of Psychiatry, University of Cambridge, UK

Historical context

From its first descriptions, schizophrenic psychosis had a longitudinal dimension. Thomas Clouston (Clouston, 1892; Murray, 1994; Murray and Jones, 1995) recognized a syndrome of 'developmental insanity' in which developmental physical abnormalities were associated with early-onset psychotic phenomena, particularly in men. Kraepelin (1896) and Bleuler (1908, 1911) noted that people who developed the psychotic syndrome were often different from their peers before psychosis began. The notion that there may be psychological differences predating psychosis was initially incorporated into psychodynamic formulations of the disorder. However, during the 1980s, a new causal paradigm emerged: the 'neurodevelopmental hypothesis' of schizophrenia (Murray and Lewis, 1987; Weinberger, 1987), which proposed a subtle deviance in early brain development, the full adverse consequences of which were not manifest until adolescence or early adulthood. The evidence for this hypothesis has been discussed in Chapter 5.

Central to a neurodevelopmental model of schizophrenia is the identification of manifestations characterizing those at risk during childhood and adolescence – before the overt symptoms of the illness appear. We might expect people who later develop schizophrenia to show either neurological or behavioural abnormalities during childhood or adolescence. Accordingly, information about childhood development and schizophrenia has been gleaned from a wide variety of sources since the 1960s including school records (Watt et al., 1978; Cannon et al., 1999), child guidance clinic records (Robins, 1966; Hartman et al., 1984; Ambelas, 1992;

Hollis, 1995; Cannon et al., 2001), conscript assessment records (David et al., 1997; Malmberg et al., 1998; Davidson et al., 1999) and even childhood 'home movies' (Walker and Lewine, 1990; Walker et al., 1993, 1994). Although these samples are biased to varying degrees, as a body of evidence they point to many social, behavioural, motor and intellectual precursors of schizophrenia (Rutter, 1984; Jones, 1999; Marenco and Weinberger, 2000). This review will focus on evidence of childhood developmental deficits preceding schizophrenia taken from two robust sources of prospective information: genetic high-risk cohorts and general population birth cohorts.

Genetic high-risk cohorts

In the genetic high-risk design, risk is determined by the individual's genetic relatedness to an affected proband. Individuals with a higher than normal genetic loading for schizophrenia, by virtue of having at least one affected first-degree relative (usually a parent), are identified and studied longitudinally. Individuals with one schizophrenic parent have a slightly greater than 10% risk of developing schizophrenia; this is 10–12 times higher than the risk in the general population. This design entails determining whether a given measure, assessed at one time point, predicts later manifestation of schizophrenia and related disorders. These high-risk studies permit the opportunity to observe the developmental course of schizophrenia. The identification of developmental precursors of schizophrenia entails the hope that characteristics assessed early in life can be used to differentiate offspring who develop psychopathology from those who do not.

We will review the literature about childhood development in children at genetic risk for schizophrenia and developmental precursors and predictors of adult schizophrenia. The high-risk studies recruit children at different times in the lifespan (Table 6.1). Two studies, the Fish High-Risk Study (Fish et al., 1992) and the Jerusalem Infant Development Study (JIDS; Marcus et al., 1981, 1993; Hans et al., 2000), began follow-up from infancy; others, such as the New York High Risk Project (NYHRP) and the Israeli High Risk Study, began in early and middle childhood. Studies that began in adolescence, such as the Copenhagen High Risk Study and the Edinburgh High Risk Study are less informative about childhood development. So far, only a few studies have followed high-risk samples into adulthood, notably the high-risk study of Barbara Fish (Fish et al, 1992), the Copenhagen High Risk Study (Cannon and Mednick, 1993), the Israeli High Risk study (Cannon et al., 2002) and the NYHRP (Erlenmeyer-Kimling et al., 2000).

Table 6.1. Genetic high-risk studies of schizophrenia reviewed in Chapter 6

High-risk study	Age at recruitment	Age at last assessment	Completed (C) or ongoing (O)
New York Infant Development Study	Birth	27–34 years	C
Jerusalem Infant Development Study (JIDS)	Birth	14–21 years	O
Copenhagen Obstetric High Risk Study	Birth	1 year	C
New York High Risk Project (NYHRP)	Mean 9 years	Mean 30 years	O
Israeli High Risk Project	Mean 11 years	35–36 years	C
Copenhagen High Risk Study	Mean 15 years	Mean 42 years	C
Finnish Adoptive Study of Schizophrenia	Mean 16 years	21–23 years	O
Edinburgh High Risk Study	Mean 21 years	Mean 24 years	O

What do we need to know about childhood developmental markers of schizophrenia from genetic high-risk studies?

There are a number of questions that can be examined using genetic high-risk studies:

- which childhood developmental impairments are associated with genetic risk for schizophrenia?
- which childhood developmental impairments predict later schizophrenia among those at genetic risk?
- what is the nature of the relationship: subgroup, dose–response or other?
- what about the false positives (i.e. those with childhood developmental impairments who do not develop schizophrenia); can they provide us with information about interactive risk factors or protective factors?
- are the findings from high-risk studies regarding childhood development generalizable to the majority of schizophrenia?

Studies with information from infancy

New York Infant Development Study

Barbara Fish began the New York Infant Development Study in 1952 and identified at birth 12 offspring of chronic schizophrenic mothers and 12 controls from similar low socioeconomic status backgrounds. Developmental assessments were made at 10 points between birth and age 2 years. Subsequent assessments were carried out at ages 9–10, 15–16, 18–19 and 20–22 years. The last assessment of current psychiatric status to date was in 1991, at ages 27–34 years. From her detailed infant observations, Fish noted abnormal timing and pattern of acquisition of milestones and growth retardation among the high-risk group (Fish, 1960; Fish and Hagin, 1973).

She invented the term *pandysmaturation* (PDM) to describe this constellation of infant developmental abnormalities (Fish, 1987) and considered this a marker in infancy for an inherited neurointegrative defect in schizophrenia, as in Meehl's 'schizotaxia' hypothesis (Meehl, 1962, 1989). Of the seven high-risk children diagnosed with PDM, all seven have been diagnosed (nonblindly) with schizophrenia or schizotypal personality disorder in adulthood (Fish, 1987). Fish partially replicated her findings in the JIDS (see below) and concluded that the findings of pandysmaturation may provide a strategy for looking at at-risk individuals before adult psychopathology becomes evident (Fish et al., 1992).

The Jerusalem Infant Development Study

The JIDS recruited high-risk and control children at birth (1973–77), and detailed information is, therefore, available from infancy on all subjects. The sample sizes vary at each assessment as siblings have been recruited to increase the numbers in the offspring groups. At the latest follow-up assessment, the sample comprised 24 offspring of schizophrenic parents, 25 offspring of parents with other mental illness and 16 offspring of parents with no mental illness. However, the subjects have not yet reached the peak risk period for schizophrenia so one cannot yet identify predictors of later schizophrenia with any degree of certainty. The subjects have been followed up at school age (7–13 years) (Marcus et al., 1993) and in adolescence (14–21 years) (Hans et al., 1999).

Neurobehavioural assessments

A global measure of poor neurobehavioural functioning was derived from factor analysis of 20 adolescent neurobehavioural variables. This resulted in two principal components: cognitive–attentional and motoric. The sample were divided into good and poor functioning by an Epanechnikov kernel procedure. The offspring of schizophrenic parents were three times more likely to be defined in this way as poorly functioning compared with offspring of nonschizophrenic parents (Hans et al., 1999). Of the offspring of schizophrenic parents, 40% showed consistently poor functioning at all three assessments. Although the JIDS offspring are still early in the period of risk for schizophrenia, seven subjects have already received diagnoses in the schizophrenia spectrum. Four are offspring of schizophrenic parents (one schizophrenia, two schizotypal personality disorder and two paranoid personality disorder); all four showed a consistently poor pattern of neurobehavioural functioning at both school age and adolescence, and three out of four also showed poor infant functioning and probable pandysmaturation (Fish et al., 1992). These findings from the current assessment of the JIDS support the hypothesis that global neurodevelopmental deficits may be premorbid indicators of genetic vulnerability to schizophrenia.

Copenhagen Obstetric High Risk Project

The Copenhagen Obstetric High Risk Project differs from the others in that it did not involve tracing or interviewing subjects (Mednick et al., 1971). A perinatal register from the University Hospital in Copenhagen, containing information on obstetric histories and 1-year developmental checks on children born between 1959 and 1961, was linked with the Danish Central Psychiatric Register. The sample for this study comprised 83 children born to a schizophrenic parent, 83 children born to a parent with personality disorder and 83 children born to normal parents. Retarded motor reflexes in the neonatal period and retarded 1-year development among the schizophrenia offspring (late in attaining milestones) were observed among the high-risk schizophrenia group. Low birthweight was significantly related to 1-year developmental status among the offspring of schizophrenic parents only.

Studies with information from middle childhood

Israeli High Risk Study

The Israeli High Risk study began in 1964 with the aim of capitalizing on a unique child-rearing circumstance found nowhere else in the world: the children's house in the kibbutz. A professional child-care worker, or metapelet, was responsible for rearing the children in a communal children's house, although the children usually spent some part of the day with their parents. The study aimed to identify a group of children at genetic risk for schizophrenia who were being raised on kibbutzim and to follow them over time. It was theorized that the stability and continuity afforded the group-raised children would have a favourable effect on their development. Such children would be less likely than those raised in the nuclear family to suffer the unpredictable behaviour and frequent absences of a mentally ill parent (for discussion see Mirsky et al., 1995).

Children were first identified at mean age 11 years and assessed again at mean age 17 years with a 15-year follow-up at ages 25–26 years and a 25-year follow-up in the early–mid thirties. Fifty index children at high risk for schizophrenia (offspring of high-risk parents) and 50 control children were identified. The initial data from the first and second round of interviews provided numerous instances of the ways in which index children differed from controls (Marcus et al., 1985). The differences involved virtually every area of functioning and included soft neurological signs such as clumsiness, poor left–right orientation and motor overflow, impaired visual motor coordination and greater distractibility, lower sociometric rankings by peers and impaired interpersonal relations, work and play activities, self-esteem and mood.

Circumstances of rearing and later psychopathology

In order to examine the effects of kibbutz and family rearing, the sample was recruited so that the 50 high-risk (index) and 50 control children could be subdivided into equal groups of 25 as follows: the kibbutz index (KI) group and the town index (TI) group, the kibbutz control (KC) group and the town control (TC) group.

At follow up in 1981 when aged 26 (Mirsky et al., 1985), the KI group (23 interviewed) had the highest incidence of psychiatric disorder: three schizophrenia, three other schizophrenia spectrum, five major affective, four minor affective, one other diagnosis and seven with no diagnosis. Corresponding figures for the 23 members of the TI group interviewed were two schizophrenia, one other schizophrenia spectrum, one major affective, no minor affective, three other diagnosis and 16 with no diagnosis. There were a total of four minor diagnoses for the control groups and 40 control cases with no diagnosis. Although one could not conclude that the kibbutz environment was associated with significantly more schizophrenia than the nuclear family, there appeared to be more psychopathology in the KI group compared with the TI group.

At the last follow-up, no new cases of schizophrenia were found (Mirsky et al., 1995). However 44% of the KI group had a severe axis 1 disorder compared with 16% in the TI group ($p = 0.03$). Only 8% of the pooled control group (KC + TC) had an axis 1 disorder ($p = 0.0007$). The authors concluded that kibbutz rearing in high-risk children increases the risk of major psychiatric disorder – though not necessarily schizophrenia. What are the potential mechanisms for this effect? One possibility is that conformity to kibbutz norms is greatly encouraged and deviant or odd behaviours are not tolerated; therefore, differences between children vulnerable to schizophrenia and controls would be exaggerated in the 'hot house' atmosphere of the kibbutz and would add to their feelings of isolation and loneliness. Another stress for the kibbutzim-reared child may lie in the forced conformity and intolerance for deviation involved in the mandatory military experience.

Other childhood predictors of later schizophrenia

The social and behavioural profile (at 11 and 17 years) of the index child who develops schizophrenia spectrum disorder was antisocial personality; did not get on with parents, teachers or peers; was rated low in social desirability by peers; low self-esteem, suspicious and withdrawn; and poor communication skills (Hans et al., 1992). Poor attention skills at age 11 (on average) were highly related to development of schizophrenia spectrum disorders in adulthood.

Protective factors

Index cases who were free of any diagnosis at the last follow-up had the highest 'sense of coherence' scores of any group, suggesting that positive self-esteem may be a protective factor for subjects at risk of schizophrenia (Mirsky et al., 1995). The future affective disorder cases had the highest intelligence quotient (IQ) of all subjects (Mirsky et al., 1995). Higher IQ may also serve as a protective factor among high-risk children in that affective disorder rather than schizophrenia developed.

The New York High Risk Project

NYHRP (Erlenmeyer-Kimling et al., 1995, 1997) was set up to look for endophenotypic markers for the genetic susceptibility to schizophrenia and began recruiting subjects in 1971–72 (sample A) with a second round of recruitment in 1977–79 (sample B). Children were recruited at ages 7–12 years (mean 9.5 years). The samples comprised 79 offspring of schizophrenic parents, 57 offspring of parents with affective disorder (40% were psychotic) and 133 offspring of parents with no mental illness. There has been some reclassification of parents originally diagnosed as schizophrenic as suffering from affective illness. Children have been assessed at six evaluation rounds, about 3 years apart, between ages 7 and 12 and ages 26 and 30 years. The last assessment was in 1994–95 (mean age 30.1 years) when full diagnostic assessments were carried out. At that time, 15% ($n = 12$) of the 79 offspring of schizophrenic parents, 7% ($n = 4$) of the 57 offspring of the affectively ill parents and 0.8% ($n = 1$) of the 133 offspring of normal parents fulfilled diagnostic criteria for schizophrenia-related psychoses (Erlenmeyer-Kimling et al., 1995, 1997).

Neuropsychological predictors

At the baseline assessment at age 7–12 years, a neuropsychological battery was administered to the children (Erlenmeyer-Kimling et al., 2000). Models containing the variables 'attention deviance', 'memory' and 'gross motor' were significantly related both to high-risk status and to risk of later developing a schizophreniform psychosis. These mediating neurobehavioural variables may be phenotypic indicators of the genetic liability to schizophrenia-related psychoses and in combination with high-risk status may predict future development of schizophrenia-related psychoses.

Combination of impairment on all three variables together achieved better classification among the offspring of schizophrenic parents with respect to false-positive rate, positive value and overall accuracy than any of the variables individually (Erlenmeyer-Kimling et al., 2000). For a model containing all three variables, sensitivity in identifying the future development of schizophrenia-related psychoses among offspring of schizophrenic parents was 50%, with a specificity of 89.6%, positive predictive value of 46.2% and overall accuracy of 83.5%. The false-positive rate was 10.4%. The nonpsychotic offspring of schizophrenic parents who were among the 10% falsely classified when all three variables were combined are of interest because they appear to be carriers of some of the susceptibility genes for schizophrenia and may yield information about some of the other factors that may be needed for the development of overt illness. False-positive subjects may have experienced less exposure to environmental factors that interact with susceptibility genes to result in full clinical expression of the illness. Among the offspring of affectively ill parents, no subjects were predicted to develop schizophrenia-related psychosis by all three models.

It is likely that deficits in attention, memory and gross motor skills reflect only some of the phenotypic indicators of a large complex of susceptibility genes. There is still a significant effect of family background on schizophrenia-related psychoses when the influence of these three mediating variables is controlled. Other measures, such as functional brain imaging or more refined neuropsychological batteries, may have been better predictors if they had been carried out during childhood.

Impaired attention in childhood appears to remain as a stable trait through childhood and into adulthood in those at risk of schizophrenia in the NYHRP (Cornblatt and Erlenmeyer-Kimling, 1985; Cornblatt et al., 1992; Erlenmeyer-Kimling and Cornblatt, 1992). Unaffected offspring in this group showed abnormal childhood attentional deficits, which were associated with later personality traits of social indifference and insensitivity (Cornblatt et al., 1992). Children of parents with affective psychosis also displayed some attentional impairment but not to the extent of schizophrenia-risk children (Cornblatt and Erlenmeyer-Kimling, 1985; Cornblatt et al., 1992) and the attentional impairments in this group were not related to the later behavioural disturbances (Cornblatt et al., 1992).

Behavioural predictors

Childhood behavioural problems in the NYHRP were rated from a parent interview at the first assessment when the children were aged 7–12 years (Amminger et al., 1999). A childhood behaviour measure, reflecting mainly externalizing behaviours, was derived from this interview using factor analysis. Items reflecting other behaviours such as social withdrawal did not yield sufficiently high loadings to be included in the analysis. No differences between the offspring groups were found with regard to childhood behaviour but, after exclusion of subjects who later developed substance abuse, subjects who developed adulthood schizophrenia-related psychoses (from sample A) displayed significantly more behavioural problems in childhood than those with adulthood affective disorders or anxiety disorders or those with substance abuse only or no disorder.

Cognitive predictors: intelligence

Intelligence scores (on Wechsler Intelligence Scale for Children (WISC) and Adult Intelligence Scale (WAIS)), were lower in the offspring of schizophrenia parents than in the offspring of affective disorder parents at the first assessment (mean age 9.4 years) but not at the second assessment (mean age 15.2 years) (Ott et al., 1998). Overall intelligence quotient (IQ) as measured in adulthood could not be conclusively linked with later schizophrenia. However, a low score on the measure of scatter (the variability in performance between subtests at the individual level) was a significant predictor of later schizophrenia-related psychoses. The authors speculate that low levels of scatter indicate a flattening of the cognitive profile in the pre-schizophrenic state, possibly related to inflexibility of cognitive functioning, but without deficiencies of particular abilities.

Studies with information from adolescence

Copenhagen High Risk Study

The Copenhagen High Risk Study is the largest high risk study in schizophrenia conducted to date and began in 1962 by recruiting 207 offspring of schizophrenic mothers and 104 offspring of control mothers when the children were, on average, 15 years. The study has followed subjects right through the risk period for schizophrenia – up to 42 years of age on average. At the last assessment (Mednick et al., 1987), 40 (19%) of the high-risk offspring fulfilled diagnostic criteria for an axis I functional psychotic illness; 42 (20%) fulfilled diagnostic criteria for cluster A personality disorder and a further 42 (20%) fulfilled diagnostic criteria for other axis I and II disorders. Among the low-risk offspring, only three (2.8%) fulfilled diagnostic criteria for an axis I functional psychotic illness; five (4.8%) fulfilled diagnostic criteria for cluster A personality disorder; and 33 (32%) fulfilled diagnostic criteria for other axis I and II disorders.

Although the recruitment in the mid-teens meant that there were no assessments of the sample in childhood, nevertheless some childhood data are available from obstetric records and from teacher reports. Mednick et al. (1987) reported that high-risk subjects who later developed schizophrenia had experienced more, and more severe, perinatal complications than those who did not. Teacher reports were available for this sample at age 15 (Olin and Mednick, 1996). Teachers more frequently judged both males and females later diagnosed with schizophrenia to be emotionally labile and more susceptible to future breakdown. They more frequently rated males as disruptive, anxious, lonely and rejected by peers and more likely to have repeated a grade. In contrast, they rated females as nervous and withdrawn. In a reanalysis of this project, Cannon et al. (1990) separated those with predominantly negative symptom schizophrenia from those with predominantly positive symptom schizophrenia. The former in their adolescence were rated by teachers to be passive, socially isolated and unresponsive to praise, while the latter were rated as overactive, irritable, distractible and aggressive.

Finnish Adoptive Family Study of Schizophrenia

The Finnish Adoptive Study of Schizophrenia focused on family environment as a risk factor for later schizophrenia (Tienari et al., 1987). It is not informative about childhood development but has given interesting information on gene–environment interaction in schizophrenia.

A nationwide sample was collected of all women who had been hospitalized because of schizophrenia between 1960 and 1979 in Finland ($n = 19\,447$). Through linkage with adoption registers, it was found that 264 of these schizophrenic mothers had given up 291 offspring for adoption. A total of 179 offspring of 164 index schizophrenic mothers comprised the final sample of index cases. Subjects were recruited at a mean age of 16 years. Index cases were matched with control adoptees (adopted-away offspring of parents who had not been hospitalized with psychosis) and their adoptive families. The adoptive index and control families were intensively studied in their homes with 2-day assessments, including couple and family interviews, the consensual Rorschach and the interpersonal perception method. Follow-up telephone interviews 5–7 years after the original assessment revealed that 15 adoptees had developed a psychotic illness: 13 from the index group and two from the control group. The families were divided into two groups on the basis of their globally rated family functioning: healthy and disturbed (moderately/severely). In the healthy rearing families, there was little mental illness among the adoptees regardless of whether or not the biological parent was schizophrenic. In disturbed families, the adoptees were much more disturbed, especially among the index adoptees (Tienari, 1991). The results are consistent with the hypothesis that healthy families have possibly protected the vulnerable child from developing schizophrenia, whereas in disturbed homes the vulnerable children are more sensitive to dysfunctional rearing.

A further analysis involved a narrower measure of family pathology – communication deviance – than the original global rating, and a measure of thought disorder as an indicator of vulnerability to schizophrenic illness (Wahlberg et al., 1997). This analysis also addressed the issue of reverse causality (i.e. whether a disordered child can alter the family dynamics or communication style of the parents). In a subsample of 58 index adoptees and 96 comparison subjects and their families, there was no significant relationship between index or control status of the adoptee and communication problems in the rearing parents. There was a highly significant gene–environment interaction effect; as in the families with high levels of communication deviance, a higher proportion of high-risk than comparison adoptees showed evidence of thought disorder. This is an example of genetic control of sensitivity to the environment: the extent to which genes control the degree to which individuals are sensitive to the predisposing, risk-increasing aspects of the environment (Ch. 12).

The Edinburgh High Risk Study

The Edinburgh High Risk Study recruited subjects with at least two family members with a diagnosis of schizophrenia (Hodges et al., 1999; Johnstone et al., 2000). High-risk subjects were recruited from age 16–25 years and this study is, therefore, not informative about early childhood development. The focus was on identifying neuroimaging and neuropsychological predictors of genetic vulnerability to schizophrenia. The high-risk group reported more psychiatric contacts during childhood and adolescence, and more childhood antisocial behaviour, childhood social isolation and interpersonal sensitivity than normal controls (Hodges et al., 1999). Significant neuropsychological differences between high-risk subjects and controls at baseline were observed for all tests of intellectual function and on aspects of executive function and memory (Byrne et al., 1999).

Summary of the data on childhood development from the high-risk studies

The following points summarize the data from all the high-risk studies described here.

1 Genetic high-risk studies show that 25–60% of high-risk children display some or all of the following developmental abnormalities: pandysmaturation (infancy), gross and fine motor impairment (early childhood), attentional and information processing deficits (early and middle childhood), cognitive and neuropsychological deficits (childhood and adolescence) and behavioural problems and social adjustment difficulties (adolescence). These deficits may indicate the influence of susceptibility genes for schizophrenia.

2 Pandysmaturation, motor and attentional deficits among high-risk children are predictive of later schizophrenia-related disorders, with positive predictive values of about 50%.

3 The circumstance of the child's upbringing (deviant communication within the family or kibbutz-rearing) appears to interact with genetic risk for schizophrenia and increases the risk of subsequent schizophrenia or other major psychopathology.

4 The false positives, high-risk children who have developmental impairments but do not develop schizophrenia, are interesting because they could provide information about possible protective factors or other risk factors required to precipitate the onset of schizophrenia. However the high-risk samples have not yet been followed through the entire period of risk. More information about false positives can be obtained in the following section in the discussion of the National Collaborative Perinatal Project.

5 Problems associated with the design of high-risk studies include small samples sizes, incomplete follow-up and the perennial problem of generalizability (since only 10% of schizophrenic patients have a parent with a diagnosis of

schizophrenia). The issue of generalizability can be examined by comparing the results of the genetic high-risk cohorts with general population birth cohorts (see below).

General population birth cohort studies

General population birth cohorts are a valuable source of unbiased and prospective data on childhood development that is not restricted to patients with an affected first-degree relative. These cohorts are derived from a general population of births and are unselected for specific genetic or environmental exposures. The cohort usually undergoes a comprehensive baseline assessment at birth or during early childhood and then is assessed at subsequent follow-ups. Data on child development are usually detailed and standardized. A wide range of factors can be examined within one study; confounding can be controlled and causal pathways can be explored. The recent prominence of these types of study in the psychiatric literature is a consequence of the 'coming-of-age' of birth cohorts that were established by far-sighted researchers many decades earlier (Susser, 1999). Most of these cohorts were set up to study childhood health and development and were not originally envisaged as a resource for schizophrenia research. Outcome data are usually obtained through psychiatric screening interviews in adulthood or linkage to national health care registers. The major problem with these cohorts is the difficulty in obtaining sufficient cases for analysis, stemming from the relative rarity of schizophrenia in the general population. Approaches to overcoming this problem include the use of nested case-control designs (Cannon et al., 1999) and combination of data from several similar cohorts (Jones and Done, 1997; Susser, 1999).

Medical Research Council National Survey of Health and Development (1946 British birth cohort)

Jones and colleagues (1994) reported on the Medical Research Council National Survey of Health and Development. This cohort is a stratified, random sample of births occurring in Britain during a week in March 1946 (Wadsworth 1991). In this survey, 5362 children were followed up at regular intervals, including 11 contacts up to the age of 16 years. Since that time, there have been nine contacts, with the most recent at 43 years. Cases of schizophrenia were identified on the basis of information from the cohort questionnaires, the Present State Examination at age 36, and the Mental Health Enquiry, a central independent register of psychiatric hospital admissions. Of 4746 subjects alive and living in the UK at age 16 years, 30 subsequently met the DSM-III-R criteria (American Psychiatric Association, 1987) for schizophrenia. The remaining 4716 subjects were considered not to have been at risk and were used as control subjects.

The children who later developed schizophrenia (cases) were shown to have a significant delay in achieving developmental milestones over the first 2 years of life. At age 2 they were less likely to have attained all the milestones of sitting, standing, walking and talking. Walking and talking showed the greatest differences, with the preschizophrenic group having an average delay of 1.2 months for each. Between ages 2 and 15 years, speech problems were also more frequent.

Consistently poorer results in the cognitive tests, conducted at ages 8, 11 and 15 years, were achieved by the cases when compared with the controls. Particular areas of deficit were verbal, nonverbal and mathematical skills. These differences appeared to widen in adolescence, although this was statistically uncertain. In terms of sociability, the children who later developed schizophrenia preferred to play on their own at ages 4 and 6 years, and showed a statistically significant linear trend for being more socially anxious as teenagers. There was no indication that low social class or disadvantaged home circumstances was associated with the later development of schizophrenia.

Regarding specificity of these precursors to schizophrenia and affective disorder, van Os et al. (1997) used the same birth cohort to show that female sex and lower scores on childhood cognitive tests predicted later depression in the total group of subjects. For those who developed childhood-onset affective disorder, there were also significant discriminant characteristics in later motor milestones attainment and the presence of more twitches and grimaces at 15 years of age. Only those in the adult-onset affective disorder group did not show these developmental delays and abnormal movements.

The National Child Development Study (1958 British birth cohort)

Another British birth cohort with a similar design has been reported by Done et al. (1991, 1994). The National Child Development Study followed subjects born in a week in March 1958. Data were collected at birth and at ages 7, 11, 16 and 23 years. At age 7, 15 398 subjects were traced. Cases were identified by means of the Mental Health Enquiry (see previous section) and Present State Examination diagnoses were made from ratings of medical notes. By 1994, 29 of the subjects were judged to have a 'narrow' diagnosis of schizophrenia, 29 were considered to have undergone an affective psychosis and 71 were judged to have a neurotic illness. A control group comprised a randomly selected sample (10%) of cohort members who had not received psychiatric treatment.

Ratings of motor function and neurological soft signs were made at ages 7 and 11. At age 7, the group that went on to develop narrowly defined schizophrenia and affective psychoses was significantly more abnormal than controls on coordination and clumsiness (Crow et al., 1995). At age 11, differences in hand preference/relative hand skill, coordination and central nervous system (CNS) impairment were apparent for the schizophrenia group compared with controls. However, some abnormalities in coordination, CNS impairment and tics and twitches were also associated with later development of affective psychosis.

Poorer educational achievement was found in the group who went on to develop schizophrenia. This encompassed a wide range of tasks and there was no change in the relative difference between the cases and controls over the age range 7 to 16 (Crow et al., 1995). Only minor cognitive deficits were measured for the preaffective psychosis subjects, but there were more marked abnormalities in the neurotic group and evidence of a decline in function in the females with age. Social disadvantage did account for some of the difference within this group.

1966 Northern Finland Birth Cohort

The Northern Finland Birth Cohort was started in 1966 and prospectively followed 12 058 children born in that year (Isohanni et al., 2000). Data have currently been collected up until age 31 on 11 017 members of the cohort who were living in Finland at the age of 16. Later achievement of developmental milestones (standing, walking or becoming potty trained) in the first year predicted the highest risk of future psychoses, while earlier attainment of these skills held a lower risk than expected. The relationship between age of acquiring motor milestones and risk of psychoses later in life appeared linear (Isohanni et al., 2000, 2001). Adolescents who performed at school below their expected grade were three times more likely to develop schizophrenia than those in their normal grade (Isohanni et al., 1998). However, a small subgroup of boys who had a fourfold increased risk of developing schizophrenia compared with comparison subjects had excellent school performance (Isohanni et al., 1999). Hence, both scholastically poor and excellent performers in this cohort appear to have an increased risk of schizophrenia.

Helsinki 1951–1960 Birth Cohort

The Helsinki 1951–1960 Birth Cohort is an example of a nested case-control study within a birth cohort of all children born over a 10-year period in Helsinki between the beginning of 1951 and the end of 1960 (Cannon et al., 1999). Those with schizophrenia (cases) were identified by using three national health-care databases and controls were taken as the next child with the same year of birth listed in the child health archives. School records were ultimately traced for 400 cases and 403 controls. School performance was compared between cases and controls for the 4 years of schooling common to all (ages 7–11). There were no differences in the mean rank in class for academic subjects between cases and controls at age 11, but those who developed schizophrenia were then less likely to progress and go on to further education at high school. The preschizophrenia group had significantly poorer performances in nonacademic subjects such as sports and handicrafts, supporting the notion of motor coordination deficits preceding schizophrenia.

Swedish Conscript Cohort

A Swedish cohort of male conscripts (David et al., 1997) found strong relationships between lower IQ scores measured at age 18 and later development of schizophrenia. Lack of sociability and increased sensitivity in childhood and adolescence (Malmberg et al., 1998) similarly conveyed an increased risk of later disease. All individuals who had a learning disability, a major neurological condition or an onset of schizophrenia before age 18 were excluded from this population at risk. The strength of these associations may, therefore, be underestimated.

Israeli Draft Board Conscript Cohort

The Israeli Draft Board assesses all Israeli males at 16 or 17 years for their eligibility to military service. Physical and psychiatric status, cognition, personality and behavioural traits are assessed. Data from these assessments on male adolescents between 1985 and 1991 have been used and linked with the National Psychiatric Hospitalization Case Registry between 1970 and 1995 to identify a group with schizophrenia (Davidson et al., 1999). Compared with matched controls, healthy males at draft assessment who went on to develop schizophrenia had significantly lower scores on all measures. A linear association between increasing risk for schizophrenia and poorer cognitive performance was found. A poorer ability to function independently, fewer social relationships and decreased organizational ability were behavioural characteristics significantly associated with the preschizophrenic group compared with controls.

The National Collaborative Perinatal Project: the Philadelphia cohort

From 1959 to 1966, the National Collaborative Perinatal Project (NCPP) enrolled for study 9236 offspring of 6753 mothers who delivered at two inner city hospital obstetric wards in Philadelphia. In 1996, a search of the Penn Longitudinal Database showed that 3.7% of the cohort members had ever had a psychotic illness (194 with schizophrenia or schizoaffective disorder and 145 with affective or drug-induced psychosis) and 9.3% had ever had a nonpsychotic diagnosis. A chart review of 144 showed that 72 fulfilled criteria for DSM-IV schizophrenia (American Psychiatric Association, 1994) or schizoaffective disorder (cases). This cohort study is unique in that it also allows investigation of childhood development among the siblings of schizophrenic patients, as the 72 cases had 63 unaffected siblings who were also NCPP study participants. Siblings of schizophrenic patients are a group at genetic high risk for schizophrenia who have not developed the condition. In a sense they can be viewed as false positives: a proportion of the siblings may display the same endophenotypic traits as the probands but have escaped developing the condition. They can be used to study possible markers of genetic liability to schizophrenia that are distinct from the precursors of the condition itself. The sibling design can also allow examination of possible interactive risk factors or protective factors for schizophrenia.

Childhood developmental variables as predictors of schizophrenia or sibling status

Motor variables

Two measures of childhood motor coordination were derived from standardized neurological and psychological examinations conducted at 8 months, 4 years and 7 years of age: unusual movements (all time points) and motor coordination (age 7 only). Motor coordination was a significant predictor of both adult schizophrenic status and unaffected sibling status (Rosso et al., 2000). 12.5% of siblings but only 4.4% of normal controls were deviant on tests of motor coordination at 7 years of age. Unusual movements at age 4 and 7 predicted adult schizophrenia status but not unaffected sibling status. The authors speculate that motor coordination problems index a familial or genetic liability to the disorder, while unusual movements were specific to those who had developed the disorder.

Cognitive functioning

Standardized tests of cognitive functioning were administered to the cohort: the Stanford–Binet intelligence test at age 4 and the WISC at age 7 years. Both subjects with schizophrenia and their unaffected siblings performed worse than controls on the cognitive tests at both ages (Cannon et al., 2000). There was an inverse linear relationship between IQ and risk of schizophrenia versus sibling status, in that the lower the childhood IQ the greater the chance of being a schizophrenic proband rather than an unaffected sibling.

Language abnormalities

At age 7, 29% of the cohort (21 schizophrenia, 17 siblings and 2047 controls) were administered a speech, language and hearing examination by a speech pathologist (Bearden et al., 2000). This test assessed expressive and receptive language ability as well as speech mechanism and production. A measure of speech intelligibility was obtained from the child's performance on this test. Speech was coded as abnormal if the child received a rating of 3 or greater on this speech intelligibility summary variable. Subjects were also administered a quantitative measure of language ability: the Auditory–Vocal Association Test, which assesses expressive language ability and word association. This test was administered to 76% of the cohort. Abnormal speech at age 7 years was a highly significant predictor of schizophrenia outcome (Bearden et al., 2000). Both schizophrenia subjects and siblings performed more poorly than controls on the Auditory–Vocal Association Test at age 7 years.

Behavioural deviance

Global social maladjustment was derived from assessments made by a clinical psychologist at 8 months, 4 years and 7 years (Bearden et al., 2000). Behaviour was rated as normal or abnormal. There were no differences between schizophrenia subjects and controls on behavioural measures at the 8 month or 4 year assessments (Bearden et al., 2000). However at age 7, social maladjustment was a significant predictor of schizophrenia. Unaffected siblings did not show any abnormality on this measure. Focal deviant behaviours, such as meaningless laughter or hand motions, excessive crying, echolalia, stereotyped behaviour, speech difficulties, thumb-sucking, nail biting, were examined at 4 and 7 years. Deviant behaviour at both 4 and 7 years of age was a significant predictor of later schizophrenia and unaffected sibling status (Bearden et al., 2000).

The role of obstetric complications

The well-established role of obstetric complications (OCs) in the development of both childhood handicaps and adult schizophrenia (Ch. 5) gives rise to the question of their contribution to childhood developmental precursors of schizophrenia. The relationship between developmental deficits and later schizophrenia in the NCPP was adjusted for the presence of OCs. Unusual movements at age 4 years were associated with hypoxia-related OCs among schizophrenic patients (Rosso et al., 2000). However, apart from this, there were no significant relationships between OCs and motor coordination deficits, cognitive test results, language abnormalities or behavioural deviance and later schizophrenia. The results suggest that childhood developmental impairments in schizophrenia may represent relatively stable indicators of genetic aetiological influences and are not caused solely by obstetric influences.

The Dunedin Multidisciplinary Health and Developmental Survey

Cannon et al. (2002) have investigated childhood developmental precursors to later schizophreniform disorder and other psychiatric outcomes in the Dunedin Multidisciplinary Health and Development Study. This 1-year (1972–73) birth cohort of 1037 children has been assessed six times between ages 3 and 13 years on a range of measures including motor development; language development; IQ; and psychological, social and behavioural adjustment. At age 26, psychiatric status was ascertained using the Diagnostic Interview Schedule and diagnostic criteria for DSM-IV and this yielded two groups with psychotic illnesses (schizophreniform disorder ($n = 36$; 3.7%) and mania ($n = 20$; 2%)) and one group with nonpsychotic illness (anxiety/depression ($n=278$; 28.5%)). All those with the psychiatric outcomes at age 26 assessed in this study (schizophreniform disorder, mania and anxiety/depression) showed significant impairment in emotional and social/interpersonal development throughout childhood. However, neuromotor, language and cognitive developmental impairments in childhood were only seen in schizophreniform disorder. The relationship between developmental impairment and schizophreniform disorder was independent of effects of sex, socioeconomic status, OCs or maternal factors. These results provide evidence for a pandevelopmental childhood impairment that occurs early in childhood and appears to be specific for schizophreniform disorder. In the same sample, Poulton et al. (2000) have shown that self-reported psychotic symptoms at age 11 predicted a very high risk of a schizophreniform disorder at age 26 years (odds ratio 16.4; 95% confidence interval 3.9–67.8). At age 11 years, psychotic symptoms did not predict mania or depression, suggesting specificity of prediction to schizophreniform disorder. Early childhood developmental impairments were related to self-reported psychotic symptoms at age 11 as well as to schizophreniform disorder at age 26, indicating continuity of the syndrome across the lifespan (Cannon et al., 2002).

Summary of information on developmental markers in schizophrenia from birth cohort studies

The following points summarize the data obtained on developmental markers for schizophrenia.

1 There is strong and consistent evidence of delays in attaining developmental milestones, cognitive and language deficits and abnormalities in social functioning in childhood among individuals who go on to develop schizophrenia or schizophreniform disorder in adulthood.

2 These developmental effects can be noted from infancy and persist throughout childhood, adolescence and early adulthood, providing support for life span models of schizophrenia.

3 Early-emerging neuromotor, receptive language and cognitive developmental deficits appear to be specific to schizophrenia (or at least schizophreniform disorder), while childhood social and emotional problems may be a more general marker of risk for a range of psychiatric illnesses in adulthood.

4 The relationship between developmental impairments and later schizophrenia appears to be linear: a dose-response relationship – with little evidence for a 'developmental' subgroup.

5 Both genetic high-risk and birth cohort studies show remarkable confluence of results, suggesting that results of the former are relevant to the majority of those with schizophrenia.

6 These developmental deficits do not appear to be mediated by obstetric or maternal factors and the most likely unifying mechanism is a genetic one (Jones and Murray, 1991).

Conclusions

The developmental epidemiology of schizophrenia points to early causes of this syndrome. Knowledge of the developmental precursors to schizophrenia may suggest the timing and content of preventive interventions (Ch. 20). This is not yet feasible because the predictive power of any models in current cohort studies is so low owing to the combination of modest relative risks, involving fairly common childhood characteristics, and, thankfully, a relatively rare adult outcome. With lifetime odds in the general population of 99% for not getting schizophrenia, it is a much safer proposition to identify who will not get the disorder than it is those who will. Nevertheless, prevention research can be conceptualized as true experiments in altering the course of development, thereby providing insight into the aetiology and pathogenesis of disordered outcomes (Cicchetti and Cannon, 1999).

What is the nature of the relationship?

There is evidence for dose–response relationships between risk for schizophrenia and timing of developmental milestones, cognitive functioning and behaviour. Findings from the birth cohort studies suggest that many children at 100% risk for schizophrenia (i.e. those who later develop schizophrenia) are showing small effects, not scoring as highly as they would have done if they had not been subject to some abnormal developmental mechanism. Thus, the whole population of children at 100% risk is shifted relative to the population at zero risk. So too, precipitating factors such as drugs, for instance cannabis consumption, have a dose–response relationship with later risk of schizophrenia (Andreasson et al., 1987). Once a child suffers a developmental perturbation in any domain, then its micro- or social environment is changed and the development of brain and mind will also be affected. This might further impinge upon the environment, setting up what has been termed a 'self-perpetuating cascade of abnormal development' (Jones et al., 1994). The limitations of currently available statistical methods and study designs do not allow us easily to test such 'cascade' models. Further discussions of developmental models in schizophrenia have been set out in detail by us in previous publications (Jones, 1999; Tarrant and Jones, 1999a,b).

Further investigation of developmental markers in schizophrenia will require extremely large samples that incorporate genetic information and this will pose a major challenge for traditional cohort designs. Statistical methods that can encompass dynamic developmental processes rather than merely cross-sectional processes need further development and application. This will not be an endeavour for epidemiology alone. It is increasingly evident that understanding the complex molecular mechanisms underlying brain growth, connectivity and maturation will be crucial to understanding the aetiology of schizophrenia.

Acknowledgements

Dr Cannon was supported by a Wellcome Trust Advanced Research Training Fellowship. Support was also provided by the Theodore and Vada Stanley Foundation and the EJLB Foundation.

REFERENCES

Ambelas A (1992) Preschizophrenics: adding to the evidence, sharpening the focus. British Journal of Psychiatry 160, 401–404.

American Psychiatric Association (1987) Diagnostic and Statistical Manual III–Revised. Washington, DC: American Psychiatric Press.

American Psychiatric Association (1994) Diagnostic and Statistical Manual of Mental Disorders IV, 4th edn. Washington, DC: American Psychiatric Press.

Amminger GP, Pape S, Rock D et al. (1999) Relationship between childhood behavioral disturbance and later schizophrenia in the New York High Risk Project. American Journal of Psychiatry 156, 525–530.

Andreasson S, Allebeck P, Engstrom A, Rydberg U (1987) Cannabis and Schizophrenia. A longitudinal study of Swedish conscripts. Lancet ii, 1483–1486.

Bearden CE, Rosso IM, Hollister JM, Sanchez LE, Hadley T, Cannon TD (2000) A prospective cohort study of childhood behavioural deviance and language abnormalities as predictors of adult schizophrenia. Schizophrenia Bulletin 26, 395–410.

Bleuler E (1908) Die Prognose der Dementia Praecox – Schizophreniegruppe. Allgemeine Zeitschrift für Psychiatrie 65, 436–464. [Translated in: Cutting J, Shepherd M (1987) The Clinical Roots of the Schizophrenia Concept. Cambridge, UK: Cambridge University Press, pp. 59–74.

Bleuler E (1911) Dementia praecox oder Gruppe der Schizophrenien. Leipzig: Deuticke.

Byrne M, Hodges A, Grant E, Owens DGC, Johnstone EC (1999) Neuropsychological assessment of young people at high genetic risk for developing schizophrenia compared with controls: preliminary findings of the Edinburgh High Risk Study. Psychological Medicine 29, 1161–1173.

Cannon M, Jones P, Huttunen MO et al. (1999) School performance in Finnish children and later development of schizophrenia: A population-based longitudinal study. Archives of General Psychiatry 56, 457–463.

Cannon M, Walsh E, Hollis C et al. (2001) Predictors of later schizophrenia and affective psychosis among attendees at a child psychiatry department. British Journal Psychiatry 178, 420–426.

Cannon M, Caspi A, Moffitt TE et al. (2002) Evidence for early, specific, pan-developmental impairment in schizophreniform disorder: results from a longitudinal birth cohort. Archives of General Psychiatry 59, 449–457.

Cannon TD, Mednick SA (1993) The Schizophrenia High Risk Study in Copenhagen: three decades of progress. Acta Psychiatrica Scandinavica 87(Suppl. 370), 33–47.

Cannon TD, Mednick SA, Parnas J (1990) Antecedents of predominantly negative and predominantly positive symptom schizophrenia in a high-risk population. Archives of General Psychiatry 47, 622–32.

Cannon TD, Bearden CE, Hollister JM, Rosso IM, Sanchez LE, Hadley T (2000) Childhood cognitive functioning in schizophrenia patients and their unaffected siblings: a prospective cohort study. Schizophrenia Bulletin 26, 379–393.

Cicchetti D, Cannon TD (1999) Neurodevelopmental processes in the ontogenesis and epigenesis of psychopathology. Development and Psychopathology 11, 375–393.

Clouston TS (1892) Clinical lectures on mental diseases, 3rd edn. London: Churchill.

Cornblatt BA, Erlenmeyer-Kimling L (1985) Global attentional deviance as a marker of risk for schizophrenia: specificity and predictive validity. Journal of Abnormal Psychology 94, 470–486.

Cornblatt BA, Lenzenweger MF, Dworkin RH, Erlenmeyer-Kimling L (1992) Childhood attentional dysfunctions predict social deficits in unaffected adults at risk for schizophrenia. British Journal of Psychiatry 161, 59–64.

Crow TJ, Done DJ, Sacker A (1995) Childhood precursors of psychosis as clues to its evolutionary origins. European Archives of Psychiatry and Clinical Neuroscience 245, 61–69.

David AS, Malmberg A, Brandt L, Allebeck P, Lewis G (1997) IQ and risk for schizophrenia: a population-based cohort study. Psychological Medicine 27, 1311–1323.

Davidson M, Reichenberg A, Rabinowotz J, Weiser M, Kaplan Z, Mordehai M (1999) Behavioural and intellectual markers for schizophrenia in apparently healthy male adolescents. American Journal of Psychiatry 156, 1328–1335.

Done J, Johnstone EC, Frith CD, Golding J, Shepard PM, Crow TJ (1991) Complications of pregnancy and delivery in relation to psychosis in adult life: data from the British Perinatal Mortality Survey. British Medical Journal 302, 1576–1580.

Done DJ, Crow TJ, Johnstone EC, Sacker A (1994) Childhood antecedents of schizophrenia and affective illness: social adjustment at ages 7 and 11. British Medical Journal 309, 699–703.

Erlenmeyer-Kimling L, Cornblatt BA (1992) A summary of attentional findings in the New York High Risk Project. Journal of Psychiatric Research 26, 405–426.

Erlenmeyer-Kimling L, Squires-Wheeler E, Adamo UH, Bassett AS, Cornblatt BA, Kesterbaum CJ (1995) The New York High Risk Project, psychoses and cluster A personality disorders in offspring of schizophrenic parents at 23 years of follow-up. Archives of General Psychiatry 52, 857–865.

Erlenmeyer-Kimling L, Adamo UH, Rock D, Roberts SA, Bassett AS, Squires-Wheeler E (1997) The New York High Risk Project: prevalence and comorbidity of axis I disorders in offspring of schizophrenic parents at 25 year follow-up. Archives of General Psychiatry 54, 1096–1102.

Erlenmeyer-Kimling L, Rock D, Roberts SA et al. (2000) Attention, memory and motor skills as childhood predictors of schizophrenia-related psychoses: the New York High Risk Project. American Journal of Psychiatry 157, 1416–1422.

Fish B (1960) Involvement of the central nervous system in infants with schizophrenia. Archives of Neurology 2, 115–121.

Fish B (1987) Infant predictors of the longitudinal course of schizophrenic development. Schizophrenia Bulletin 13, 395–409.

Fish B, Hagin R (1973) Visual-motor disorders in infants at risk for schizophrenia. Archives of General Psychiatry 28, 900–904.

Fish B, Marcus J, Hans SL, Auerbach JG, Perdue S (1992) Infants at risk for schizophrenia: sequelae of a genetic neurointegrative defect. A review and replication analysis of pandysmaturation in the Jerusalem Infant Development Study. Archives of General Psychiatry 49, 221–235.

Hans SL, Marcus J, Henson L, Auerbach JG, Mirsky AF (1992) Interpersonal behaviour of children at risk for schizophrenia. Psychiatry 55, 314–335.

Hans SL, Marcus J, Nuechterlain KH, Asarnow RF, Styr B, Auerbach JG (1999) Neurobehavioural deficits at adolescence in children at risk for schizophrenia: the Jerusalem Infant Development Study. Archives of General Psychiatry 56, 741–748.

Hans SL, Auerbach JG, Asarnow JR, Styr B, Marcus J (2000) Social adjustment of adolescents at risk for schizophrenia: the Jerusalem Infant Development Study. Journal of the American Academy of Child and Adolescent Psychiatry 39, 1407–1414.

Hartman E, Milofsky E, Vaillant G (1984) Vulnerability to schizophrenia: prediction of adult schizophrenia using childhood information. Archives of General Psychiatry 41, 1050–1056.

Hodges A, Byrne M, Grant E, Johnstone E (1999) People at risk of schizophrenia: sample characteristics of the first 100 cases in the Edinburgh High-Risk Study. British Journal of Psychiatry 174, 547–553.

Hollis C (1995) Child and adolescent (juvenile onset) schizophrenia. A case control study of premorbid developmental impairments. British Journal of Psychiatry 166, 489–495.

Isohanni I, Jarvelin MR, Nierminen P et al. (1998) School performance as a predictor of psychiatric hospitalisation in adult life. A 28 year follow-up in the Northern Finland 1966 Birth Cohort. Psychological Medicine 28, 967–974.

Isohanni I, Jarvelin MR, Jones P, Jokelainen J, Isohanni M (1999) Can excellent school performance be a precursor of schizophrenia? A 28-year follow-up in the Northern Finland 1966 birth cohort. Acta Psychiatrica Scandinavica 100, 17–26.

Isohanni M, Jones P, Kemppainen L et al. (2000) Childhood and adolescent precursors of schizophrenia in the Northern Finland 1966 Birth Cohort – a descriptive life-span model. European Archives of Psychiatry and Clinical Neuroscience 250, 311–319.

Isohanni M, Jones PB, Moilanen K, Rantakallio P, Veijola J (2001) Early developmental milestones in adult schizophrenia and other psychoses. A 31 year follow-up of the North Finland 1966 Birth Cohort. Schizophrenia Research, 52, 1–19.

Johnstone E, Abukmeil SS, Byrne M et al. (2000) Edinburgh high-risk study – findings after four years: demographic, attainment and psychopathological issues. Schizophrenia Research 46, 1–15.

Jones PB (1999) Longitudinal approaches to the search for the causes of schizophrenia: past, present and future. In: Search for the Causes of Schizophrenia, Vol. IV Balance of the Century, Gattaz WF, Häfner H, eds. Darmstadt: Steinkopf and Berlin: Springer.

Jones PB, Done DJ (1997) From birth to onset: a developmental perspective of schizophrenia in two national birth cohorts. In: Neurodevelopment and Adult Psychopathology, Keshavan MS, Murray RM, eds. Cambridge, UK: Cambridge University Press, pp. 119–136.

Jones PB, Murray RM (1991) The genetics of schizophrenia is the genetics of neurodevelopment. British Journal of Psychiatry 158, 615–623.

Jones P, Rodgers B, Murray R, Marmot M (1994) Child developmental risk factors for adult schizophrenia in the British 1946 birth cohort. Lancet 344, 1398–1402.

Kraepelin E (1896) Dementia praecox. In: Psychiatrie, 5th edn. Leipzig: Barth, pp. 426–441. Translated in Cutting J, Shepherd M (1987) The Clinical Roots of the Schizophrenia Concept. Cambridge, UK: Cambridge University Press, pp. 13–24.

Malmberg A, Lewis G, David A, Allebeck P (1998) Premorbid adjustment and personality in people with schizophrenia. British Journal of Psychiatry 172, 08–313.

Marcus J, Auerbach J, Wilkinson L, Burack CM (1981) Infants at risk for schizophrenia: the Jerusalem Infant Development Study. Archives of General Psychiatry 38, 703–713.

Marcus J, Hans SL, Lewow E (1985) Neurological findings in high risk children: childhood assessment and 5 year follow-up. Schizophrenia Bulletin 11, 85–100.

Marcus J, Hans SL, Auerbach JG, Auerbach AG (1993) Children at risk for schizophrenia. The Jerusalem Infant Development Study II: neurobehavioural deficits at school age. Archives of General Psychiatry 50, 797–809.

Marenco S, Weinberger DR (2000) The neurodevelopmental hypothesis of schizophrenia: following a trail of evidence from cradle to grave. Development and Psychopathology 12, 501–527.

Mednick SA, Mura E, Schulsinger F, Mednick B (1971) Perinatal conditions and infant development in children with schizophrenic parents. Social Biology 18, S103–S113.

Mednick SA, Parnas J, Schulsinger F (1987) The Copenhagen High Risk project. 1962–1986. Schizophrenia Bulletin 13, 485–495.

Meehl PE (1962) Schizotaxia, schizotypy, schizophrenia. American Psychologist 17, 827–838

Meehl PE (1989) Schizotaxia revisited. Archives of General Psychiatry 46, 935–944.

Mirsky AF, Silberman EK, Latz A, Nagler S (1985) Adult outcomes of high-risk children: differential effects of town and kibbutz rearing. Schizophrenia Bulletin 11, 150–154.

Mirsky AF, Kugelmass S, Ingraham LJ, Frenkel E, Nathan M (1995) Overview and summary: twenty-five year follow-up of high-risk children. Schizophrenia Bulletin 21, 227–239.

Murray RM (1994) Neurodevelopmental schizophrenia: the rediscovery of dementia praecox. British Journal of Psychiatry 165, 6–12.

Murray RM, Jones P (1995) Schizophrenia: disease or syndrome? Discussion. In: Search for the Causes of Schizophrenia, Vol. III, Gattaz WF, Häfner H, eds. Berlin: Springer-Verlag, pp. 186–192.

Murray RM, Lewis SW (1987) Is schizophrenia a neurodevelopmental disorder? British Medical Journal 295, 681–682.

Olin SS, Mednick SA (1996) Risk factors of psychosis: identifying vulnerable populations premorbidly. Schizophrenia Bulletin 22, 223–240.

Ott SL, Spinelli S, Rock D, Roberts S, Amminger GP, Erlenmeyer-Kimling L (1998) The New York High Risk Project: social and general intelligence in children at risk for schizophrenia. Schizophrenia Research 31, 1–11.

Poulton R, Caspi A, Moffitt TE, Cannon M, Murray RM. Harrington H-L (2000) Children's self-reported psychotic symptoms and adult schizophreniform disorder: a 15-year longitudinal study. Archives of General Psychiatry 57, 1053–1058.

Robins LN (1966) Deviant Children Grown Up. A Sociological and Psychiatric Study of Sociopathic Personality. Baltimore, MD: Williams & Wilkins.

Rosso IM, Bearden CE, Hollister JM et al. (2000) Childhood neuromotor dysfunction in schizophrenia patients and their unaffected siblings: a prospective cohort study. Schizophrenia Bulletin 26, 367–378.

Rutter M (1984) Psychopathology and development: 1. Childhood antecedents of adult psychiatric disorder. Australian and New Zealand Journal of Psychiatry 18, 225–234.

Susser E (1999) Life course cohort studies in schizophrenia. Psychiatric Annals 29, 161–165.

Tarrant CJ, Jones PB (1999a) Precursors to schizophrenia: do biological markers for schizophrenia have specificity? Canadian Journal of Psychiatry 44, 335–349.

Tarrant CJ, Jones PB (1999b) The specificity of developmental precursors of schizophrenia and affective disorders. Psychiatric Annals 29, 137–144.

Tienari P (1991) Interaction between genetic vulnerability and family environment: the Finnish adoptive family study of schizophrenia. Acta Psychiatrica Scandinavica 84, 460–465.

Tienari P, Sorri A, Lahti I et al. (1987) Genetic and psychosocial factors in schizophrenia: the Finnish Adoptive Family Study. Schizophrenia Bulletin 13, 477–484.

van Os J, Jones PB, Lewis G, Wadsworth M, Murray R (1997) Developmental precursors of affective illness in a general population birth cohort. Archives of General Psychiatry 54, 625–631.

Wadsworth MEJ (1991) The Imprint of Time. Childhood history and adult life. Oxford: Clarendon Press.

Wahlberg K-E, Wynne LC, Oja H et al. (1997) Gene-environment interaction in vulnerability to schizophrenia: findings from the Finnish Adoptive Family Study of Schizophrenia. American Journal of Psychiatry 154, 355–362.

Walker E, Lewine RJ (1990) Prediction of adult-onset schizophrenia from childhood home movies of the patients. American Journal of Psychiatry 147, 1052–1056.

Walker EF, Grimes KE, Davis DM, Smith AJ (1993) Childhood precursors of schizophrenia: facial expressions of emotion. American Journal of Psychiatry 150, 1654–1660.

Walker E, Savoie T, Davis D (1994) Neuromotor precursors of schizophrenia. Schizophrenia Bulletin 20, 441–451.

Watt NF (1978) Patterns of childhood social development in adult schizophrenics. Archives of General Psychiatry 35, 160–165.

Weinberger DR (1987) Implications of normal brain development for the pathogenesis of schizophrenia. Archives of General Psychiatry 44, 660–669.

7

Prodrome, onset and early course of schizophrenia

Heinz Häfner

Central Institute of Mental Health, Mannheim, Germany

The first treatment contact of persons falling ill with schizophrenia is usually preceded by incipient psychosis with a mean duration of 1 year or more and a prodromal phase of several years (Table 7.1). The length of these early phases of illness is a predictor of an unfavourable short- and long-term illness course (Crow et al., 1986; Loebel et al., 1992; McGorry et al., 1996; Wyatt et al., 1998). Hope exists that early detection and early intervention will enable us to prevent, delay or alleviate psychosis onset (McGorry et al., 1996). However, the prognostic significance of untreated psychosis or disorder is confounded by disease-related prognostic indicators: an insidious versus an acute type of onset (Verdoux et al., 2001).

The prodrome

Historical context

As early as 1861, Wilhelm Griesinger described a melancholic prodromal phase of psychotic illness. Kraepelin (1893) observed a gradual deterioration of mental functioning, disturbances of attention and daydreaming before the emergence of psychotic symptoms and 'advanced dementia' in dementia praecox. According to Mayer-Gross (1932), difficulties with thinking and concentration as well as loss of acitivity marked an insidious onset and persisted without other symptoms of the illness for long periods of time before the first psychotic symptoms appear. Eugen Bleuler (1911) called the prephase characterized by irritability, introversion, eccentricity and changes of mood 'latent schizophrenia'. He believed that the illness could come to a halt at any stage of this early development and turn into a neurosis.

Harry Stack Sullivan (1927) supplemented Eugen Bleuler's psychodevelopmental approach by a psychodynamic model. He explained the hysteric, neuraesthenic and obsessive-compulsive symptoms, which often preceded the onset of psychosis for lengthy periods of time, as dysfunctional ways of coping with more profound

Table 7.1. Duration of the prodromal and psychotic prephase until first contact according to nine selected studies with different diagnostic definitions and methods of assessment

Author	Number	Duration from first sign (years)	Duration from first psychotic symptom (years)
Gross (1969) Germany	290	3.5	
Lindelius (1979) Sweden	237		4.4[a]
Huber et al. (1979) Germany	502	3.3	
Loebel et al. (1992) USA	70	2.9	1.0
Beiser et al. (1993) Canada	70	2.1	1.0
McGorry et al. (1996) Australia	200	2.1	1.4
Lewine (1980) USA	97		1.9
Häfner et al. (1995) Germany	232	5.0[b]	1.1
Johannessen et al. (1999) Norway	43		2.2

Notes:

[a] Age at first psychotic symptoms or marked personality changes indicative of mental illness.

[b] Prodromal phase until appearance of first psychotic symptom only.

Source: modified from Häfner et al. (1998a).

disturbances in the prodromal illness phase. But he did not succeed in developing, on this basis, reliable prognostic indicators and effective ways of early intervention.

Cameron (1938) was the first to assess the mean duration of untreated psychosis: 32.4% of the patients experienced their first psychotic symptoms within 6 months of first admission for schizophrenia, 17.5% within 6 months to 2 years and 48.1% 2 years or more before first admission for schizophrenia. He described a prodromal phase characterized by social withdrawal, reduced work performance, affective flattening and bizarre beliefs as well as a continuous transition to ideas and delusions of persecution. After Cameron, the research efforts into the early course of schizophrenia were interrupted for almost half a century.

Assessment of prodromal signs and symptoms

First attempts at defining and systematically assessing prodromal signs were made in the context of a targeted antipsychotic therapy of relapses of schizophrenia. An advantage of this procedure was that its prognostic efficiency could be prospectively validated (Carpenter and Heinrichs, 1983; Birchwood et al., 1989; Cutting and Dunne, 1989; Hirsch and Jolley, 1989; Gaebel et al., 1993). The results, however, were inconsistent, mainly because of (i) differences in the type of prodromal sign included and in the definitions of a psychotic relapse and (ii) insufficient monitoring of their development over time. Nevertheless, various items from the early scales for the identification of early signs and symptoms of psychotic relapses have been integrated in subsequent instruments for the assessment of onset and early course (Häfner et al., 1992; Maurer and Häfner, 1995; Yung et al., 1998).

The domains in which changes in incipient psychosis can basically occur are:
- biological (e.g. increase in morphological brain anomalies, dopamine activity, neurophysiological (electroencephalographic changes, changes in evoked potentials))
- neuropsychological (attention, memory)
- observed behaviour
- self-experienced signs or symptoms.

The difficulty in generating biological indicators of a psychosis onset lies in the fact that current knowledge of the disease process is still limited and that such changes have a continuous nature. Most of the biological findings associated with psychosis are trait factors that appear to be indicators of lifetime risk and may not be causally involved in onset. For example, studying the 1966 North Finland birth cohort until age 32 years, Isohanni et al. (1999) found that a greater number of deviant biological and behavioural abnormalities in childhood and adolescence did not correlate with an earlier illness onset. Cornblatt et al. (1998) showed in adolescents and young adults in their first episodes of schizophrenia that biological abnormalities, attention and social skills deficits, cognitive dysfunction and abnormal eye tracking preceding the clinical symptoms did not correlate significantly with the patient's clinical state. These 'behavioural markers', Cornblatt and Keilp (1994) demonstrated, 'remained constant across development' (Cornblatt et al., 1998). One likely explanation is that they are expressions of early premorbid neurodevelopmental disorders.

For these reasons, schizophrenia and psychosis continue to be defined exclusively in clinical terms. Psychosis onset is currently depictable only at the level of self-experienced symptoms and observable behaviour. Nonetheless, the monitoring of the neuropsychological and neurophysiological indicators of the disorder from the earliest possible timepoint on is a highly promising approach to modelling the early course of schizophrenia. Efforts to this end are underway at various sites (McGorry et al., 1996; Klosterkötter et al., 1997; Bilder; 1998; Cornblatt et al., 1998; Salokangas et al., 1999). The question whether most of the prodromal symptoms emerge additionally or merely aggravate persisting developmental impairments and anomalies can only be answered in this way.

The instruments for the assessment of symptoms of schizophrenia based on the DSM-IV (American Psychiatric Association, 1994) or ICD-10 (World Health Organization, 1992) almost invariably fail to provide a comprehensive list of the prodromal signs. Using the nine prodromal syndromes (social isolation or withdrawal; marked impairment in role functioning; markedly peculiar behaviour; marked impairment in personal hygiene; blunted, flat or inappropriate affect; digressive, vague or metamorphic speech; odd or bizarre ideation; unusual perceptional experiences; marked lack of initiative, interest or energy (McGorry et al., 1995) listed in the DSM-III-R (American Psychiatric Association, 1987) that are artificially generated on the basis of the full-blown disorder, Jackson et al. (1995) analysed their comparative frequencies and diagnostic efficiencies in a sample of 313 first episodes of functional psychosis. Individual prodromal symptoms were relatively poor at distinguishing between diagnoses and were not pathognomonic of schizophrenia. McGorry et al. (1995) studied the prevalence of these nine prodromal symptoms prospectively in a large representative sample ($n=2525$) of Australian school children at mean ages of 16, 14 and 12 years. The prevalences ranged from 8 to 51%, indicating a high frequency in the healthy population and a low specificity for schizophrenia.

On the basis of several retrospective long-term longitudinal studies, Huber and his colleagues generated a list of 'basic disturbances' (Huber, 1966, 1997; Gross, 1969, 1989; Huber et al., 1979, 1980; Klosterkötter et al., 1994, 1996, 1997), which as self-experienced phenomena are close to the negative syndrome, precede the first psychotic epsiode and follow it as residual symptoms. In a follow-up of 502 first hospital admissions diagnosed according to the criteria of Bleuler and Schneider for schizophrenia, with an average duration of 22.4 years, the authors found a prodromal phase of 3 months to 3 years (Huber et al., 1979) in only 36.6%, whereas in another 15% intermittent prodromal symptoms had been present (Gross, 1969). The comparatively small number presumably resulted from the extremely long period of retrospection. The most frequent prodromal and residual symptom was cenaesthesia, a construct of the authors encompassing changes in bodily perception such as congestion in the head, tremor, oppression on the chest, dizziness, weakness, palpitations, etc.

On the basis of their findings, Huber and Gross constructed the Bonn Scale for the Assessment of Basic Symptoms (BSABS: Gross et al., 1987). It includes subscales on dynamic deficiency; cognitive disturbances of thought, perception and motor action; cenaesthesias; and disturbances of the central autonomic nervous system (sleep disturbances etc.). Each single item is rated by its closeness to positive symptoms in three degrees: (i) characteristic, i.e. the phenomenon observed is sufficiently similar to certain full-blown psychotic symptoms; (ii) accompanied by a sense of strangeness, splitting or restlessness; and (iii) associated with a delusional explanation. The BSABS is useful in depicting transition from attenuated positive symptoms to a full-blown psychosis (Klosterkötter et al., 2001). However, because its terminology differs from that in the DSM-III, DSM-IV, ICD-9 and ICD-10, comparisons with other scales are difficult.

In contrast to Chapman and his colleagues (McGhie and Chapman, 1961; Chapman, 1966; Chapman and Chapman, 1980, 1987), who produced their list of early symptoms studying first-episode cases of schizophrenia retrospectively, Huber and colleagues (Gross et al., 1987) constructed theirs on the basis of post-psychotic residual symptoms. Nevertheless, several of the BSABS items have proven useful and have been included in the instrument for a Comprehensive Assessment of At Risk Mental States (CAARMS; Yung and McGorry, 1996; Yung et al., 1998) and the semi-structured interview IRAOS (Häfner et al., 1992). Yung and McGorry (1996) listed the nine most important prodromal symptoms from previous publications: reduced attention and concentration; reduced energy, motivation and anergia; depressive mood; sleeping disturbances; anxiety; social withdrawal; mistrust; social dysfunctioning; and irritability.

Phase models of early illness course

Conrad (1958) studied 107 young German soldiers returning from the frontline because of a psychosis. Proceeding from gestalt psychology, he distinguished four phases of developing schizophrenia.

1 *Trema*, characterized by depression, anxiety, tension, irritability and mysterious experiences, and likened by Conrad to stagefright.

2 The transition from *trema* to *apopheny*, corresponding to the transition from the nonspecific prodromal phase to incipient psychosis, which was presumed to be marked by predelusional mood. Conrad referred to delusional mood (Jaspers calls it *Wahnstimmung*) as 'the most important notion of classic psychiatry', denoting the peculiarly threatening, but vague, experience of changed meaning that the person affected cannot explain. Although not showing clear delusional content, it is frequently reported to precede full-blown delusional phenomena.

3 *Anastrophae*, in which these new experiences become attributed to external causes: delusions and hallucinations. Reality control and insight into illness are lost.

4 The *apocalypse* phase, corresponding to full-blown psychosis. This refers to a complete loss of structure in perception, experience and thought.

Following Conrad, Docherty et al. (1978) proposed six stages of progressive decompensation, which they believed to explain how both first episodes and relapses evolve: (i) overextension, (ii) restricted consciousness, (iii) disinhibition, (iv) psychotic disorganization, (v) psychotic resolution and (vi) equilibrium. Their aim was to use this model for preventive intervention. Hambrecht and Häfner (1993) tested Conrad's phase model on IRAOS data from the ABC (Age, Beginning and Course) Schizophrenia Study. In 76% of the cases, *trema* preceded *apopheny* (i.e. a prodromal phase led to an incipient psychosis). Significant transitions to the other phases could not be proven. Both Conrad and Docherty and colleagues proceeded from the assumption that a majority of the cases of incipient schizophrenia run through these presumed regular sequences of phases, but this has not yet been shown to be the case.

Prospective validation of prodromal and attenuated psychotic symptoms

The predictive efficiency of prodromal symptoms must be validated prospectively against the actual psychosis onset. A shortened version of the BSABS has been subjected to a prospective validation in a high-risk group (Klosterkötter et al., 2001): 160 patients up to age 50 with various diagnoses in need of psychiatric treatment who were referred to five German psychiatric outpatient university departments for diagnostic clarification. The patients were suspected of suffering from schizophrenia but had not yet developed psychotic symptoms. They were interviewed using the BSABS and Present State Examination (PSE) 9 on admission and re-examined 9.5 years later on average. At the initial assessment, 110 patients reported prodromal symptoms.

Almost 50% of the total sample and 70% of the patients with 'prodromal' symptoms subsequently developed a schizophrenic episode fulfilling the DSM-IV criteria: women an average of 4.3 years later and men 6.7 years later. The item list as a whole showed an extremely high predictive power with a sensitivity of 0.98, a negative predictive power of 0.98, but a clearly lower specificity (0.59) and positive predictive power (0.70). In this study, the single symptoms that were most predictive of an early diagnosis of schizophrenia were not true prodromes but attenuated positive symptoms (Table 7.2). The state approach (Yung et al., 1998) used in this study reflects two fundamental issues. First, if the aim is to predict an imminent psychosis onset and not only the lifetime risk, a distinction must be made between persistent trait markers and truly prodromal symptoms (Cornblatt et al., 1998). Second, the extremely high psychosis risk in this group leads to a high predictive efficiency of the BSABS symptoms, but the results are not valid for the general population or even clinical groups because the inclusion criteria defining the risk are not clear.

A recent study by Yung et al. (1998) of individuals with an imminent psychosis onset was the first to use an indicator of change in patients in need of early intervention. The following trait factors were used: age of risk 16 to 30 years, and schizotypal personality or a first-degree relative with a history of psychotic disorder. Attenuated psychotic symptoms and BLIPS (Brief Limited Intermittent Psychotic Symptoms; Yung et al., 1998) were selected as state indicators, and the criterion 'any change in mental state and functioning, which results in a loss of 30 points or more in the Global Assessment of Functioning (GAF) scale for at least one month' was selected as an indicator of the processlike accumulation of the disorder. Of 119 individuals referred for treatment to the PACE clinic in Melbourne, 20 fulfilled the criteria and were followed up at monthly intervals. Eight (40%) of these patients

Table 7.2. Diagnostic efficiency indices of prodromal symptoms that occur at least in a quarter of patients who later developed schizophrenia (sensitivity >0.25) and have a good positive predictive power (>0.70)

Item No.	Prodromal symptoms	Sensitivity	Specificity	Positive predictive power	Negative predictive power	False-positive predictions (%)	False-negative predictions (%)
C.1.1	Interference of thought	.42	.91	.83	.62	4.4	28.8
C.1.2	Obsessional perseveration of thought	.32	.88	.71	.57	6.3	33.8
C.1.3	Pressure of thought	.38	.96	.91	.62	1.9	30.6
C.1.4	Subjective blocking of thought	.34	.86	.71	.57	6.9	32.5
C.1.6	Disturbances of receptive speech	.39	.91	.82	.61	4.4	30.0
C.1.15	Disturbances of discrimination between ideas and perception, phantasy and memory contents	.27	.95	.84	.57	2.5	36.3
C.1.17	Tendency to delusion of reference	.39	.89	.78	.60	5.6	30.0
C.2.11	Derealisation	.28	.90	.73	.56	5.0	35.6
	Optic perception disturbances	.46	.85	.75	.62	7.5	26.9
	Acoustic perception disturbances	.29	.89	.72	.53	5.6	35.0

Source: Klosterkötter et al. (2001).

developed a frank psychosis according to BPRS (brief psychiatric rating scale) criteria within 6 months, five patients as early as the first month. The conclusion from this study (Yung et al., 1998) is that, at least in this particular sample, attenuated and transient psychotic symptoms, together with an indicator of a rapid deterioration in the patient's mental state, are powerful predictors of an imminent psychosis onset at least in individuals with a high lifetime risk.

Onset and early course

Defining onset and early course

The end of the early illness phase or prodrome is usually defined by first treatment contact or first admission. But this event is also determined by the patient's help-seeking behaviour and the availability of care. A suitable illness-related event to mark the end of the early illness phase is the climax of the first psychotic episode, operationalized as the maximum level of positive symptoms (Häfner et al., 1995). Illness onset is more difficult to define. One factor is the diagnostic criteria used. For example, the C criterion of a DSM-III-R or DSM-IV diagnosis of schizophrenia (i.e. persistence of at least 6 months of cognitive and social impairment) increases the proportion of insidious onsets and excludes acute-onset psychoses. For this reason, no course-related criteria should be used in assessing onset.

The best way of assessing the onset of schizophrenia would be a prospective design, for example the study of how developmental delays and cognitive and social impairments (Done et al., 1994a,b; Jones and Done, 1997; van Os et al., 1997; Isohanni et al., 1999) are transformed into a prodromal phase of schizophrenia (Nuechterlein et al., 1992; Dohrenwend et al., 1995). A prospective population study is not practical because of the low incidence rate and the rather poor predictive power of developmental antecedents (Jones, 1999). In addition, the prodromal phase cannot be assessed prospectively because schizophrenia starts with nonspecific signs in about 75% of all schizophrenics. What can be investigated by a prospective design, until we are able to diagnose the disorder earlier, are risk factors for psychosis, without drawing a precise distinction between premorbid traits and mutable prodromal signs.

A Swedish conscript study (Malmberg et al., 1998) among 50 087 young men aged 18 to 20 years showed that the items 'having fewer than two friends', 'preference for socializing in small groups', 'feeling more sensitive than others' and 'not having a steady girlfriend' were associated with a high relative risk (odds ratio 30.7) for developing schizophrenia in a period of risk of 15 years. But in the total sample, a positive response to all four items predicted psychosis only in 3%, because of the high prevalence of these features in the general population. A similar finding has been reported from an Israeli conscript study (Davidson et al., 1999). Davidson et al.

(1999) and Rabinowitz et al. (2000) conducted a similar controlled study of Israeli male conscripts aged 16–17 years born during a 7-year period. Using the National Hospitalization Psychiatric Case Register, the authors identified 692 individuals who had been hospitalized for schizophrenia for the first time in a 9-year period following the initial testing. The results for these individuals, who were compared with the entire conscript population and matched controls, pointed in the same direction as the results of the Swedish study. With effect sizes ranging from 0.40 to 0.58, the young males diagnosed with schizophrenia fared significantly worse than the controls in all tests of cognitive functioning. The same was true for behavioural functioning although, as in the Swedish study, it was poor social functioning, with an effect size difference of 1.25, that turned out to be the main indicator of risk.

Rabinowitz et al. (2000) also tested the effect of time that elapsed from initial testing to first admission and found that the shorter this period was the more the probands differed from controls on IQ test scores (Raven's Progressive Matrices) and on social functioning in particular. The distribution of the differences on these two dimensions of assessment showed a significant linear trend. A significant relationship between these two measures and age at illness onset as an indicator of a greater severity of illness in persons with a lower age at illness onset did not emerge. It is, therefore, reasonable to assume that the more pronounced cognitive and social impairment in the group with a short latency between illness onset and first admission was accounted for by a higher proportion of individuals in advanced stages of the prodromal phase or early illness.

Selecting probands at an increased lifetime risk for schizophrenia (e.g. persons with an increased familial load, severe perinatal brain damage (Isohanni et al., 1999) or mental disorder in need of treatment and suspected to be schizophrenic (Klosterkötter et al., 2001)) improves the chances of finding prodromal cases and making correct predictions. But by enriching the psychosis risk in this way, the pool of persons at risk for schizophrenia in the general population is reduced to a small high-risk group, at the cost of the external validity of the results. This might be a correct design for intervention studies because in this way it might be possible to increase the proportion of individuals who will benefit from treatment (Yung et al., 1998). However, the only way to obtain generally valid results at present is to study onset and early course retrospectively in large, population-based samples of first episodes of schizophrenia from the entire age range of illness.

Assessment of onset

Caution is needed to reduce psychosis-related memory distortion and recall deficits. At present, the first episode is the closest we can get to onset. Patients must be interviewed immediately after the psychosis has remitted sufficiently. The time matrix must be structured by anchor events, such as birthdays or holidays spent abroad (Häfner et al., 1992). No ideal solution has yet been found for discriminating between nonspecific initial symptoms and premorbid antecedents of schizophrenia or symptoms of other causes. In the ABC Schizophrenia Study, a hierarchical model reflecting the different degrees of specificity of three symptom categories was used, as initial signs of the disorder qualified only phenomena that were new at a certain point in time. Nonspecific symptoms were required to have persisted continuously from that time on, and negative symptoms were required to have been present either continuously or recurrently up until the psychosis. Positive symptoms were counted in all instances, even if transient.

Systematic retrospective analysis of onset and early course: the ABC Study

The ABC Schizophrenia Study is a population-based sample of 232 first-illness episodes (representing 84% of first treatment episodes). The Instrument for the Retrospective Assessment of the Onset of Schizophrenia (IRAOS), a semi-structured interview (Häfner et al., 1992, 1999), was designed for the assessment of individual social development, premorbid adjustment, onset of prodromal signs and symptoms, functional impairment and social disability. The test construction has been described elsewhere (Häfner et al., 1992). In addition to the closed questions on prodromal items, interviewees are also asked open-ended questions about the prodrome and the time of emergence of the disorder. The IRAOS was used by psychiatrists and psychologists to interview the patients and their significant others and in a modified version to evaluate other sources of information such as medical case records. The information obtained was arranged in a time matrix with the help of individual anchor events.

Perception of prodromal signs and symptoms by others is an important precondition for an early recognition of the illness. Hambrecht and Häfner (1997) studied the ABC first-episode sample of patients with schizophrenia and the family members who were in sufficiently close contact with the patients during the period of onset and early illness. Both the patients, in their first psychotic episodes, and family members went through an IRAOS interview simultaneously. The authors found a surprisingly high degree of agreement between the estimates of the time of illness onset between the patients and their family members. Single phenomenon positive symptoms, such as delusions and hallucinations, were frequently observed by the significant others with, on average, only 1 month's delay. Nonspecific and negative symptoms, such as depression or loss of energy, were frequently noticed by the family members with a delay of 6 months and noted in psychiatric case records or school records with a delay of 15 months. The less-specific symptoms were in many cases misinterpreted. Abnormal behaviour, too, was seen differently: attempted suicide was mostly regarded as an immediate sign of illness and dated almost correctly, but social withdrawal and passivity were often for a long time considered as part of normal development by significant others.

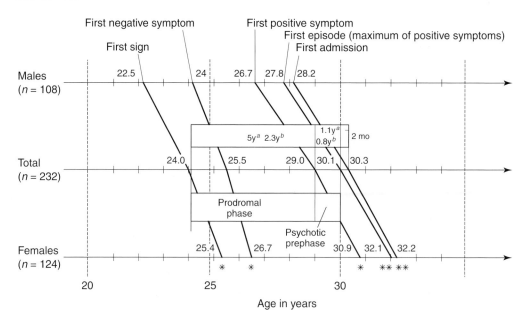

Fig. 7.1.   Mean age values at five definitions of onset until first admission for patients with first-episode schizophrenia ($n=232$) of broad definition. [a]Mean; [b]median; *$p=0.05$; **$p=0.01$.

Stages of illness onset

Figure 7.1 depicts mean age for men and women at the appearance of the first illness sign, no matter what type, and of further milestones of early illness course. The prodromal phase, from onset to first psychotic symptom, had a mean duration of 5 years. The psychotic prephase, from the first positive symptom to the maximum of positive symptoms, had a duration of 1.1 years. First admission took place some 2 months later, mostly precipitated by the psychosis. Survival analysis with first admission as the target event revealed a distribution of the durations of early illness course, which was markedly skewed to the left (Fig. 7.2). Of those with broadly defined schizophrenia, 33% took less than 1 year to develop. Only 18% had an acute type of onset of 4 weeks or less and 68% had a chronic type of onset of 1 year or more. Only 6.5% started with positive symptoms: 20.5% presented both positive and negative symptoms within the same month; and 73% presented negative or nonspecific symptoms, thus experiencing a prodromal phase. The accumulation of the three clinical symptom categories in the early course is illustrated in Figure 7.3, based on the mean number of symptoms per year and, in the last year before first admission, per month. Nonspecific and negative symptoms started to increase early; positive symptoms appeared fairly late in the early course, showing an exponential increase until the climax of

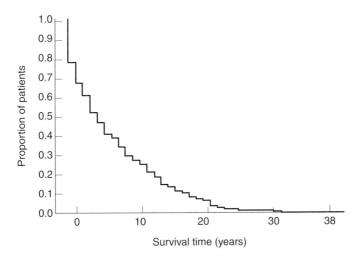

Fig. 7.2.   Survival function for the duration of the early course (first admission sample; $n = 267$).
Survival time was mean 6.29 years (SD $\pm$ 6.84 years): median 4.38 years and maximum
37.92 years.

the first psychotic episode. In the psychotic episode, all three symptom categories
accumulated rapidly and reached a maximum, followed by an almost parallel
decrease.

Gender differences

In Figure 7.1, a significant gender difference is visible in the mean age at illness
onset, as defined by the milestones of early course. The earlier onset in men has
been widely reported (for review see Angermeyer and Kühn, 1988; Lewine, 1988).
This difference is not an artefact from differences in diagnostic definitions or
gender differences in the early course (Loranger, 1984; Castle et al., 1998; Häfner et
al., 1998b; Seeman and Lang, 1990). The analysis of pooled data from 10 centres of
the World Health Organization (WHO) DOSMED (Determinants of Outcome of
Severe Mental Disorders) study (Hambrecht et al., 1992) showed a mean age difference of 3.4 years and, hence, some consistency across countries and cultures. In
familial cases, this sex difference appears to be absent (DeLisi et al., 1994; Albus and
Maier, 1995) almost exclusively because of women's reduced age at onset. Könnecke
et al. (2000) found in a replication study that pre- and perinatal complications also
significantly reduced the gender difference in age at onset but the effect was weaker
than that seen for familial load. The mean age at onset for women with neither of
these risk factors was several years later than that of men with or without these risk
factors or that of women with these risk factors.

The distributions of illness onset according to three definitions until age 59 years

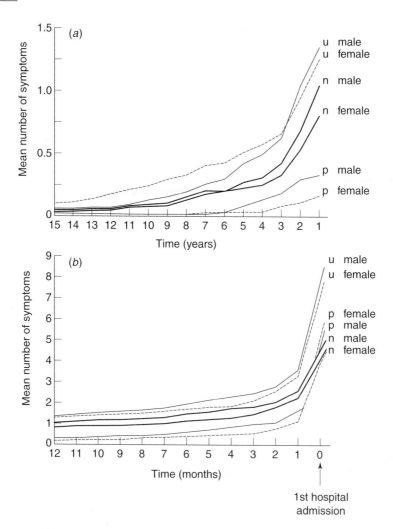

Fig. 7.3.   Cumulative numbers of positive (p), negative (n) and unspecific (u) symptoms of onset until first hospital admission for schizophrenia (108 males; 124 females. (*a*) Mean number of symptoms per year; (*b*) mean number of symptoms per month in the year preceding first hospital admission. (From Häfner et al., 1995.)

showed steep increases for both men and women in adolescence and young adulthood. Male onsets peaked at age 15 to 25 years, female onsets, showing a slightly slower increase, at age 15 to 29 years. At the age of decreasing oestrogen secretion (45 to 50 years), women showed a second peak of onsets, lower than the first one. This second peak has also been demonstrated on the pooled data from the WHO DOSMED study (Hambrecht et al., 1992), the Danish national case-register (Häfner et al., 1998c) and the Camberwell case register (Castle et al., 1998). For further discussion of late-onset schizophrenia see Chapter 9.

Possible explanations for gender difference

The explanation of the sex difference in age at illness onset as a protective effect of oestrogen (e.g. Seeman and Lang, 1990) was supported by a sensitivity-attenuating effect of oestrogen on central dopamine D_2 receptors in animal experiments (Häfner et al., 1991; Gattaz et al., 1992). Further evidence was provided by the finding that schizophrenic symptoms become milder with increasing oestrogen plasma levels in the menstrual cycle (Riecher-Rössler et al., 1994a,b). Cohen et al. (1999) found a significant relationship between age of menarche and age at onset in women, but not a comparable relation in men: the earlier the age at menarche, the later the age at first psychotic symptom and the age at first hospitalization. In a controlled intervention study of first-onset schizophrenia treated with oestrogen substitution in two different doses on the one hand and neuroleptic standard therapy on the other, Kulkarni et al. (1999) provided preliminary evidence that women with higher doses of oestrogen substitution showed a more rapid decrease in positive symptoms than women with lower doses or placebo controls.

A comparison of the ABC first-episode sample with controls matched for age, sex and place of residence showed that more women (52%) than men (28%) were married at illness onset, which could be explained by the fact that women in the general population married on average 2.5 years earlier, and female patients on average became ill 4 years later than men. But already in the early illness course, women suffered divorces and partnership losses in the same way as their male counterparts with an earlier illness onset, so that the proportion married was 33% (men: 17%) 5 years later. The WHO DOSMED and the ABC Schizophrenia Study included illness onsets only until age 54 and 59 years, respectively. Schizophrenia incidence was long presumed to decrease with increasing age. First-contact rates for late- and very-late-onset illness were studied by Castle et al. (1998) on the basis of OPCRIT computer program DSM-III-R diagnoses of schizophrenia using data from the Camberwell case register. First admissions for schizophrenia beyond age 60 years showed a highly significant female preponderance, which was well in accordance with a study of van Os et al. (1995), which, based on the Dutch national case register, showed an increase in first admission rates from about 10/100 000 in the age group 60 to 65 years to 25/100 000 in the age group 90 years and over. A reason for this inconsistency is the ongoing controversy about which delusional disorders and late paraphrenias should be included in late-onset schizophrenia and which should be classified separately. Another reason is the lack of population studies of the elderly, with the consequence that information on incidence is almost invariably based on service utilization data.

What symptoms mark the onset of schizophrenia?

The ten most frequent initial symptoms (except one sex-related item: worrying) were equally frequent in both men and women and mainly belonged to two

Table 7.3. The ten most frequent earliest signs of schizophrenia (independent of the course) reported by the patients[a]

	Total (%) (n=232)	Men (%) (n=108)	Women (%) (n=124)	p value
Restlessness	19	15	22	
Depression	19	15	22	
Anxiety	18	17	19	
Trouble with thinking and concentration	16	19	14	
Worrying	15	9	20	*
Lack of self-confidence	13	10	15	
Lack of energy, slowness	12	8	15	
Poor work performance	11	12	10	
Social withdrawal, distrust	10	8	12	
Social withdrawal, communication	10	8	12	

Notes:

[a] Based on closed questions, multiple counting possible. All items tested for sex differences.

* $p \leq 0.05$.

Source: modified from Häfner et al. (1995).

symptom dimensions: an affective depressive and a negative dimension (Table 7.3). The early occurrence of indicators of functional impairment (such as trouble with thinking and concentration, and loss of energy) pointed to early consequences of the disorder in terms of social functioning and risk of stagnation or decline in social status. The earliest positive symptom (delusions) appeared an average of 14.3 months, the first hallucination 8.7 months and the first formal thought disorder 8.2 months before first admission. The cumulative prevalence of delusions in the early illness course was 96%, that of auditory hallucinations 69% and of psychotic thought disorder 62%. This result reflects the selective influence positive symptoms have as the leading diagnostic criteria for schizophrenia on the type of patients included in or excluded from study samples of schizophrenia. Arranging the earliest symptoms by their time of emergence in a time matrix of up to 60 months before first admission, we found four depressive symptoms: depressed mood, suicide attempt, loss of self-confidence, and feelings of guilt. These tended to occur 5 to 3 years before first admission (Fig. 7.4). In the second time window, 4 to 2 years before first admission, all the negative symptoms appeared. It was only in the last year before first admission that positive symptoms emerged. This finding gives the impression of a regular sequence of phases in the early illness course reminiscent of the models of Conrad (1958) and Docherty et al. (1978). However, these data are based on group means and, therefore, this sequence is not necessarily valid for individual patients.

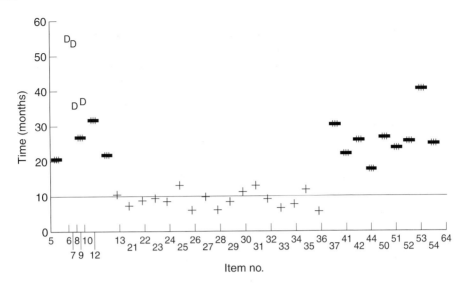

Fig. 7.4.   The time differences for positive and negative symptoms from first onset of symptoms until first hospitalization with schizophrenia diagnosis (first-episode sample, $n = 232$). The *x*-axis shows IRAOS items: D, depression; 7, suicide attempts; 8, loss of self-confidence; 10, feelings of guilt; positive symptoms (17 items) indicated by $+$; negative symptoms (13 items) indicated by horizontal bar. (From Häfner and Maurer, 1999.)

Early illness course as a prognostic indicator of later course

Depressive mood was common; 81% of the 203 patients without schizoaffective psychosis had suffered from depressive mood for at least 2 weeks before first admission: 39% continuously, 34% recurrently and 8% only once. A comparison of 57 patients with schizophrenia with 57 population controls matched on age, sex and place of residence showed that three depressive symptoms were highly significantly more frequent in patients than in controls, with odds ratios ranging from 3 to 5. Because of its comparative rareness, the 40% excess of attempted suicide did not reach statistical significance but arguably has clinical relevance.

The further course and predictive efficiency of early (prodromal) symptoms was studied in a representative subsample of 115 first episodes at six cross-sections over 5 years after first admission. Patients with schizophrenia who suffered from depressive mood in the early illness course showed significantly higher on scores of depressive, positive, negative and nonspecific symptoms in the first episode than nondepressed patients. After remission of the first episode, the mean score for depressive symptoms remained more or less stable. Neither positive nor nonspecific symptoms could be predicted by the presence of depressive symptoms in the early illness course. In contrast, absence of depressive symptoms in the early course was correlated with affective flattening in the 5 years following first admission. This

Table 7.4. Social role performance at the emergence of the first sign of mental disorder and at first admission (at onset and end of the early course)

	At first sign of mental disorder			At first admission		
	Schizophrenics ($n=57$)	Controls ($n=57$)	p value	Schizophrenics ($n=57$)	Controls ($n=57$)	p value
Age (years)	24.0	24.0		30.0	30.0	
School education (%)	65	61	NS	93	95	NS
Occupational training (%)	37	44	NS	63	65	NS
Employment (%)	33	42	NS	44	58	<0.01
Own income (%)	37	42	NS	49	74	<0.01
Own accommodation (%)	46	51	NS	63	75	NS
Marriage or stable partnership (%)	47	58	NS	25	68	<0.001

finding means that depression is a predictor of a severe first episode and of a low score for negative symptoms after remission, whereas a low score for depressive symptoms predicts more affective flattening. Because of the early emergence of negative symptoms and functional impairment, most patients with schizophrenia started to suffer from social disability (≥ 2 on the Disability Assessment Schedule (DAS)) 24 to 51 months before first admission, long before they received appropriate treatment. Two years before first admission, 57% of the patients were considerably impaired in the (DAS) domains of work performance, household chores, communication and leisure activities.

The effect of early social disability on the further illness course can only be judged against a baseline (i.e. the level of social development at illness onset). In the ABC first-episode sample, no significant differences were observable in the fulfilment of six main social roles between patients and controls at the age of illness onset: rate of persons with completed school education, completed occupational training, age at first job, having one's own income and accommodation, and being married or in a stable partnership. By the time of first admission, patients with schizophrenia had fallen significantly behind the controls in several roles, most markedly in marriage or stable partnership (Table 7.4). In sum, patients with schizophrenia were not yet markedly socially disadvantaged before illness onset.

Age and level of social development are highly significantly correlated. Men fall ill with schizophrenia 3 to 4 years earlier and, in our population of origin (Germany), marry 2.5 years later than women. Their level of social development at illness onset, in the social role of marriage in particular, was, therefore, considerably lower than that of the women. In addition, young men with schizophrenia showed a significant excess of socially adverse behaviour at first admission: for example self-neglect, lack of interest in finding a job, deficits in hygiene, aggressive behaviour and an elevated cumulative prevalence of alcohol and drug abuse until first admission. Female patients, in contrast, showed a significant excess of 'social conformity'. The socially adverse male behaviour is reflected in all population studies in the form of elevated rates of conduct disorders, aggressiveness, antisocial personality, alcohol and drug abuse. In schizophrenia, it is, therefore, classified as sex-specific illness behaviour and not as a direct expression of the disorder (Häfner et al. 1995). In a model of stepwise logistic regression, level of social development at the first psychotic symptom and socially adverse behaviour at the end of the pre-phase turned out to be the only factors significantly predicting 5-year social outcome. The traditional prognostic indicators age, sex, symptomatology (CATEGO total score) and type of illness onset merely acted indirectly via the level of social development at illness onset and illness behaviour. The symptom-related illness course showed no sex difference.

It seems that the social course of schizophrenia is largely determined by functional impairment and social disability in the early illness course and by the consequences they have on further social development after illness onset. In early-onset illness, the result is social stagnation at a low level of social development; in late-onset illness, when a comparatively high level of social development has been attained, social decline occurs. The more favourable social course of the disorder observed in women has to do with a higher level of social development, related to a later illness onset and socially more adaptive illness behaviour. It does not appear to be related to women having a milder form of the disorder.

Comorbidity of schizophrenia and alcohol and drug abuse

In the ABC study, the lifetime prevalence of alcohol abuse (based on the IRAOS: for at least 1 month, the patient had times of heavy drinking, problems with family owing to drinking, missed work because of drinking or showed withdrawal symptoms like morning shakes) until age at first admission was 24% for the first-episode sample and 12% for controls (Hambrecht and Häfner, 1996; Häfner et al., 1999), and that of drug abuse (based on the IRAOS: consumption of illegal drugs more than once a week over at least 1 month) was 14% for patients and 7% for controls (relative risk 2). Studies on the topic almost invariably show a preponderance of men: we found a cumulative prevalence of any type of misuse of 39% in men and of 22% in women. At 88%, cannabis was the most frequently abused substance, followed by alcohol at 58%. Thirty-five per cent of the patients with drug abuse and 18% of those with alcohol abuse started the abuse in the same month as the onset of schizophrenia. In this small group, the precipitation of illness onset by substance abuse cannot be excluded, especially since these patients were significantly younger at illness onset than nonabusing patients. In contrast, we could not support the neurobiologically more probable hypothesis of a drug-related precipitation of a psychotic episode in our study. Only in 3% did the onset of both abuse and psychosis occur in the same month, and only in about 4% did psychosis onset follow onset of abuse with a time span of less than 1 year. The longest interval between onset of drug abuse and onset of first psychotic symptom was 5.7 years. However, presence of alcohol and drug abuse in the early illness course was a predictor of an elevated score for positive symptoms in both the psychotic episode and in the 5 years following first admission. Positive symptoms of all three types – delusions, hallucinations and thought disorder – were increased, with hallucinations and thought disorders showing the highest values (see also Addington and Addington, 1998). In contrast, substance abuse significantly reduced affective flattening, probably in the context of a dysfunctional self-therapy, with a latency of several years. At the same time, substance and drug abuse may have contributed to a poorer compliance with antipsychotic therapy, which could have led to an increased level of positive symptoms.

Implications for studies using onset as a design variable

The fact that an early illness course of several years' duration exists before the first treatment contact has consequences for the interpretation of research results based on first admission as the definition of illness onset. This holds, for example, for reports of a significant excess of first admissions for schizophrenia from the lowest social class and poor, disintegrated neighbourhoods of big cities as well as for their possible interpretation by social causation and social selection hypotheses (Faris and Dunham, 1939; Kohn, 1969; Eaton, 1999). The social disadvantage of patients with schizophrenia at the time of first admission might simply be a consequence of the preceding early-illness course. In a retrospective assessment of premorbid behaviour, too, possible contamination with the prodromal phase has to be taken into account.

Conclusions

Onset and early course might be of far greater importance for further illness course and social outcome than any of the later stages of illness. Since negative symptoms and functional impairment usually emerge in the prodromal phase, they lead to social consequences, depending on the patient's level of social development at illness onset. A diagnosis of schizophrenia as a precondition for antipsychotic therapy is currently possible only after psychotic symptoms have emerged. It is not yet possible to predict in the prodromal phase whether or when psychotic symptoms will emerge. Attempts to develop early recognition inventories and to validate them in controlled prospective studies will, therefore, be a focal point of future research.

REFERENCES

Addington J, Addington D (1998) Effect of substance abuse in early psychosis. British Journal of Psychiatry 172 (Suppl. 33), 134–136.

Albus M, Maier W (1995) Lack of gender differences in age at onset in familial schizophrenia. Schizophrenia Research 18, 51–57.

American Psychiatric Association (1987) Diagnostic and Statistical Manual III–Revised. Washington, DC: American Psychiatric Press.

American Psychiatric Association (1994) Diagnostic and Statistical Manual IV, 4th edn. Washington, DC: American Psychiatric Press.

Angermeyer MC, Kühn L (1988) Gender differences in age at onset of schizophrenia. European Archives of Psychiatric and Neurological Science 237, 351–364.

Beiser M, Erickson D, Flemming JAE, Iacono WG (1993) Establishing the onset of psychotic illness. American Journal of Psychiatry 150, 1349–1354.

Bilder RM (1998) The neuropsychology of schizophrenia – What, when, where, how? In: Schizophrene Störungen. State of the art II, Fleischhacker WW, Hinterhuber H, Meise U, eds. Innsbruck: Verlag Integrative Psychiatrie, pp. 155–171.

Birchwood M, Smith J, Macmillan F et al. (1989) Predicting relapse in schizophrenia: the development and implementation of an early signs monitoring system using patients and families as observers. Psychological Medicine 19, 649–656.

Bleuler E (1911) Dementia praecox oder Gruppe der Schizophrenien. In: Handbuch der Psychiatrie, Aschaffenburg G, ed. Leipzig: Deuticke; pp. 1–420.

Cameron DE (1938) Early schizophrenia. American Journal of Psychiatry 95, 567–578.

Carpenter W, Heinrichs D (1983) Early intervention, time limited targeted pharmacotherapy for schizophrenia. Schizophrenia Bulletin 9, 533–542.

Castle DJ, Wessely S, van Os J, Murray RM (1998) Psychosis in the Inner City. East Sussex: Psychology Press.

Chapman JP (1966) The early symptoms of schizophrenia. British Journal of Psychiatry 112, 225–251.

Chapman LJ, Chapman JP (1980) Scales for rating psychotic and psychotic-like experiences as continua. Schizophrenia Bulletin 6, 476–489.

Chapman LJ, Chapman JP (1987) The search for symptoms predictive of schizophrenia. Schizophrenia Bulletin 13, 497–503.

Cohen RZ, Seeman MV, Gotowiec A, Kopala L (1999) Earlier puberty as a predictor of later onset of schizophrenia in women. American Journal of Psychiatry 156, 1059–1064.

Conrad K (1958) Die beginnende Schizophrenie. Versuch einer Gestaltanalyse des Wahns. Stuttgart: Thieme-Verlag.

Cornblatt B, Keilp J (1994) Impaired attention, genetics, and the pathophysiology of schizophrenia. Schizophrenia Bulletin 20, 31–46.

Cornblatt B, Obuchowski M, Schnur D, O'Brien JD (1998) Hillside study of risk and early detection in schizophrenia. British Journal of Psychiatry 172(Suppl. 33), 26–32.

Crow T, MacMillan JF, Johnson AL, Johnstone EC (1986) A randomized controlled trial of prophylactic neuroleptic treatment. British Journal of Psychiatry 148, 120–127.

Cutting J, Dunne F (1989) Subjective experience of schizophrenia. Schizophrenia Bulletin 15, 217–231.

Davidson M, Reichenberg A, Rabinowitz J, Weiser M, Kaplan Z, Mark M (1999) Behavioral and intellectual markers for schizophrenia in apparently healthy male adolescents. American Journal of Psychiatry 156, 1328–1335.

DeLisi LE, Bass N, Boccio A, Shilds G, Morganti C, Vita A (1994) Age of onset in familial schizophrenia. Archives of General Psychiatry 51, 334–335.

Docherty JP, van Kammen DP, Siris SG, Marder SR (1978) Stages of onset of schizophrenic psychosis. American Journal of Psychiatry 135, 420–426.

Dohrenwend BP, Shrout PE, Link BG, Skodol AE, Stueve A (1995) Life events and other possible psychosocial risk factors for episodes of schizophrenia and major depression: A case-control study. In: Does Stress Cause Psychiatric Illness? Mazure CM, ed. Washington, DC: American Psychiatric Press, pp. 43–65.

Done DJ, Crow TJ, Johnstone EC, Sacker A (1994a) Childhood antecedents of schizophrenia and affective illness: social adjustment at ages 7 and 11. British Medical Journal 309, 699–703.

Done DJ, Sacker A, Crow TJ (1994b) Childhood antecedents of schizophrenia and affective illness: intellectual performance at ages 7 and 11. Schizophrenia Research 11, 96–97.

Eaton WW (1999) Evidence for universality and uniformity of schizophrenia around the world: assessment and implications. In: Search for the Causes of Schizophrenia, Vol. IV: Balance of the Century, Gattaz WF, Häfner H, eds. Darmstadt: Steinkopff and Berlin: Springer, pp. 21–33.

Faris RE, Dunham W (1939) Mental Disorders in Urban Areas. An ecological study of schizophrenia and other psychoses. Chicago: University of Chicago Press.

Gaebel W, Frick U, Köpcke W et al. (1993) Early neuroleptic intervention in schizophrenia: are prodromal symptoms valid predictors of relapse? British Journal of Psychiatry 163(Suppl.), 8–12.

Gattaz WF, Behrens S, de Vry J, Häfner H (1992) Östradiol hemmt Dopamin-vermittelte Verhaltensweisen bei Ratten – ein Tiermodell zur Untersuchung der geschlechtsspezifischen Unterschiede bei der Schizophrenie. Fortschritte der Neurologie Psychiatrie 60, 8–16.

Griesinger W (1861) Pathologie und Therapie psychischer Krankheiten, 2nd edn. Stuttgart: Adolph Krabbe.

Gross G (1969) Prodrome und Vorpostensyndrome schizophrener Erkrankungen. In: Schizophrenie und Zyklothymie, Huber G, ed. Thieme; Stuttgart, pp. 177–187.

Gross G (1989) The basic symptoms of schizophrenia. British Journal of Psychiatry 155(Suppl. 7), 21–25.

Gross G, Huber G, Klosterkötter J, Linz M (1987) Bonner Skala für die Beurteilung von

Basissymptomen (BSABS: Bonn Scale for the Assessment of Basic Symptoms). Berlin: Springer.

Häfner H, Maurer K (1999) Methodological aspects of onset research in schizophrenia: the Mannheim study. In: One World, One Language – Paving the Way to Better Perspectives for Mental Health, López-Ibor JJ, Lieh-Mak F, Visotsky HM, Maj M, eds. Seattle, WA: Hogrefe and Huber Publishers, pp. 170–183.

Häfner H, Behrens S, de Vry J, Gattaz WF (1991) An animal model for the effects of estradiol on domapine-mediated behavior: implications for sex differences in schizophrenia. Psychiatry Research 38, 125–134.

Häfner H, Riecher-Rössler A, Hambrecht M et al. (1992) IRAOS: an instrument for the retrospective assessment of the onset of schizophrenia. Schizophrenia Research 6, 209–223.

Häfner H, Maurer K, Löffler W et al. (1995) Onset and early course of schizophrenia. In: Search for the Causes of Schizophrenia, Vol. III., Gattaz WF, Häfner H, eds. Berlin: Springer-Verlag, pp. 43–66.

Häfner H, an der Heiden W, Löffler W, Maurer K, Hambrecht M (1998a) Beginn und Frühverlauf schizophrener Erkrankungen. In: Frühdiagnostik und Frühbehandlung psychischer Störungen, Klosterkötter J, ed. Berlin: Springer for Bayer-ZNS-Symposium XIII, pp. 1–28.

Häfner H, an der Heiden W, Behrens S et al. (1998b) Causes and consequences of the gender difference in age at onset of schizophrenia. Schizophrenia Bulletin 24, 99–113.

Häfner H, Hambrecht M, Löffler W, Munk-Jørgensen P, Riecher-Rössler A (1998c) Is schizophrenia a disorder of all ages? A comparison of first episodes and early course across the life-cycle. Psychological Medicine 28, 351–365.

Häfner H, Maurer K, Löffler W, an der Heiden W, Könnecke R, Hambrecht M (1999) Onset and prodromal phase as determinants of the course. In: Search for the Causes of Schizophrenia, Vol. IV: Balance of the Century, Gattaz WF, Häfner H, eds. Darmstadt: Steinkopf and Berlin: Springer, pp. 1–24.

Hambrecht M, Häfner H (1993) 'Trema, Apophänie, Apokalypse' – Ist Conrads Phasenmodell empirisch begründbar? Fortschritte der Neurologie Psychiatrie 61, 418–423.

Hambrecht M, Häfner H (1996) Substance abuse and the onset of schizophrenia. Biological Psychiatry 40, 1155–1163.

Hambrecht M, Häfner H (1997) Sensitivity and specificity of relatives' reports on the early course of schizophrenia. Psychopathology 30, 12–19.

Hambrecht M, Maurer K, Häfner H, Sartorius N (1992) Transnational stability of gender differences in schizophrenia? European Archives of Psychiatry and Clinical Neuroscience 242, 6–12.

Hirsch SR, Jolley AG (1989) The dysphoric syndrome in schizophrenia and its implications for relapse. British Journal of Psychiatry 155(Suppl. 5), 46–50.

Huber G (1966) Reine Defektsyndrome und Basisstadien endogener Psychosen. Fortschritte der Neurologie Psychiatrie 34, 409–426.

Huber G (1997) The heterogeneous course of schizophrenia. Schizophrenia Research 28, 177–185.

Huber G, Gross G, Schüttler R (1979) Schizophrenie. Berlin: Springer.

Huber G, Gross G, Schüttler R, Linz M (1980) Longitudinal studies of schizophrenic patients. Schizophrenia Bulletin 6, 592–605.

Isohanni M, Isohanni I, Järvelin MR, Jones P, Mäkikyrö T, Rantakallio P (1999) Childhood and adolescent predictors of schizophrenia. In: Proceedings of the XI World Congress of Psychiatry, Hamburg, 6–11 August, 1999.

Jackson HJ, McGorry PD, Dudgeon P (1995) Prodromal symptoms of schizophrenia in first-episode psychosis: prevalence and specificity. Comprehensive Psychiatry 36, 241–250.

Johannessen JO, Larsen TK, McGlashan T (1999) Duration of untreated psychosis: An important target for intervention in schizophrenia? Nordic Journal of Psychiatry 53, 275–283.

Jones PB (1999) Longitudinal approaches to the search for the causes of schizophrenia: Past, present and future. In: Search for the Causes of Schizophrenia, Vol. IV, Balance of the Century, Gattaz WF, Häfner H, eds. Darmstadt: Steinkopff and Berlin: Springer, pp. 91–119.

Jones P, Done DJ (1997) From birth to onset: a developmental perspective of schizophrenia in two national birth cohorts. In: Neurodevelopmental and Adult Psychopathology, Keshavan MS, Murray RM, eds. Cambridge, UK: Cambridge University Press, pp. 119–136.

Klosterkötter J, Albers M, Steinmeyer EM, Hensen A, Saß H (1994) The diagnostic validity of positive, negative, and basic symptoms. Neurological Psychiatry and Brain Research 2, 232–238.

Klosterkötter J, Ebel H, Schultze-Lutter F, Steinmeyer EM (1996) Diagnostic validity of basic symptoms. European Archives of Psychiatry and Clinical Neuroscience 246, 147–154.

Klosterkötter J, Ebel H, Schultze-Lutter F, Steinmeyer EM (1997) Early self-experienced neuropsychological deficits and subsequent schizophrenic diseases: An 8-year average follow-up prospective study. Acta Psychiatrica Scandinavica 95, 390–404.

Klosterkötter J, Hellmich M, Steinmeyer EM, Schultze-Lutter F (2001) Diagnosing schizophrenia in the initial prodromal phase. Archives of General Psychiatry 58, 158–164.

Kohn M (1969) Class and Conformity: a study of values. Homewood, IL: Dorsey Press.

Könnecke R, Häfner H, Maurer K, Löffler W, an der Heiden W (2000) Main risk factors for schizophrenia: increased familial loading and pre- and perinatal complications antagonize the protective effect of oestrogen in women. Schizophrenia Research 44, 81–93.

Kraepelin E (1893) Psychiatrie. Ein kurzes Lehrbuch. Leipzig: Ambrosius Abel.

Kulkarni J, Burger H, Reidel A, Taffe J, de Castella A (1999) Clinical estrogen trials in patients with schizophrenia. In: Proceedings of the XI World Congress of Psychiatry, Hamburg, 6–11 August, 1999.

Lewine RJ (1980) Sex differences in age of symptom onset and first hospitalization in schizophrenia. Am J Orthopsychiatry 50, 316–322.

Lewine RRJ (1988) Gender and schizophrenia. In: Handbook of Schizophrenia, Vol. 3, Nasrallah HA, ed. Amsterdam: Elsevier, pp. 379–397.

Lindelius R (1979) A study of schizophrenia. Acta Psychiatrica Scandinavica Suppl. 216.

Loebel AD, Lieberman JA, Alvir JMJ, Mayerhoff DI, Geisler SH, Szymanski SR (1992) Duration of psychosis and outcome in first-episode schizophrenia. American Journal of Psychiatry 149, 1183–1188.

Loranger AW (1984) Sex difference in age of onset of schizophrenia. Archives of General Psychiatry 41, 157–161.

Malmberg A, Lewis G, David A, Allebeck P (1998) Premorbid adjustment and personality in people with schizophrenia. British Journal of Psychiatry 172, 308–313.

Maurer K, Häfner H (1995) Methodological aspects of onset assessment in schizophrenia. Schizophrenia Research 15, 265–276.

Mayer-Gross W (1932) Die Klinik. In: Handbuch der Geisteskrankheiten, Vol. 9: Die Schizophrenie, Bumke O, ed. Berlin: Springer, pp. 293–578.

McGhie A, Chapman J (1961) Disorders of attention and perception in early schizophrenia. British Journal of Medicine and Psychology 34, 103–115.

McGorry PD, McFarlane C, Patton GC et al. (1995) The prevalence of prodromal features of schizophrenia in adolescence: a preliminary survey. Acta Psychiatrica Scandinavica 92, 241–249.

McGorry PD, Edwards J, Mihalopoulos C, Harrigan SM, Jackson JH (1996) EPPIC: An evolving system of early detection and optimal management. Schizophrenia Bulletin 22, 305–326.

Nuechterlein KH, Dawson ME, Gitlin M et al. (1992) Developmental processes in schizophrenic disorders: longitudinal studies of vulnerability and stress. Schizophrenia Bulletin 18, 387–425.

Rabinowitz J, Reichenberg A, Weiser M, Mark M, Kaplan Z, Davidson M (2000) Cognitive and behavioural functioning in men with schizophrenia both before and shortly after first admission to hospital. British Journal of Psychiatry 177, 26–32.

Riecher-Rössler A, Häfner H, Dütsch-Strobel A et al. (1994a) Further evidence for a specific role of estradiol in schizophrenia? Biological Psychiatry 36, 492–495.

Riecher-Rössler A, Häfner H, Stumbaum M, Maurer K, Schmidt R (1994b) Can estradiol modulate schizophrenic symptomatology? Schizophrenia Bulletin 20, 203–214.

Salokangas RKR, Honkonen T, Stengard E (1999) Discharged schizophrenic patients in the community – implications for service development. In: WPA Section Symposium From Epidemiology to Clinical Practice, Turku/Finland, 1–4 August, 1999.

Seeman MV, Lang M (1990) The role of estrogens in schizophrenia gender differences. Schizophrenia Bulletin 16, 185–194.

Sullivan HS (1927) The onset of schizophrenia. American Journal of Psychiatry 84, 105–134.

van Os J, Howard R, Takei N, Murray R (1995) Increasing age is a risk factor for psychosis in the elderly. Social Psychiatry and Psychiatric Epidemiology 30, 161–164.

van Os J, Jones PB, Lewis G, Wadsworth M, Murray RM (1997) Developmental precursors of affective illness in a general population birth cohort. Archives of General Psychiatry 54, 625–631.

Verdoux H, Liraud F, Bergey C, Assens F, Abalan F, van Os J (2001) Is the association between duration of untreated psychosis and outcome confounded? A two year follow-up study of first-admitted patients. Schizophrenia Research 49, 231–241.

World Health Organization (1992) International Classification of Diseases, 10th draft. Geneva: World Health Organization.

Wyatt RJ, Damiani LM, Henter ID (1998) First-episode schizophrenia. British Journal of Psychiatry 172(Suppl. 33), 77–83.

Yung AR, McGorry PD (1996) The prodromal phase of first-episode psychosis: past and current conceptualisations. Schizophrenia Bulletin 22, 353–370.

Yung AR, Phillips LJ, McGorry PD et al. (1998) Prediction of psychosis. British Journal of Psychiatry 172(Suppl. 33), 14–20.

8

The value of first-episode studies in schizophrenia

Mary Clarke[1] and Eadbhard O'Callaghan[2]

[1]St John of God Hospital, Stillorgan, Ireland
[2]University College Dublin and Stanley Foundation Research Centre, Blackrock, Ireland

When Eve Johnstone and colleagues (1976), and later Weinberger et al. (1979a,b) reported that patients with schizophrenia showed evidence of morphological brain abnormality, many interested researchers expressed considerable scepticism (Gelenburg, 1976; Jellinek, 1976; Marsden, 1976). Were the abnormalities attributable to medication, institutionalization, ageing or simply an epiphenomenon?

There is now considerable evidence that schizophrenia is a brain disease characterized by abnormalities in cerebral structure and function (Waddington, 1993; Carpenter and Buchanan, 1994; Weinberger, 1995; Harrison, 1999). Studies using neuroimaging, neuropathology and neurophysiological approaches have now localized these changes to the frontotemporal regions of the brain (Bogerts et al., 1990; DeLisi et al., 1991; Degreef et al., 1992; Bilder et al., 1992; Hoff et al., 1992; Sweeney et al., 1992; Saykin et al., 1994; Salisbury et al., 1998). But why did it take over a decade to lay the sceptics' doubts to rest? Because of sampling: schizophrenia has a high prevalence but low incidence, so most research studies are either cross-sectional in design (mixing incident and prevalent cases) or focus on individuals who have been ill and receiving treatment for many years (Lieberman et al., 1992). The so-called 'convenience sample' favours those with established chronic illness at the expense of patients with good outcome psychotic illness who do not remain in contact with services. Therefore, the powerful effects of medication, hospitalization and the chronic schizophrenic process itself are further concentrated in typical research samples.

A complementary methodology is to study patients longitudinally from the earliest phases of the illness. This methodology enables us to address at least two issues about many of the physical and social phenomena associated with schizophrenia identified in cross-sectional studies. What is their temporal relationship to the onset of the illness? Are they static or progressive over the course of the disease? Screening the general population would be an ideal methodology to identify individuals at the earliest stage of illness but would be very expensive, time consuming and, given the relatively low incidence of the disorder, yield very few cases. Follow-up of high-risk groups such as those with a family history of schizophrenia is undoubtedly more efficient and has proved very useful (McNeil and Kaij, 1987; Erlenmeyer-Kimling et al., 1997). However, the sample generated loses the representative pattern inherent in a population-based model. Researchers have turned to the 'practical solution' in a new generation of studies termed 'first-episode' or 'first-onset' studies: 'a sample offering a unique opportunity to more completely understand the nature of schizophrenia by examining subjects before extended neuroleptic treatment and the development of chronic symptoms' (Kirch et al., 1992).

Advantages of first-episode studies

First-episode studies offer a number of advantages. Reasonable sample sizes can be collected so that hypotheses about the aetiology and course of the disorder can be tested. Relevant risk factors may be more accurately evaluated earlier rather than later in the illness (Keshavan and Schooler, 1992). The relative homogeneity within the sample with respect to illness history and neuroleptic exposure facilitates the assessment of numerous biologic variables. Indeed, some patients will never have been exposed to neuroleptic medication at the time of assessment. Finally, as many of the changes seen in the course of schizophrenia probably develop during the early stages of the illness (Shepherd et al., 1989), longitudinal studies will inform us about the course and diversity of this illness.

Contemporary first-episode studies can be broadly divided into two groups: first, epidemiological approaches that have collected 'all incident cases' from a defined region and focused on areas such as incidence, risk factors and outcome; second, smaller studies that have concentrated on specialized fields such as neuro-imaging.

Studies of incident first-episode cases

Time trends in incidence

First-episode incidence studies have indicated that schizophrenia may be a 'disappearing' disease (Eagles and Whalley, 1985; Der et al., 1990; Harrison and Mason, 1993; Brewin et al., 1997). The multicentre World Health Organization (WHO) Ten Country Study showed little variation between countries for narrowly defined schizophrenia, yet the incidence rates for broadly defined schizophrenia were nearly twice as high in developing countries as in the developed world (Jablensky et al., 1992). However, the data refer to the administrative incidence or first-contact incidence of the disorder. Admission rates may be influenced by factors such as increasing deinstitutionalization and changes in diagnostic practice (Kendell et al., 1993). If data concerning the actual onset of the disease are carefully collected, it should be possible over a period of time to provide figures on the true incidence of the disorder. This will establish whether there are indeed real changes in the incidence of the disorder over time and if the incidence varies between different countries. In turn, incident figures can then be more precisely linked to variation in the occurrence of underlying risk factors. Further exploration of these issues can be found in Chapter 3.

Risk factors and comorbidity

It can be difficult to establish whether some of the ascertained risk factors for schizophrenia are true independent risk factors or merely early manifestations of the disease process. For example 50% of those with schizophrenia have a lifetime history of substance abuse or dependence (Mueser et al., 1990; Reiger et al., 1990; Dixon et al., 1991). Comorbid substance abuse is associated with a younger age at onset of psychotic symptoms (Addington and Addington, 1998; Cantwell et al., 1999) and a poorer prognosis (Owen et al., 1996; Swofford et al. 1996; Kovasznay et al., 1997). First-episode studies indicate that this problem exists at first presentation, with approximately one-third reporting a history of comorbid substance or alcohol abuse (Cantwell et al., 1999). But is there a causal relationship between the two disorders or do individuals with schizophrenia use drugs as a means to self-medicate? First-episode studies have examined the temporal relationship between the onset of symptoms, both prodromal and psychotic, and substance misuse. One such study showed that substance misuse preceded the first symptom in approximately one-third of cases, followed it in another third and emerged within the same month in the final third (Hambrecht and Häfner, 1996). Therefore, a simple unidirectional causal model seems unlikely.

Gender effects

Gender effects in schizophrenia are well described but not fully understood. Gender differences are reported for age at onset of symptoms, treatment response, course of illness and outcome. One of the most consistent findings in psychiatric epidemiology is that males are hospitalized at an earlier age than females (Angermayer and Kuhn, 1988). This is uniform both in different countries and across different cultures (Häfner et al., 1989; Hambrecht et al., 1992). However, does this reflect true differences in age at symptom onset or are men simply more likely to come to treatment earlier? First-episode studies confirm that males have a younger age at onset of psychotic symptoms than females (Häfner et al. 1993; Szymanski et al., 1996). There are several possible explanations for this effect; males may be more likely to have a history of obstetric complications than females

(O'Callaghan et al., 1992; Kirov et al., 1996; Verdoux et al., 1997), and there is some evidence that patients with a history of obstetric complications have an earlier onset of symptoms than those without such complications. Alternatively, the protective effect of oestrogen in females (Seeman and Lang, 1990; Häfner et al., 1993; Szymanski et al., 1995), the later age at illness onset in females and the enhanced pharmacological responsivity to medication (Szymanski et al., 1996) may influence the gender differences in outcome.

Course and outcome

In the past, outcome was assessed by studying the easily accessible populations of long-stay patients or by focusing on series of consecutive hospital admissions. Studies confined to long-stay patients are likely by the very nature of the sample to represent the severe end of the disease spectrum. Outcome results based on consecutive hospital admissions are difficult to interpret. These samples tend to over-represent readmissions as distinct from first-episode cases. This causes a number of difficulties for prognostic research. Most of the clinical deterioration in schizophrenia has been observed to occur early, usually in the first 5 years of the illness (Kraepelin, 1919; Ciompi, 1980; Huber et al., 1980; Shepherd et al., 1989; Eaton, 1992a,b; Mason et al., 1996). Therefore, in order to capture the true diversity in the course of the disorder, it is of fundamental importance to study patients from the earliest phases of the illness (Andreasen et al., 1990b). Furthermore, it becomes increasingly difficult to test hypotheses about predictors such as employment or marital status in a meaningful way, as they may be consequences of the disease process rather than independent prognostic variables. Moreover, given the propensity of neuroleptic medication to induce both psychological and neurological side effects, it is preferable to perform baseline assessments, ideally before patients have been medicated or as close as possible to the commencement of treatment. Finally, since illness chronicity is an important predictor of future outcome, the relative proportions of first-episode compared with readmission patients in any sample is likely to influence strongly the reported outcome (Shepherd et al., 1989; Harrison and Mason, 1993).

Consequently, the patient population should consist of a cohort that is homogeneous with regard to stage of illness (Keshavan and Schooler, 1992; Ram et al., 1992). The first strategy was the long-term follow-back studies (Bleuler, 1978; Ciompi, 1980). These studies retrospectively identified first-admission patients from hospital records and reassessed them, often many years later. The principal methodological shortcoming to this approach is the retrospective nature of both the diagnoses and the prognostic data. Such limitations can best be overcome by prospective first-episode outcome studies. These studies have variously concentrated on the short-term treatment response, on outcome predictors or have described relapse rates or mortality by suicide (Johnstone et al., 1992; Tohen et al., 1992; Geddes et al., 1994; Gupta et al., 1997; Wiersma et al., 1998).

Patients with a first episode of schizophrenia usually respond well to treatment (MacMillan et al., 1986; Scottish Schizophrenia Research Group, 1988; Lieberman et al., 1996; Robinson et al., 1999). Male sex, obstetric complications, more severe positive symptoms at baseline and parkinsonian side effects of treatment have been shown to predict a poor response to treatment (Alvir et al., 1999; Robinson et al., 1999). Other studies have reported that treatment response in first-episode psychosis is positively correlated with cortical grey matter volumes (Zipursky et al., 1998) and abnormalities in the lateral and third ventricles (Lieberman et al., 1993a); however, the findings have not been entirely consistent (Robinson et al., 1999).

Those variables that predict treatment response may not follow through to predicting relapse. In a 5-year follow-up study, relapse (measured by ratings on the Clinical Global Impression Scale and the Schedule for Affective Disorders and Schizophrenia Change Version) was associated with medication noncompliance and poorer premorbid adaptation (Robinson et al., 1999). In another study, longer duration of subsequent hospitalization was associated with greater severity of neurological soft signs at baseline (Johnstone et al., 1990). Recently, a lot of interest has focused on the relationship between the initial duration of untreated psychosis (DUP) and outcome, with some studies reporting that a longer DUP is associated with an increased risk of relapse (Crow et al., 1986) and poorer symptomatic and functional outcome (Johnstone et al., 1990; Loebel et al., 1992). This has led to an interest in early intervention programmes (Birchwood et al., 1997). However, it is possible that the effect of DUP may be mediated by its association with known prognostic indicators such as family history and educational attainment (Verdoux et al., 1998) or its relationship with baseline symptomatology (Larsen et al., 1996a).

Relapse rates of between 34 and 55% have been reported over the first year of illness (Scottish Schizophrenia Research Group, 1988; Birchwood et al., 1992). In a 15-year follow-up, the relapse rate only increased slightly to 67%, with 11% dying by suicide (Wiersma et al., 1998). In general, the findings from longitudinal studies support the idea that most of the clinical deterioration occurs during the first 5 years (Mason et al., 1995) and that males have a poorer outcome than females. Several explanations for differences in outcome between males and females have been proposed, including methodological issues (such as lack of control for potential confounds like age at onset, marital status and premorbid adjustment), differences in brain structure and function, the presence of oestrogen (which may exert a neuroleptic-like effect) and pharmacokinetic dissimilarities (Angermayer et al., 1990). An 8-year follow-up of first-admission patients with schizophrenia, controlling for the confounders of age at onset, marital status and premorbid adjustment, showed that females spent fewer days in hospital and survived longer in the community before readmission (Angermeyer et al., 1990).

Abnormalities in cerebral structure and function at the time of first presentation

The principal structural brain abnormalities seen in schizophrenia on magnetic resonance imaging (MRI) are enlargement of the lateral and third ventricles, with some loss of brain tissue (Lawrie and Abukmeil, 1998). These changes are concentrated in the temporal lobe and particularly affect medial temporal lobe structures (Lawrie and Abukmeil, 1998; Nelson et al., 1998).

MRI studies have demonstrated that the abnormalities seen in chronic patients are also present at the time of first presentation (Bogerts et al., 1990; DeLisi et al., 1991; Degreef et al., 1992; Lieberman et al., 1993b; Nopoulos et al., 1995; Lim et al., 1996; Barr et al., 1997; Whitworth et al., 1998; Zipursky et al., 1998). Similarly, frontal lobe abnormalities, such as functional metabolic hypoactivity, appear to be already present not only at the first psychotic episode but also in the neuroleptic naive state, as shown by magnetic resonance spectroscopy (MRS) (Pettegrew et al., 1991), single photon emission computed tomography (SPECT) (Andreasen et al., 1992) and positron emission tomography (PET) (Buchsbaum et al., 1992; Gur et al., 1995).

Evidence for brain abnormalities in schizophrenia goes beyond neuroimaging. Both newly medicated and neuroleptic-naive patients show neuropsychological deficits, principally in the areas of memory and executive functioning, indicative of left temporal hippocampal dysfunction, although features consistent with a broader impairment may be seen (Bilder et al., 1992; Hoff et al., 1992; Saykin et al., 1994; Kenny et al., 1997; Binder et al., 1998; Hutton et al., 1998a; Mohamed et al., 1999). Neurophysiological studies show that the abnormalities in smooth pursuit eye movements and saccadic rhythm in patients with established schizophrenia are also present near the onset of the disorder (Lieberman et al., 1993b; Hutton et al., 1998b). Similarly, examination of neuroleptic-naive first-episode patients has shown that abnormalities in P300 amplitude are present prior to the administration of neuroleptic medication in the early phase of the disorder (Hirayasu et al., 1998). Furthermore, first-episode patients, even if neuroleptic naive, show an excess of neurological soft signs (Sanders et al., 1994; Gupta et al., 1995).

Controversy existed over whether tardive dyskinesia in schizophrenics was solely a consequence of antipsychotic drug treatment or whether it reflected an intrinsic aspect of the disease process. First-episode studies have demonstrated that dyskinetic movements are present in patients with schizophrenia who have never been exposed to neuroleptic medication (Chatterjee et al., 1995; Chakos et al., 1996;

Gervin et al., 1998; Puri et al., 1999). Findings with regard to spontaneous extra-pyramidal signs are not as consistent (Chatterjee et al., 1995; Puri et al., 1999).

Interpretation of the changes

Reduced volumes of limbic temporal lobe structures, neurological dysfunction and dyskinetic movements have been shown to be present at the time of first presentation, which supports the assumption that these abnormalities are not simply a consequence of illness chronicity or neuroleptic treatment. However, precise dating of these changes is difficult as, for many patients, a substantial period elapses between the onset of psychotic symptoms and actual presentation to the psychiatric services (Loebel et al., 1992; Beiser et al., 1993; Larsen et al., 1996a). On balance, the available research would suggest that many of these deficits probably antedate the onset of overt illness, since studies have demonstrated that children who develop schizophrenia, both in high-risk and more representative samples, have deficits in cognitive functioning (Mirsky et al., 1985; Parnas and Schulsinger, 1986; Done et al., 1994; Jones et al., 1994; Davidson et al., 1999) and also display neuromotor abnormalities (Walker et al., 1994, 1999). Developmental abnormalities in high-risk children are discussed in detail in Chapter 6.

Static versus progressive change?

Longitudinal first-episode studies have addressed the issue of the progression of these abnormalities (Bilder et al., 1992; Goldberg et al., 1993; Waddington et al., 1996). Follow-up MRI studies in first-episode patients are still in an early stage of development and the findings are equivocal, with some studies demonstrating that these changes are static (Jaskiw et al., 1994; Vita et al., 1997), while others show progression (DeLisi et al., 1997). Longitudinal neuropsychological studies of first-episode patients do not support the view of a progressive decline but instead show stability with perhaps even some improvement over time (McCreadie et al., 1989; Censits et al., 1997; Gold et al., 1999; Hoff et al., 1999). This contrasts with the finding from cross-sectional studies that progressive cognitive deterioration ensues in the long term (Bilder et al., 1992). In the only published follow-up study of neurological soft signs, in 18 patients with first-episode schizophrenia, neurological soft signs tended to increase, especially in those with a family history or a non-remitting course (Madsen et al., 1999a).

However there are numerous difficulties in interpreting these studies. Lack of statistical power because of small numbers, lack of suitable control subjects and differing follow-up periods constitute some of the core problems. These sometimes conflicting findings, specially in imaging studies, could potentially be explained by a subgroup of patients that have deteriorating course (Davis et al., 1998). They could also represent the effects of different quantities of medication (Madsen et al., 1999b) or could be an artifact of the control groups.

Methodological issues in first-episode studies

Control groups

One of the most critical methodological issues in first-episode studies is the selection of the control group, particularly when the differences being measured are likely to be small. The issue of control selection has received particular attention in imaging studies, where it has been debated that the use of medical patients with 'normal scans' rather than healthy community members as control subjects may influence the outcome of computed tomography (CT) studies in schizophrenia (Smith and Iacono, 1986; Raz et al., 1988a,b; Smith et al., 1988, 1998; Pfefferbaum et al., 1990). The selection of an appropriate control group poses a number of challenges. First, control subjects are frequently not sampled from the same population as the cases, thus leading to a potentially misleading effect estimate. Second, control groups occasionally comprise patients with other psychiatric illness, again leading to the possibility of inaccurate results. Finally, there is often failure to collect adequate information on potentially important confounding variables, such as handedness, socioeconomic status, migrant status and length of education. For example, matching for handedness may be important when lateralized differences are being explored, as left-handed people may have significant differences in brain hemispheric asymmetry compared with right-handed people (Zipursky et al., 1990). Furthermore, others have noted a relationship between social class or educational status and brain structural variables (Pearlson et al., 1989; Andreasen et al., 1990a). However, controls are now being recruited in an increasingly sophisticated manner, often from the same population base as cases, and sufficient information is being collected to take into account the potential effects of confounding variables (de Myer et al., 1988; Pfefferbaum et al., 1990).

Definition of the first episode

What exactly is a first episode of schizophrenia? When does it begin and end? Although in some individuals this is very clear, others make a very gradual transition from an 'odd' premorbid personality to prodromal symptoms before the emergence of any definite psychotic symptoms (Larsen et al., 1996b). The prodromal period is discussed in Chapter 7. Keshavan and Schooler (1992) reviewed first-episode studies and concluded that there were marked inconsistencies in the delineation of a number of key variables, including illness onset, and recommended that in order for future studies to be meaningfully compared it is necessary to operationalize some of these definitions. To date, however, there is still no standardized definition of onset. In practice, most date onset from the appearance of the first psychotic symptom (Loebel et al., 1992; Beiser et al., 1993). However, some authors would argue that onset should be defined only when the full criteria for the syndrome are met (Haas and Sweeney, 1992). Nonetheless, it has been suggested that it may prove unrealistic to produce a 'gold standard' definition of onset or episode of a psychotic illness (Kirch et al., 1992); rather, the method used should be explicitly outlined, both to aid in the interpretation of any findings and also to facilitate comparison of results across different studies.

Study population

The study findings are also likely to be influenced by the source from which the cases were recruited. For example, a group of cases drawn from a well-defined 'epidemiological' population base may constitute a markedly different sample from that derived from a tertiary or specialist referral centre. Although tertiary referral settings do offer some advantages (for example individuals who may be more willing to participate in research), the generalizability of any findings may be consequently limited, since such a sample may be preselected on the basis of factors such as poor prognosis or treatment resistance. (Lieberman et al., 1993a). Furthermore, the distribution of diagnoses within such an incident sample may be dramatically different. This point is particularly well illustrated when the diagnoses of private- and public-based first-episode studies are compared; in the McLean project, 74% of the incident sample had a diagnosis of affective psychosis, whereas in most other studies the majority have schizophrenia or schizophreniform psychosis (Tohen et al., 1992). Therefore, sources other than a catchment area service are unlikely to be representative of the distribution of schizophrenia as a whole.

Another issue that has particular relevance for an epidemiological enquiry is the percentage of patients treated either exclusively as outpatients or entirely within primary care. Though data on these figures are rather sparse, nonetheless there is evidence that some patients (2.5%) are managed entirely by their general practitioners and are never seen by the psychiatric services (Watts, 1973). Other groups that may miss referral to the psychiatric services are the homeless, though there are conflicting reports as to whether there are large numbers of untreated individuals with schizophrenia among this group (Munk-Jørgensen and Mortensen, 1993; Geddes and Kendell, 1995).

The inclusion and exclusion criteria that are applied at intake are also likely to influence significantly the findings of the study. These criteria vary from group to group but commonly include age, treatment history, comorbid substance abuse and prior neurological illness or head injury. Samples are frequently defined by strict age limits. This will affect both the reported age at onset of psychosis and, depending on the upper age limit applied, may also influence the gender distribution, as females have a bimodal peak for age at onset. Although comorbid substance abuse may confound the investigation of a number of the biological variables, for example the neurology of the disorder (Browne et al., 2000), excluding individuals with a history of substance abuse or dependence may lead to a number of biases. At least one-third of the potential sample and possibly more males (Bromet et al., 1992) would be automatically excluded. Furthermore, the age-at-onset figures may be affected and the outcome in such cohorts may appear more optimistic than truly justified.

The diagnostic dilemma

The question of whether a diagnosis can be validly assigned at the time of first presentation has been extensively debated. There are still some important differences between ICD-10 (World Health Organization, 1992) and DSM-IV (Spitzer et al., 1995) that may result in two quite different populations of 'first-episode schizophrenia'. ICD-10 requires psychotic symptoms to be present for at least most of the time over a period of a month. Because of concerns about the reliability of assessment, prodromal symptoms are acknowledged but not included in the diagnostic criteria. DSM-IV takes a different approach, only requiring active symptoms for a week, or less if treated, but specifies a minimum time period of 6 months, and this may include prodromal symptoms. Therefore, for any given sample, the diagnostic breakdown may be markedly influenced by one's choice of operational criteria. One solution is to use a polydiagnostic approach and apply several sets of diagnostic criteria simultaneously, thus allowing for more meaningful comparisons to be made across different studies.

Schizophrenic disorders have been shown to be a relatively stable broad diagnostic category in both the short (86.5–88.9% stable over 6 months) (Fennig et al., 1994) and long term (78% stable over 7 years) (Chen et al., 1996). However, figures overall may vary depending on the criteria used (Ganguli and Brar, 1992; Biehl et al., 1986). Nevertheless, both ICD-10 and DSM-IV have been shown to have high predictive validity, and that of ICD-10 is enhanced by adding a 6-month duration criterion (Mason et al., 1997). As a diagnosis of schizophrenia may not remain stable over time, ideally longitudinal studies should include all new cases of psychosis at recruitment rather than restricting intake to those who fulfil diagnostic criteria for schizophrenia at the point of entry. Similarly, to ensure maximum follow-up, all these individuals should be included in any longitudinal assessments.

Conclusions and future directions

The first-episode approach is but one strategy to address the enigma of schizophrenia. It may not be the optimal approach, but it is likely to answer questions that cross-sectional studies never will. The early phases of the illness represent an important period, both from a research viewpoint and also in relation to the outcome of the illness and any one individual's future prognosis. Although the first-episode strategy has helped to clarify some important concepts, many questions remain unanswered. Does the incidence of the disorder vary both temporally and geographically? What is the relationship if any between risk factors? How do genetic and environmental risk factors interact? What are the true or independent predictors of outcome? Do secondary prevention programmes work?

Despite extensive research into genetic and possible environmental 'risk factors' associated with schizophrenia, most fundamental issues remain unclear. Many 'aetiological' studies are plagued by power limitations, but multicentre first-episode strategies could provide cohorts to evaluate risk factors without compromising sampling methodology. These, in turn, can be linked with longitudinal studies that assess the impact of these variables on outcome.

Other factors also likely to influence outcome are compliance and familial expressed emotion. Though there is an extensive literature on compliance, few studies have looked at compliance at first presentation, where it may be possible to separate patient-related factors from treatment- and medication-related variables and tailor intervention accordingly. Evaluating 'premorbid' attitudes to psychotropic medication, both from the patient and the family perspective, may be another useful area to explore. Similarly, baseline assessments of insight and family expressed emotion at first presentation may provide a clearer picture as to how these variables influence the course and outcome of the disorder (Huguelet et al., 1995; Linszen et al., 1997).

REFERENCES

Addington J, Addington D (1998) Effect of substance misuse in early psychosis. British Journal of Psychiatry 172(Suppl. 33), 134–136.

Alvir JM, Woerner MG, Gunduz H et al. (1999) Obstetric complications predict treatment response in first episode schizophrenia. Psychological Medicine 29, 621–627.

Andreasen VC, Ehrhardt JC, Swayze VW et al. (1990a) Magnetic resonance imaging of the brain in schizophrenia – the pathophysiological significance of the structural abnormalities. Archives of General Psychiatry 47, 35–44.

Andreasen NC, Flaum M, Swayze VW et al. (1990b) Positive and negative symptoms in schizophrenia: a critical reappraisal. Archives of General Psychiatry 45, 79–91.

Andreasen NC, Rezai K, Alliger R et al. (1992) Hypofrontality in neuroleptic naïve patients and in patients with chronic schizophrenia. Archives of General Psychiatry 49, 943–958.

Angermayer MC, Kuhn L (1988) Gender differences in age at onset of schizophrenia: an overview. European Archives of Psychiatry and Neurological Science 237, 351–364.

Angermayer MC, Kuhn L, Goldstein JM (1990) Gender and the course of schizophrenia: differences in treated outcomes. Schizophrenia Bulletin 16, 293–307.

Barr WB, Ashtari M, Bilder RM et al. (1997) Brain morphometric comparison of first-episode schizophrenia and temporal lobe epilepsy. British Journal of Psychiatry 170, 515–519.

Beiser M, Erickson D, Fleming J, Iacono WG (1993) Establishing the onset of psychotic illness. American Journal of Psychiatry 159, 1349–1354.

Biehl H, Maurer K, Schubart C et al. (1986) Prediction of outcome and utilization of medical services in a prospective study of first onset schizophrenics. Results of a prospective 5-year follow-up study. European Archives of Psychiatry and Neurological Science 236, 139–147.

Bilder RM, Lipschutz-Broch L, Reiter G et al. (1992) Intellectual deficits in first-episode schizophrenia: evidence for progressive deterioration. Schizophrenia Bulletin 18, 437–448.

Binder J, Albus M, Hubmann W et al. (1998) Neuropsychological impairment and psychopathology in first-episode schizophrenic patients related to the early course of illness. European Archives of Psychiatry and Clinical Neuroscience 248, 70–77.

Birchwood M, Cochrane R, MacMillan J et al. (1992) The influence of ethnicity and family structure on relapse in first episode schizophrenia. British Journal of Psychiatry 163, 783–790.

Birchwood M, McGorry P, Jackson H (1997) Early intervention in schizophrenia. British Journal of Psychiatry 170, 2–5.

Bleuler M (1978) The long term course of the schizophrenic psychoses. In: The Nature of Schizophrenia, Wynne LC, Cromwell RL, Matthysse S, eds. New York: Wiley, pp. 631–640.

Bogerts B, Ashtari M, Degreef G et al. (1990) Reduced temporal limbic structure volumes on magnetic resonance images in first episode schizophrenia. Psychiatry Research 35, 1–13.

Brewin J, Cantwell R, Dalkin T et al. (1997) Incidence of schizophrenia in Nottingham. A comparison of two cohorts, 1978–80 and 1992–94. British Journal of Psychiatry 171, 140–144.

Bromet EJ, Schwartz JE, Fennig S et al. (1992) The epidemiology of psychosis: the Suffolk County Mental Health Project. Schizophrenia Bulletin 18, 243–255.

Browne S, Clarke M, Gervin M et al. (2000) Determinants of neurological dysfunction in first episode schizophrenia. Psychological Medicine 30, 1433–1441.

Buchsbaum MS, Haier RJ, Potkin SG et al. (1992) Frontostriatal disorder of cerebral metabolism in never medicated schizophrenics. Archives of General Psychiatry 49, 935–942.

Cantwell R, Brewin J, Glazebrook C et al. (1999) Prevalence of substance misuse in first episode psychosis. British Journal of Psychiatry 174, 150–153.

Carpenter WT, Buchanan RW (1994) Schizophrenia. New England Journal of Medicine 330, 681–690.

Censits DM, Ragland JD, Gur RC et al. (1997) Neuropsychological evidence supporting a neurodevelopmental model of schizophrenia: a longitudinal study. Schizophrenia Research 24, 289–298.

Chakos MH, Alvir JM, Woerner MG et al. (1996) Incidence and correlates of tardive dyskinesia in first episode of schizophrenia. Archives of General Psychiatry 53, 313–319.

Chatterjee A, Chakos M, Koreen A et al. (1995) Prevalence and clinical correlates of extrapyramidal signs and spontaneous dyskinesia in never-medicated schizophrenic patients. American Journal of Psychiatry 152, 1724–1729.

Chen YR, Swann AC, Burt DB (1996) Stability of diagnosis in schizophrenia. American Journal of Psychiatry 153, 682–686.

Ciompi L (1980) Catamnestic long term study on the course of life and aging of schizophrenics. Schizophrenia Bulletin 6, 606–618.

Crow TJ Cross AJ, Johnstone EC et al. (1986) A randomised controlled trial of prophylactic neuroleptic medication. British Journal of Psychiatry 148, 120–127.

Davidson M, Reichenberg A, Rabinowitz J et al. (1999) Behavioral and intellectual markers for schizophrenia in apparently healthy male adolescents. American Journal of Psychiatry 156, 1328–1335.

Davis KL, Buchsbaum MS, Shihabuddin L et al. (1998) Ventricular enlargement in poor-outcome schizophrenia. Biological Psychiatry 43, 783–793.

Degreef G, Ashtari M, Bogerts B et al. (1992) Volumes of ventricular system subdivisions measured from magnetic resonance images in first episode schizophrenic patients. Archives of General Psychiatry 49, 531–537.

DeLisi LE, Hoff AL, Schwartz JE et al. (1991) Brain morphology in first episode schizophrenia-like psychotic patients: a quantitative magnetic resonance imaging study. Biological Psychiatry 29, 159–175.

DeLisi LE, Sakuma M, Tew W et al. (1997) Schizophrenia as a chronic active brain process: a study of progressive brain structural change subsequent to the onset of schizophrenia. Psychiatry Research 74, 129–140.

de Myer MK, Gilmor RL, Hendrie HC et al. (1988) Magnetic resonance brain images in schizophrenic and normal subjects: influence of diagnosis and education. Schizophrenia Bulletin 14, 21–32.

Der G, Gupta S, Murray R (1990) Is schizophrenia disappearing? Lancet 335, 513–516.

Dixon L, Haas G, Weiden PJ et al. (1991) Drug abuse in schizophrenic patients: clinical correlates and reasons for use. American Journal of Psychiatry 148, 224–230.

Done DJ, Crow TJ, Johnstone EV, Sacker A (1994) Childhood antecedents of schizophrenia and affective illness. British Medical Journal 309, 699–703.

Eagles JM, Whalley LJ (1985) Decline in the diagnosis of schizophrenia among first admissions to Scottish mental hospitals from 1969–1978. British Journal of Psychiatry 146, 151–154.

Eaton WW, Mortensen PB, Herrman H et al. (1992a) Long-term course of hospitalization for schizophrenia: Part I. Risk for rehospitalization. Schizophrenia Bulletin 18, 217–228.

Eaton WW, Bilker W, Haro JM et al. (1992b) Long-term course of hospitalization for schizophrenia: Part II. Change with passage of time. Schizophrenia Bulletin 18, 229–241.

Erlenmeyer-Kimling L, Adamo UH, Rock D (1997) The New York High-Risk Project. Prevalence and comorbidity of axis I disorders in offspring of schizophrenic parents at 25-year follow-up. Archives of General Psychiatry 54, 1096–1102.

Fennig S, Kovasznay B, Rich C et al. (1994) Six-month stability of psychiatric diagnoses in first-admission patients with psychosis. American Journal of Psychiatry 151, 1200–1208.

Ganguli R, Brar J (1992) Generalizability of first-episode studies in schizophrenia. Schizophrenia Bulletin 18, 463–469.

Geddes JR, Kendell RE (1995) Schizophrenic subjects with no history of admission to hospital. Psychological Medicine 25, 859–868.

Geddes J, Mercer G, Frith CD et al. (1994) Prediction of outcome following a first episode of schizophrenia. A follow-up study of Northwick Park first episode study subjects. British Journal of Psychiatry 165, 664–668.

Gelenburg AJ (1976) Cerebral ventricular size and cognitive impairment in chronic schizophrenia. Lancet ii, 1304.

Gervin M, Browne S, Lane A et al. (1998) Spontaneous abnormal involuntary movements in first-episode schizophrenia and schizophreniform disorder: baseline rate in a group of patients from an Irish catchment area. American Journal of Psychiatry 155, 1202–1206.

Gold S, Arndt S, Nopoulos P et al. (1999) Longitudinal study of cognitive function in first episode and recent onset schizophrenia. American Journal of Psychiatry 156, 1342–1348.

Goldberg TE, Hyde TM, Kleinman JE (1993) Course of schizophrenia: neuropsychological evidence for a static encephalopathy. Schizophrenia Bulletin 19, 797–804.

Gupta S, Andreasen NC, Arndt S et al. (1995) Neurological soft signs in neuroleptic-naive and neuroleptic-treated schizophrenic patients and in normal comparison subjects. American Journal of Psychiatry 152, 191–196.

Gupta S, Andreasen NC, Arndt S et al. (1997) The Iowa Longitudinal Study of Recent Onset Psychosis: one-year follow-up of first episode patients. Schizophrenia Research 17, 1–13.

Gur RE, Mozley PD, Resnick SM et al. (1995) Resting cerebral glucose metabolism in first-episode and previously treated patients with schizophrenia relates to clinical features. Archives of General Psychiatry 52, 657–667.

Häfner H, Riecher A, Maurer K et al. (1989) How does gender influence age at first hospitalisation for schizophrenia. A transnational case register study. Psychological Medicine 19, 903–918.

Häfner H, Riecher-Rossler A, An der Heiden W et al. (1993) Generating and testing a causal explanation of the gender difference in age at first onset of schizophrenia. Psychological Medicine 23, 925–940.

Hambrecht M, Häfner H (1996) Substance abuse and the onset of schizophrenia. Biological Psychiatry 40, 1155–1163.

Hambrecht M, Maurer K, Häfner H (1992) Transnational stability of gender differences in schizophrenia? An analysis based on the WHO Study on determinants of outcome of severe mental disorders. European Archives of Psychiatry and Clinical Neuroscience 242, 6–12.

Harrison PJ (1999) The neuropathology of schizophrenia. A critical review of the data and their interpretation. Brain 122, 593–624.

Harrison, G, Mason P (1993) Schizophrenia – falling incidence and better outcome? British Journal of Psychiatry 163, 535–541.

Haas GL, Sweeney JA (1992) Premorbid and onset features of first-episode schizophrenia. Schizophrenia Bulletin 18, 373–386.

Hirayasu Y, Asato N, Ohta H et al. (1998) Abnormalities of auditory event-related potentials in schizophrenia prior to treatment. Biological Psychiatry 43, 244–253.

Hoff AL, Riordan H, O'Donnell D, et al. (1992) Anomalous lateral sulcus asymmetry and cognitive function in first-episode schizophrenia. Schizophrenia Bulletin 18, 257–272

Hoff AL, Sakuma M, Wieneke M et al. (1999) Longitudinal neuropsychological follow up of patients with first episode schizophrenia. American Journal of Psychiatry 156, 1336–1341.

Huber G, Gross G, Schuttler R et al. (1980) Longitudinal studies of schizophrenic patients. Schizophrenia Bulletin 6, 592–605.

Huguelet P, Favre S, Binyet S et al. (1995) The use of the Expressed Emotion Index as a predictor of outcome in first admitted schizophrenic patients in a French speaking area of Switzerland. Acta Psychiatrica Scandinavica 92, 447–452.

Hutton SB, Crawford TJ, Puri BK et al. (1998b) Smooth pursuit and saccadic abnormalities in first-episode schizophrenia. Psychological Medicine 28, 685–692.

Hutton SB, Puri BK, Duncan LJ et al. (1998a) Executive function in first-episode schizophrenia. Psychological Medicine 28, 463–473.

Jablensky A, Sartorius N, Ernberg G et al. (1992) Schizophrenia: manifestations, incidence, and course in different cultures. A World Health Organization ten country study. Psychological Medicine Monograph Supplement 20. Cambridge, UK: Cambridge University Press.

Jaskiw GE, Juliano DM, Goldberg TE et al. (1994) Cerebral ventricular enlargement in schizophreniform disorder does not progress. A seven year follow-up study. Schizophrenia Research 14, 23–28.

Jellinek EH (1976) Cerebral atrophy and cognitive impairment in chronic schizophrenia. Lancet ii, 1202–1203.

Jones P, Rodgers B, Murray R (1994) Childhood developmental risk factors from schizophrenia in the British 1946 birth cohort. Lancet 344, 1398–14021.

Johnstone EC, Crow TJ, Frith CD et al. (1976) Cerebral ventricular size and cognitive impairment in chronic schizophrenia. Lancet 2, 924–926.

Johnstone EC, Macmillan FJ, Frith CD, Benn DK, Crow TJ (1990) Further investigation of the predictors of outcome following first schizophrenic episodes. British Journal of Psychiatry 157, 182–189.

Johnstone EC, Frith CD, Crow TJ et al. (1992) The Northwick park 'Functional Psychosis Study: diagnosis and outcome. Psychological Medicine 22, 331–346.

Kendell RE, Malcolm DE, Adams W (1993) The problems of detecting changes in the incidence of schizophrenia. British Journal of Psychiatry 162, 212–218.

Kenny JT, Friedman L, Findling RL et al. (1997) Cognitive impairment in adolescents with schizophrenia. American Journal of Psychiatry 154, 1613–1615.

Keshavan MS, Schooler NR (1992) First-episode studies in schizophrenia: criteria and characterization. Schizophrenia Bulletin 18, 491–513.

Kirch DG, Keith SJ, Matthews SM (1992) Research on first-episode psychosis: report on a National Institute of Mental Health Workshop. Schizophrenia Bulletin 18, 179–184.

Kirov G, Jones PB, Harvey I et al. (1996) Do obstetric complications cause the earlier age at onset in male than female schizophrenics? Schizophrenia Research 20, 117–124.

Kovasznay B, Fleischer J, Tanenberg-Karant et al. (1997) Substance use disorder and the early course of illness in schizophrenia and affective psychosis. Schizophrenia Bulletin 23, 195–201.

Kraepelin E (1919) Dementia Praecox and Paraphrenia. [Translated by Barclay RM.] Edinburgh: E and S Livingstone.

Larsen TK, McGlashan TH, Moe LC (1996a) First-episode schizophrenia: I. Early course parameters. Schizophrenia Bulletin 22, 241–256.

Larsen TK, McGlashan TH, Johannessen JO et al. (1996b) First-episode schizophrenia: II. Premorbid patterns by gender. Schizophrenia Bulletin 22, 257–269.

Lawrie SM, Abukmeil SS (1998) Brain abnormality in schizophrenia. A systematic and quantitative review of volumetric magnetic resonance imaging studies. British Journal of Psychiatry 172, 110–120.

Lieberman JA, Alvir JM, Woerner M, et al. (1992) Prospective study of psychobiology in first-episode schizophrenia at Hillside Hospital. Schizophrenia Bulletin 18, 351–371.

Lieberman J, Jody D, Geisler S et al. (1993a) Time course and biologic correlates of treatment response in first-episode schizophrenia. Archives of General Psychiatry 50, 369–376.

Lieberman, JA, Jody D, Alvir JM et al. (1993b) Brain morphology, dopamine, and eye-tracking abnormalities in first-episode schizophrenia: prevalence and clinical correlates. Archives of General Psychiatry 50, 357–368.

Lieberman JA, Alvir JM, Koreen A et al. (1996) Psychobiologic correlates of treatment response in schizophrenia. Neuropsychopharmacology 14(Suppl. 3), 13S–21S.

Lim KO, Tew W, Kushner M et al. (1996) Cortical grey matter volume deficit in patients with first episode schizophrenia. American Journal of Psychiatry 153, 1548–1553.

Linszen DH, Dingemans PM, Nugter MA et al. (1997) Patient attributes and expressed emotion as risk factors for psychotic relapse. Schizophrenia Bulletin 32, 119–130.

Loebel AD, Lieberman JA, Alvir JM et al. (1992) Duration of psychosis and outcome in first-episode schizophrenia. American Journal of Psychiatry 149, 1183–1188.

MacMillan JF, Crow TJ, Johnson Al et al. (1986) Northwick Park Study of first episodes of schizophrenia. II Short term outcome in trial entrants and trial eligible patients. British Journal of Psychiatry 148, 128–133.

Madsen AL, Vorstrup S, Rubin P et al. (1999a) Neurological abnormalities in schizophrenic patients: a prospective follow-up study 5 years after first admission. Acta Psychiatrica Scandinavica 100, 119–125.

Madsen AL, Karle A, Rubin P et al. (1999b) Progressive atrophy of the frontal lobes in first-episode schizophrenia: interaction with clinical course and neuroleptic treatment. Acta Psychiatrica Scandinavica 100, 367–374.

Marsden CD (1976) Cerebral atrophy and cognitive impairment in chronic schizophrenia. Lancet ii, 1079.

Mason P, Harrison G, Glazebrook C et al. (1995) Characteristics of outcome in schizophrenia at 13 years. British Journal of Psychiatry 167, 596–603.

Mason P, Harrison G, Glazebrook C et al. (1996) The course of schizophrenia over 13 years. A report from the International Study on Schizophrenia (ISoS) coordinated by the World Health Organization. British Journal of Psychiatry 169, 580–586.

Mason P, Harrison G, Croudace T et al. (1997) The predictive validity of a diagnosis of schizophrenia. A report from the International Study of Schizophrenia (ISoS) coordinated by the World Health Organization and the Department of Psychiatry, University of Nottingham. British Journal of Psychiatry 170, 321–327.

McCreadie RG, Wiles D, Grant S et al. (1989) The Scottish First Episode Schizophrenia Study. VII. Two-year follow-up. Scottish Schizophrenia Research Group. Acta Psychiatrica Scandinavica 80, 597–602.

McNeil TF, Kaij (1987) Swedish High-Risk Study: sample characteristics at age 6. Schizophrenia Bulletin 13, 373–381.

Mirsky AF, Silberman EK, Latz A, Nagler S (1985) Adult outcomes of high risk children. Schizophrenia Bulletin 11, 150–154.

Mohamed S, Paulsen JS, O'Leary D et al. (1999) Generalized cognitive deficits in schizophrenia: a study of first-episode patients. Archives of General Psychiatry 56, 749–754.

Mueser KT, Yarnold PR, Levinson DF et al. (1990) Prevalence of substance misuse in schizophrenia: Demographic and clinical factors. Schizophrenia Bulletin 16, 31–56.

Munk-Jørgensen P, Mortensen P (1993) Is schizophrenia really on the decrease? European Archives of Psychiatry and Clinical Neuroscience 242, 244–247.

Nelson MD, Saykin AJ, Flashman LA et al. (1998) Hippocampal volume reduction in schizophrenia as assessed by magnetic resonance imaging: a meta-analytic study. Archives of General Psychiatry 55, 433–440.

Nopoulos P, Torres I, Flaum M et al. (1995) Brain morphology in first-episode schizophrenia. American Journal of Psychiatry 152, 1721–1723.

O'Callaghan E, Gibson T, Colohan HA et al. (1992) Risk of schizophrenia in adults born after obstetric complications and their association with early onset of illness: a controlled study. British Medical Journal 21, 305, 1256–1259.

Owen PR, Fischer EP, Booth BM et al. (1996) Medication compliance and substance abuse among patients with schizophrenia. Psychiatric Services 47, 853–858.

Parnas J, Schulsinger H (1986) Continuity of formal thought disorder from childhood to adulthood in a high risk sample. Acta Psychiatrica Scandinavica 74, 246–251.

Pearlson GD, Kim WS, Kubos KL et al. (1989) Ventricle-brain ratio, computed tomographic density, and brain area in 50 schizophrenics. Archives of General Psychiatry 46, 690–697.

Pettegrew JA, Keshavan MS, Panchalingam K et al. (1991) Alterations in brain high energy phosphate and membrane phospholipid metabolism in first episode drug naive schizophrenics. Archives of General Psychiatry 48, 563–568.

Pfefferbaum A, Lim KO, Rosenbloom M et al. (1990) Brain magnetic resonance imaging: approaches for investigating schizophrenia. Schizophrenia Bulletin 16, 453–476.

Puri BK, Barnes TR, Chapman MJ et al. (1999) Spontaneous dyskinesia in first episode schizophrenia. Journal of Neurology, Neurosurgery and Psychiatry 66, 76–78.

Ram R, Bromet EJ, Eaton WW et al. (1992) The natural course of schizophrenia: a review of first-admission studies. Schizophrenia Bulletin 18, 185–207.

Raz NR, Raz S, Bigler E (1988a) Ventriculomegaly in schizophrenia: the role of control groups and the perils of dichotomous thinking. Psychiatry Research 26, 245–248.

Raz S, Raz N, Bigler E (1988b) Ventriculomegaly in schizophrenia: is the choice of controls important? Psychiatry Research 24, 71–77.

Reiger DA, Kaelber CT, Rae DS et al. (1990) Comorbidity of mental disorders with alcohol and other drug abuse. Journal of the American Medical Association 264, 2511–2518.

Robinson DG, Woerner MG, Alvir JM et al. (1999) Predictors of treatment response from a first episode of schizophrenia or schizoaffective disorder. American Journal of Psychiatry 156, 544–549.

Salisbury DF, Shenton ME, Sherwood AR et al. (1998) First-episode schizophrenic psychosis differs from first-episode affective psychosis and controls in P300 amplitude over left temporal lobe. Archives of General Psychiatry 55, 173–180.

Sanders RD, Keshavan MS, Schooler N (1994) Neurological examination abnormalities in neuroleptic-naive patients with first-break schizophrenia: preliminary results. American Journal of Psychiatry 151, 1231–1233.

Saykin AJ, Shtasel DL, Gur RE et al. (1994) Neuropsychological deficits in neuroleptic naive patients with first-episode schizophrenia. Archives of General Psychiatry 1, 124–131.

Scottish First Episode Schizophrenia Study V. One-year follow-up. Scottish Schizophrenia Research Group. (1988) British Journal of Psychiatry 152, 470–476.

Seeman MV, Lang M (1990) The role of oestrogens in schizophrenia gender differences. Schizophrenia Bulletin 16, 185–195.

Shepherd M, Watt D, Falloon I (1989) The natural history of schizophrenia: a five-year follow-up study of outcome and prediction in a representative sample of schizophrenics. Psychological Medicine Supplement 15. Cambridge, UK: Cambridge University Press, pp. 1–46.

Smith GN, Iacono W (1986) Lateral ventricular size in schizophrenia and choice of control group. Lancet i, 1450.

Smith GN, Iacono WG, Moreau M et al. (1988) Choice of comparison group and findings of computerised tomography in schizophrenia. British Journal of Psychiatry 153, 667–674.

Smith GN, Kopala LC, Lapointe JS et al. (1998) Obstetric complications, treatment response and brain morphology in adult-onset and early-onset males with schizophrenia. Psychological Medicine 28, 645–653.

Spitzer RL, Williams JB, Gibbon M et al. (1995) Structured Clinical Interview for DSM-IV-patient edition (SCID-P). Washington, DC: American Psychiatric Press.

Sweeney JA, Haas GL, Li S (1992) Neuropsychological and eye movement abnormalities in first-episode and chronic schizophrenia. Schizophrenia Bulletin 18, 283–293.

Swofford CD, Kasckow JW, Scheller Gilkey G et al. (1996) Substance use: a powerful predictor of relapse in schizophrenia. Schizophrenia Research 20, 145–151.

Szymanski S, Lieberman JA, Alvir JM et al. (1995) Gender differences in onset of illness, treatment response, course, and biologic indexes in first-episode schizophrenic patients. American Journal of Psychiatry 152, 698–703.

Szymanski SR, Cannon TD, Gallacher F et al. (1996) Course of treatment response in first-episode and chronic schizophrenia. American Journal of Psychiatry 153, 519–525.

Tohen M, Stoll AL, Strakowski SM et al. (1992) The McLean First-Episode Psychosis Project: six-month recovery and recurrence outcome. Schizophrenia Bulletin 18, 273–282.

Verdoux H, Geddes JR, Takei N et al. (1997) Obstetric complications and age at onset in schizophrenia: an international collaborative meta-analysis of individual patient data. American Journal of Psychiatry 154, 1220–1227.

Verdoux H, Bergey C, Assens F et al. (1998) Prediction of duration of psychosis before first admission. European Psychiatry 13, 346–352.

Vita A, Dieci M, Giobbio GM et al. (1997) Time course of cerebral ventricular enlargement in schizophrenia supports the hypothesis of its neurodevelopmental nature. Schizophrenia Research 17;23, 25–30.

Waddington JL (1993) Schizophrenia: developmental neuroscience and pathobiology. Lancet 341, 531–536.

Waddington JL, Youssef H (1996) Cognitive dysfunction in chronic schizophrenia followed prospectively over 10 years and its longitudinal relationship to the emergence of tardive dyskinesia. Psychological Medicine 26, 681–688.

Walker EF, Savoie T, Davis D (1994) Neuromotor precursors of schizophrenia. Schizophrenia Bulletin 20, 441–451.

Walker EF, Lewis N, Loewy R, Palyo S (1999) Motor dysfunction and risk for schizophrenia. Journal of Neurology, Neurosurgery and Psychiatry 66, 76–78.

Watts C (1973) Review of schizophrenics in a rural practice over 26 years. British Medical Journal i, 465–469.

Weinberger DR (1995) From neuropathology to neurodevelopment. Lancet 346, 552–557.

Weinberger DR, Torrey EF, Neophytides AN et al. (1979a) Lateral cerebral ventricular enlargement in chronic schizophrenia. Archives of General Psychiatry 36, 735–739.

Weinberger DR, Torrey EF, Neophytides AN, et al. (1979b) Structural abnormalities in the cerebral cortex of chronic schizophrenic patients. Archives of General Psychiatry 36, 935–939.

Whitworth AB, Honeder M, Kremser C et al. (1998) Hippocampal volume reduction in male schizophrenic patients. Schizophrenia Research 25;31, 73–81.

Wiersma D, Nienhuis FJ, Slooff CJ et al. (1998) Natural course of schizophrenic disorders: a 15-year followup of a Dutch incidence cohort. Schizophrenia Bulletin 24, 75–85.

World Health Organization (1992) The ICD-10 Classification of Mental and Behavioural Disorders: Clinical Descriptions and Diagnostic Guidelines. Geneva: World Health Organization.

Zipursky RB, Lim KO and Pfefferbaum A (1990) Computerised volumetric assessment of cerebral asymmetry from CT scans. Psychiatry Research 35, 3571–3589.

Zipursky RB, Zhang-Wong J, Lambe EK et al. (1998) MRI correlates of treatment response in first episode psychosis. Schizophrenia Research 27, 81–90.

9

Schizophrenia at the extremes of life

Kenneth G. D. Orr[1] and David J. Castle[2]

[1]Fremantle Hospital and Health Service, Australia
[2]Mental Health Research Institute and University of Melbourne, Australia

This chapter compares and contrasts the characteristics of patients presenting for the first time with a schizophrenia-like illness at the extremes of life. Unless otherwise stated, 'childhood onset' refers to illness onset in childhood (0–12 years) and 'adolescent onset' to onset roughly between ages 13 and 18 years (Werry, 1992). The term 'early onset' is used for both childhood- and adolescent-onset schizophrenia. Very-late-onset (or 'late paraphrenia') illness is taken as onset after the age of 60 years (Roth, 1955). The chapter details the epidemiology, gender differences, phenomenology, risk factors (including premorbid functioning), outcome and treatment for early- and very-late-onset schizophrenia in turn, pointing up areas of similarity as well as important differences in these domains. This is summarized in Tables 9.1 and 9.2. In the concluding section, we address the issue of whether the similarities outweigh the differences, how far the differences can be considered merely a reflection of the same illness impinging upon the individual at different developmental/degenerative phases of life, and to what extent the differences might point to early- and very-late-onset illnesses being, in fact, discrete entities.

Methodological concerns

Research into the prevalence and incidence of schizophrenia in early life has been infrequent and often incomplete. This is a consequence, in part, of the rarity of the disorder, particularly in childhood. It also reflects the variations in diagnostic classifications and their application and the age-dependent variations in symptomatology (Werry, 1992). Kydd and Werry (1982) have discussed the effect of changing nosological constructs, which do not incorporate aetiological principles, on the defining of childhood schizophrenia. They point out that, prior to the introduction of DSM-III (American Psychiatric Association, 1980) and ICD-8 (World Health Organization, 1967), the conflation of all presumed psychotic disorders of childhood (for example, autism and early-onset schizophrenia) into one category

Table 9.1. A comparison of early- and very-late-onset schizophrenia

	Early onset	Very late onset (>60 years)
Gender	Males>females (especially childhood onset)	Females≥males
Phenomenology	Positive, negative and disorganized symptoms all seen. Negative symptoms often prominent. Formal thought disorder common	Florid persecutory delusions; prominent hallucinations; negative symptoms and formal thought disorder rare
Premorbid functioning	Impairment across multiple domains, including social and educational	Poor social adjustment common, but premorbid occupational functioning usually unimpaired
Longitudinal course	Poor social and occupational outcome	Good preservation of affect and personality. Social outcome often impaired; few progress to dementia
Response to antipsychotic medication	Positive symptoms respond but often partially. Treatment resistance common	Positive symptoms usually respond

muddied any reasonable epidemiological approach. Häfner and Nowotny (1995) articulated the logistic difficulties of studying early-onset schizophrenia. For prospective studies, the need to screen large populations with broad inclusion criteria to ascertain cases presenting with nonspecific prodromal symptoms, as well as the need for adequate, regular follow-up, entails great costs and much endeavour.

Studies of very-late-onset schizophrenia have been impeded by changes over time in nosology and age cut-offs, and by a general reluctance, expressly in the USA, to consider that schizophrenia can indeed manifest for the first time in late life. Comparisons of studies in this population are hampered by differences in diagnostic criteria employed, age cut-offs and mode of ascertainment (e.g. hospitalized samples versus case registers).

Prevalence rates

Early-onset schizophrenia

Although rare, it has been recognized for over a century that schizophrenia at an early age exists. In his clinical sample of 1054 patients with dementia praecox, Kraepelin (1919) ascertained 3.5% had an onset before the age of 10, and 2.7% between 10 and 15 years. Beitchman (1985) estimated that the treated prevalence of schizophrenia with onset before 15 years of age was one-fiftieth the treated

Table 9.2. Putative risk factors for early- and very-late-onset schizophrenia

Putative risk factor	Early onset	Very late onset (>60 years)
Genetic	++ FH schizophrenia	+ FH schizophrenia + FH depression in some studies
Sensory impairment		+ Expressly unadjusted visual and hearing
Social isolation	+ Often consequent upon prodrome or illness itself	++ Often antedates illness onset
Premorbid personality	Shy/withdrawn; schizotypal	+ Paranoid/schizoid traits
Pregnancy and birth complications	+ Associated with early onset, expressly in males*; limited data in childhood onset	No unequivocal evidence of an association
Structural brain abnormalities	++ Grey matter reduction, generally considered to antedate illness onset; some evidence of progressive changes*	± White matter changes (probably artifactual) + Grey matter volume reduction, similar to those in early-onset schizophrenia
Neurocognitive impairment	Diffuse impairment; possibly more pronounced in attention, memory and executive function*	Diffuse impairment; nonspecific*

Notes:
FH, family history; +, positive, ++, strong positive. * Denotes that findings are based on very few studies.

prevalence of the later-onset probands. However, this is possibly an overestimate (Nicolson and Rapoport, 2000).

Gillberg (2001) emphasizes the rarity of childhood-onset schizophrenia. Using data from two population studies of autism prevalence in North Dakota (Burd et al., 1987) and western Sweden (Gillberg, 1984), the rates of childhood schizophrenia are estimated at 1.9 and 1.6 in 100 000 children, respectively. A nationwide register-based study from Denmark looking at all inpatients first diagnosed with schizophrenia confirmed the rarity of early-onset schizophrenia; indeed, only 4 and 28 probands under the age of 13 years and 15 years, respectively, received the initial diagnosis over a period of 24 years from a population of some 5 million (Thomsen, 1996). In a German population-based study (Häfner and Nowotny, 1995) ascertaining all admissions for schizophrenia over a 2-year period in a catchment population of about 1.5 million, admissions for schizophrenia before the age of 12 years were reported to 'hardly occur'.

Very-late-onset schizophrenia

It was Roth (1955) who placed very-late-onset schizophrenia on the modern psychiatric map, identifying a group of patients with florid delusions and hallucinations, but with good preservation of affect and personality, whose first onset of illness occurred usually after the age of 60. He coined the term 'late paraphrenia' for this group of patients and demonstrated a far more favourable outcome than for age-matched patients with dementia.

Harris and Jeste (1988) have reviewed the published literature on proportions of patients with schizophrenia who had a first onset of illness in late life. Despite methodological difficulties, they computed weighted mean proportions (weighting on sample size) of schizophrenia patients with a first onset after the age of around 40 years to be 23.5%, with subanalyses showing that, of late-onset cases (mostly after 40), 57.5% first manifested the illness in their fifth decade, 30.2% in their sixth decade, and 12.3% after age 60; this translates as 13%, 7%, and 3%, respectively, of all schizophrenia patients.

More recently, Castle and Murray (1993) reported rates for nonaffective psychotic disorders across all ages at onset, using data from the Camberwell Cumulative Case Register, a register of all contacts with psychiatric services from a defined inner-city London catchment area. In that study, fully 12% had their first onset of illness after age 60, with a rate of illness for DSM-III-R schizophrenia (American Psychiatric Association, 1987) being of the order of 12 per 100 000 population per year.

The discrepancy in reported rates for very-late-onset schizophrenia reflects discrepancies in definition of illness and methodological problems such as case finding; such individuals are often reclusive and paranoid, yet well preserved in terms of self-care, and are thus unlikely to come to the attention of psychiatric services. Also, such cases have often been excluded from epidemiological studies of schizophrenia and related disorders (see Castle, 1999). However, it is clear that a schizophrenia-like illness can manifest for the first time in very late life, and that the number of such cases is not trivial.

Gender differences

It is received wisdom that the lifetime morbid risk of schizophrenia is the same for males and females, albeit that males tend to have an earlier mean onset. However, it is not usually appreciated that the age-at-onset distributions for men and women with schizophrenia differ markedly from each other (see Castle et al., 1998 and Ch. 7).

In terms of the extremes of life, most studies of childhood-onset schizophrenia reveal a male excess, with ratios of the order of 2:1 to 2.5:1 (Werry and McClellan,

1992; McClellan et al., 1993). Loranger (1984) found that 7 of 100 consecutive male admissions with a DSM-III diagnosis of schizophrenia were first treated before the age of 11, compared with only 1 of 100 females. Kolvin et al. (1971a) reported a male to female ratio of 2.66:1 for childhood-onset schizophrenia, while Spencer and Campbell (1994) reported that 12 of 16 schizophrenic children with an onset of illness at less than 12 years of age were male.

However, some other studies have revealed no gender difference, or even an excess of females, amongst adolescent-onset cases of schizophrenia (Kydd and Werry, 1982; Yang et al., 1995) In part, this inconsistency may be caused by a pubertal effect in females. Indeed, Kraepelin (1919) noted an excess of males (2.4:1) in those with an onset of dementia praecox before 10 years of age but concluded that both sexes are affected in the same degree in those aged 10–15 years. In more modern studies, Hollis (1995) reported, in a sample of 61 schizophrenic patients, that the male to female ratio for the childhood-onset group (7–13) was 2.6:1 compared with 0.9:1 for the adolescent-onset group (14–17), while Galdos et al. (1993) reported a nonsignificant excess of female schizophrenia or paranoia in the age group 10–14 years.

One proposition to explain this seeming disparity in gender difference between childhood and adolescent onset reflects the propensity for boys in the later age range to display more conduct disturbance. Häfner and Nowotny (1995) conjectured that studies relying on case ascertainment from psychiatric services alone will miss a proportion of male schizophrenic patients who have been diverted into the criminal justice system.

What is more consistently reported is that very-late-onset schizophrenia is essentially a female disorder (reviewed by Castle, 1999). This female preponderance is not merely a reflection of the relative longevity in women and presumably reflects underlying differences in the ageing process as it affects male and female brains. In particular, it has been suggested that the slower rate of loss of dopamine D_2 receptors in the female brain, compared with the male, could account, in part at least, for this excess, as well as for the particular susceptibility of elderly females to the dyskinetic side effects of antipsychotic medications.

Phenomenology

Early-onset schizophrenia

Symptoms identified during the active phase of the schizophrenic illness in children and adolescents include hallucinations, delusions and disorder of thought form. Distinguishing these symptoms may be a formidable task in the young child, particularly in the presence of developmental delays in language or cognition. Therefore, diagnosis based on phenomenological grounds alone is insufficient, and clarification is reliant on consideration of intellectual level, specific developmental disorders, organicity and the psychosocial context (Parry-Jones, 1991).

Auditory hallucinations appear to be a common symptom (about 80% of affected children) and include the classic Schneiderian types (Russell et al., 1989). Visual and tactile hallucinations are less frequent. However, hallucinations can occur in children and adolescents with nonpsychotic disorders (Garralda, 1985), which can lead to possible misdiagnosis (McClellan and Werry, 1994).

Delusional beliefs are present in just over half of reported cases of childhood-onset schizophrenia (Kolvin et al., 1971b; Russell et al., 1989; Werry et al., 1991; Green et al., 1992). Delusional content of various themes has been described and their complexity varies with the maturational stage of the patient.

Formal thought disorder can be identified and is often present in the older child and adolescent with schizophrenia (Kolvin, 1971; Russell et al., 1989; Green et al., 1992; Caplan, 1994); its identification in the younger child, and in the presence of significant developmental language disorder and autistic features, can be problematic (Volkmar et al., 1988). It appears that the quality of the thought disorder, certainly in adolescent-onset schizophrenia, is similar to that manifested by adult schizophrenia patients (Makowski et al., 1997).

Negative symptoms are readily identifiable in childhood-onset schizophrenia, with inappropriate or blunted affect being described in the majority (Kolvin et al., 1971b; Russell et al., 1989; Werry et al., 1991; Spencer and Campbell, 1994). Indeed, the prevalence of negative symptoms is probably higher than in adult-onset schizophrenia (Yang et al., 1995) and certainly far higher than in very-late-onset schizophrenia (see below). Furthermore, the negative symptoms tend to show temporal stability and to be predictive of poor outcome (Remschmidt et al., 1994; Maziade et al., 1996a).

Very-late-onset schizophrenia

The original phenomenological descriptions of late paraphrenia patients by Roth (1955) and by Kay and Roth (1961) have been validated in numerous subsequent studies. The classical presentation is of florid persecutory beliefs with prominent hallucinations in the setting of preserved personality. So-called 'partition' delusions are particularly common (Howard et al., 1992). In contrast, negative symptoms such as affective flattening are rarely seen, while formal thought disorder is almost never found.

Pearlson et al. (1989) compared early- and late-onset patients with each other, as well as with early age-at-onset patients who had grown old. The late-onset group was more likely than their younger counterparts, and the early-onset elderly group, to exhibit visual, tactile and auditory hallucinations and persecutory delusions, but less likely to show affective flattening and formal thought disorder. Therefore, the phenomenological differences are not merely a consequence of the ageing process itself and might reflect true differences in underlying pathophysiology.

Risk factors

Genetic

A genetic basis to schizophrenia is well established (McGuffin et al., 1995; see also Chs. 10 and 11), but it is unlikely that the magnitude of genetic contribution for all cases is uniform. Indeed, it is probable that the risk of schizophrenia is contributed to by a number of genes of small effect (Cardno and McGuffin, 1996). It is possible that a greater dose of such genes would cause earlier clinical manifestation. This concept of a genetic dose effect would stipulate that very-early-onset schizophrenia has a stronger familial basis than the adult forms. Earlier work in this regard, which does suggest increased familiality in such cases (Kolvin et al., 1971a), is marred by methodological deficits such as the lack of blind assessments of the relatives and lack of use of structured diagnostic assessments. The Roscommon family study (Kendler et al., 1996) did not find that early age of onset characterized a group of probands with higher genetic liability. However, McGlashan and Fenton (1991), in their thorough review, concluded that the nonparanoid, earlier-onset types of schizophrenia were associated with a greater familial risk than the later-onset paranoid subtype. Pulver et al. (1990) reported an increase of familial risk in those whose disease onset was before 17 years of age, while Sham and colleagues (1994) demonstrated increased familial risk of schizophrenia in first-degree relatives in patients with an early onset of illness (<22 years). In a population-based study using nationwide registers, Suvisaari and colleagues (1998) demonstrated that early onset of schizophrenia is associated with high familial loading for the disorder. It would appear that currently the balance of evidence favours an association between familial risk and early-onset schizophrenia.

One tenable speculation is that there is an increased rate of chromosomal anomalies underpinning schizophrenia phenocopies that could appear as an early-onset disorder. It has been suggested that 22q11 deletion syndrome represents an identifiable subtype of schizophrenia (Bassett and Chow, 1999) and that this could be associated with an early onset of the disorder (Gothelf et al., 1999). In an ongoing study of childhood-onset schizophrenia at the US National Institute of Mental Health (NIMH), 5 of 47 probands exhibited cytogenetic abnormalities, including one with a sex chromosome anomaly (Kumra et al., 1998; Nicolson et al., 1999a). These authors conjecture that in certain individuals cytogenetic abnormalities may lead to an earlier age of onset of schizophrenia because they predispose brain development to greater susceptibility to added pathogenic factors, which interact to result in the disorder.

The study of familial aggregation in very-late-onset schizophrenia has been bedevilled by problems of case ascertainment and diagnostic vagaries, and the fact that many first-degree relatives will have died before going through the entire period of risk for the illness (if late-onset itself 'breeds true'). Despite these methodological pitfalls, most studies of very-late-onset schizophrenia tend to show an elevated risk for schizophrenia amongst relatives, though the degree of risk varies from study to study and mostly the studies do not include control subjects (reviewed by Castle and Howard, 1992). In one of the few prospective controlled family studies of very-late-onset schizophrenia, Howard et al. (1997) collected information on psychiatric morbidity in 269 first-degree relatives of 47 probands with late paraphrenia (onset after age 60) and compared the findings with data from 272 first-degree relatives of 42 age-matched well controls. The relatives of the late paraphrenia group did not differ from those of their well controls in terms of risk for schizophrenia, but they did show a significantly elevated risk ($p = 0.003$) of depression. Although this finding may raise the possibility of genetic heterogeneity in this particular group of disorders, many other studies have revealed a great deal of overlap between schizophrenia and affective disorders.

Pregnancy and birth complications

There is a robust relationship of small effect between pregnancy and birth complications (PBCs) generally and the development of schizophrenia (Geddes and Lawrie, 1995; see Ch. 5). PBCs might be a stronger risk factor in patients with an earlier age of onset (O'Callaghan et al., 1992; Verdoux et al., 1997; Smith et al., 1998; Rosso et al., 2000), particularly in males (McGrath and Murray, 1995; Kirov et al., 1996). A significant association has been reported between PBCs and males who exhibit the stigmata of the neurodevelopmental form: cognitive deficits, premorbid abnormalities and negative symptoms (Rifkin et al., 1994). In an elegant population-based, nested case-control study investigating patients first presenting with psychosis between the ages of 15 and 21 years (Hultman et al., 1999), the authors found that bleeding in pregnancy and multiparity were associated with a three- to fourfold increased risk for schizophrenia in males. It is the neurotoxic effects of fetal hypoxia caused by certain PBCs that may prove to be the common pathological mechanism engendering this increased risk for early-onset schizophrenia (Rosso et al., 2000).

Two recent studies have looked specifically at the association between PBCs and childhood-onset schizophrenia. In a case-control study of 36 patients using sibling comparisons, no significant difference was found between the groups in rates of PBCs (Nicolson et al., 1999b). However, in an epidemiological case-control study from Japan (Matsumoto et al., 1999) where 33 patients with childhood-onset schizophrenia aged between 8 and 13 years were compared with a control group of children with anxiety disorders, there was a significant association between PBCs and the development of schizophrenia in childhood. They found that the odds ratio for the risk of the development of schizophrenia associated with PBCs was 3.5 (95% confidence interval (CI) 1.30–9.10). This association was greatest for males, where the risk for the development of schizophrenia was about six times greater than for those male children without a history of PBCs. The authors suggest tentatively that their results are compatible with the conjecture that patients with early-onset schizophrenia are more likely to have a history of PBCs than those with a late onset.

PBCs have not, to our knowledge, been systematically investigated in very-late-onset schizophrenia. In one of the few comparative studies, Castle et al. (1997) found that 14.1% of early-onset ($<$25 years) schizophrenics had a history of PBCs, compared with only 4.5% of those with onset after age 60 (relative risk 0.29; 95% CI 0.03–2.29). These data were collected from case records and the findings require replication, but they are compatible with other studies (see above) which suggest that PBCs are a risk factor for an early onset of disorder (see Verdoux et al., 1997).

Developmental risk factors

Delayed milestones, and neuromotor and verbal dysfunction, have been described in preschizophrenic children compared with other groups (Jones et al., 1994; Walker et al., 1994; see Ch. 6). A number of studies suggest such abnormalities might be particularly common in those with an early onset of illness. For example, Hollis (1995) reported a higher risk of premorbid social, motor and language impairment in a sample of childhood- and adolescent-onset schizophrenics, compared with controls; the impairment was most marked in the childhood-onset group. Features of pervasive developmental delay, and language abnormalities, have also been noted in childhood-onset schizophrenia (Alaghband et al., 1995). Morice and Ingram (1983) showed that, compared with schizophrenia patients with a later onset of illness, those with adolescent onset showed reduced syntactic complexity of verbal language. Russell et al. (1989) noted that a quarter of their sample of children with schizophrenia had exhibited various autistic symptoms premorbidly. Recent work indicates an excess of neuromotor abnormalities in children with schizophrenia (see Jacobsen and Rapoport, 1998).

Preliminary findings from the Maudsley Early Onset Schizophrenia Study (Frangou, 1999) indicate that patients with early-onset schizophrenia (mean age at onset of first psychotic symptoms was 14 years) experienced significantly more family adversity and language problems (one-third of the sample) compared with matched healthy controls.

Premorbid social adjustment and personality

Early-onset schizophrenic subjects have often exhibited premorbid abnormal socialization. Werry et al. (1994) reported that over 50% of their childhood- and adolescent-onset schizophrenia subjects exhibited moderate to severe premorbid personality disorder, most commonly of the odd/eccentric type. Of course, such a label is questionable in such young subjects and might reflect prodromal symptoms or be an indication of the broader cerebral dysfunction noted in many such cases (see below). As a result, these features cannot readily be accepted as risk factors but rather serve as early (and nonspecific) developmental markers for the disorder.

Premorbid personality in very-late-onset schizophrenia is often described in terms that include reclusiveness, hostility and suspiciousness (see Castle and Howard, 1992). Of course, retrospective assessment of personality is difficult, but one would presume a proportion would fulfil criteria for paranoid or schizoid personality disorder. What is striking, however, is that mostly individuals with late-onset schizophrenia exhibited good premorbid educational and occupational achievement, in marked contrast to many of their early-onset counterparts. Whether this reflects the developmental stage at which the illness manifests or is a marker of different disease processes is not clear. Indeed, Retterstol (1968) stated that psychotic decompensation is an 'understandable transition' in individuals with such a personality structure, while Post (1966), amongst others, suggested that such personality traits are an attenuated manifestation of the underlying illness.

Sensory impairment

We are not aware of any robust findings of an association between sensory impairment and early-onset schizophrenia, but an association between very-late-onset schizophrenia and sensory impairment has been reported by a number of different authors. Prager and Jeste (1993) reviewed 27 published studies examining a possible association between sensory impairment and late-life psychosis. Most of these studies supported an association, but most had serious methodological problems, including the lack of age-matched nonpsychiatric control subjects. In their own case-control study, Prager and Jeste (1993) found an excess of 'corrected' visual and hearing impairment in late-onset schizophrenia patients, but not of uncorrected (constitutional) visual acuity or pure-tone audiometry. This makes interpretation of causality difficult, and the exact mechanism whereby sensory impairment contributes to very-late-onset psychosis (and not to early-onset disorder) is unclear.

Social isolation

Social isolation is often a consequence of either the premorbid or the prodromal symptoms of schizophrenia, or of the illness itself. Thus, negative symptoms lead to a lack of the will to socialize, while positive symptoms such as persecutory beliefs may lead to the individual avoiding others. Bizarre, disorganized and erratic behaviour, as well as stigma and social ostracism, also contributes to family dislocation and social isolation in schizophrenia at any time of life. Of particular interest in very-late-onset schizophrenia is whether social isolation might itself contribute to the risk of the disorder. Certainly, a history of social isolation often antedates the onset of illness, compatible with the notion that many such individuals have underlying paranoid/schizoid personality structures. However, the illness itself, as outlined above, might also cause or at least contribute to the social isolation. Sensory impairment might also play a part. Consequently, cause and effect are difficult to disentangle, and social isolation of itself should probably not be considered a major independent causal factor for the disorder.

Structural brain abnormalities
Early-onset schizophrenia

Neuroimaging studies in childhood-onset schizophrenia have been relatively sparse and beset by methodological shortcomings (Findling et al., 1995). Earlier work indicated the presence of a variety of brain abnormalities, which have also been documented in adult-onset schizophrenia. These include enlarged ventricles (Schultz et al., 1983), enlarged third ventricular volume and cerebellar abnormalities (Woody et al., 1987). Preliminary results from the Maudsley Early Onset Schizophrenia Study reveal that patients with early-onset schizophrenia had smaller cerebral, frontal lobe and hippocampal volumes compared with normal controls (Frangou, 1999).

The NIMH childhood-onset schizophrenia project aims to study brain morphology in this group in a more systematic way. If childhood and adolescent schizophrenia on the whole represents rare but contiguous manifestations of adult-onset schizophrenia then it would be expected that there would be similar structural abnormalities that may evidence progression over time. Brain magnetic resonance imaging on 21 patients with childhood-onset schizophrenia showed significantly smaller cerebral volumes and midsagittal thalamic areas, and probable larger lateral ventricles, than healthy controls (Frazier et al., 1996). A striking negative correlation between total cerebral volume and negative symptom score was also reported (Alaghband et al., 1997). Follow-up scanning after 2 years and approximately 4 years has demonstrated progression of these changes during adolescence, with these differential changes tapering off as the probands approach adulthood (mean age 19.4 years) (Rapoport et al., 1997; Jacobsen et al., 1998; Giedd et al., 1999).

The progressive changes reported have not been seen consistently in longitudinal studies of adult probands. The interpretation of this finding warrants some caution. This NIMH sample was refractory to the therapeutic effects of typical neuroleptics and thus may intrinsically have a more severe form of the illness. Furthermore, there is shifting sample size across the studies and it is not clear whether the effect of subject dropout over time was statistically accounted for. Nevertheless, it may be that research in this early-onset group will provide a window into the pathophysiology of schizophrenia and demonstrates the possibility of a limited neurodegenerative process.

Very-late-onset schizophrenia

In very-late-onset schizophrenia, neuroimaging studies have mostly concentrated on two relatively discrete phenomena, namely specific white matter changes and grey matter volumetric analysis. For the former, a number of studies have suggested an excess of white matter abnormalities in the brains of individuals with late-onset schizophrenia. This is felt to be indicative of underlying cerebral damage, mostly vascular in aetiology. However, if vascular risk factors are fastidiously controlled for, there is no true excess of such abnormalities in this group of patients, teasing at the (false) organic/functional dichotomy (Howard et al., 1995).

Probably more pertinent to the current discourse is the finding, in at least some patients with late-onset schizophrenia, of generalized volumetric brain abnormalities, notably of superior temporal gyrus (see Barta et al., 1997), akin to those found in early-onset schizophrenia patients (see above). In one of the few comparative neuroimaging studies, Pearlson et al. (1993) found similar structural abnormalities in early- and late-onset schizophrenia patients. In reviewing this somewhat conflicting literature, Pearlson (1999) concluded that emerging data support the concept that patients with early- and late-onset schizophrenia share common structural 'brain abnormalities'. The potential theoretic implications for this conclusion are detailed below.

Neurocognitive impairment

Cognitive deficits have been consistently documented in schizophrenia, but the precise nature is yet to be delineated. Findings suggest that there is an underperformance on a wide array of cognitive tasks, but that certain domains, such as attention and memory (Aleman et al., 1999), and executive performance (Goldberg et al., 1995; Goldberg and Gold, 1995) are particularly impaired.

Early-onset schizophrenia

There is persuasive evidence that preschizophrenic children have developmental trajectories that are partially shaped by underlying cognitive deficits (Jones et al., 1993, 1994). A tenable premise holds that the onset of a schizophrenic illness during childhood or adolescence is associated with more severe and/or widespread neuropsychological deviation (Fish, 1977), which may evidence limited progressive deterioration. Goldberg et al. (1988), showed lower performance intelligence quotient (IQ) scores in adolescents with psychosis than in nonpsychotic controls, while the verbal IQ was comparable in the two groups. Hoff et al. (1996), in a study of 49 patients with chronic schizophrenia, demonstrated earlier age at onset of illness to be associated with poor cognitive performance involving motor and language domains. Of course, such findings are confounded by the disruption to learning and education that an early onset of illness imposes.

A study by Basso et al. (1997) found a generalized pattern of neuropsychological deficits and diffuse cerebral dysfunction in adult patients with chronic schizophrenia of adolescent onset, which was more severe than both the adult-onset and control group. Performances were particularly poor on measures of memory and executive function. Early results from the ongoing Maudsley Early Onset Schizophrenia Study also demonstrate the presence of wide-ranging deficits in intelligence, executive function and memory (Kravariti et al., 1999). The possibility of a more specific impairment of verbal memory is being considered. Nevertheless, conclusions regarding the evidence for specific neurocognitive impairment, other than IQ, in adolescent-onset schizophrenia is hampered by the small number of published studies and the fact that they use different tasks and methodology. What is crucial in researching this area is to take into account the fact that an early-onset illness causes early disruption to educational and social development (Häfner et al., 1998).

Data specifically from childhood-onset cohorts are sparse, though difficulties in attention and information processing have been identified in such patients (Asarnow and Sherman, 1984). Asarnow and colleagues (1994a) have suggested that neuropsychological dysfunction in children with schizophrenia is contiguous with impairment in adult-onset disorder, and that the underpinning deficit is one of information processing. Neuropsychological examination of a group of children from the NIMH study with treatment-resistant very-early-onset schizophrenia (Kumra et al., 2000) indicated a pattern of cognitive deficits, including deficits in attention, learning, and abstraction, that is contiguous with that reported in adult-onset schizophrenia. These findings are tentative, given the numbers in this study were small and there was no normal control group.

Very-late-onset schizophrenia

In very-late-onset schizophrenia, there are only a handful of controlled studies reporting systematic neuropsychological testing. Almeida et al. (1995) subjected 40 very-late-onset schizophrenic patients and 33 age-matched controls to a battery of neuropsychological tests and found impairment in the patient group across all tasks, even though they were matched on premorbid IQ and schooling. The pattern of impairment was quite different from that found in patients with Alzheimer or

Lewy body dementia but was very similar to that seen in early-onset schizophrenia (see above). This again begs the question of how similar or different early- and very-late-onset schizophrenia are, in terms of aetiopathology.

Longitudinal course and outcome

Early-onset schizophrenia

As discussed earlier, historical variations in classification of childhood-onset schizophrenia, and a relative paucity of extended follow-up studies with adequate numbers, mar a robust characterization of the longitudinal course. Furthermore, a potential confounding factor is initial misdiagnosis (McClellan et al., 1993). In one study, over 50% of children who had an eventual mood disorder were initially diagnosed as having schizophrenia (Werry et al., 1991). In a 10-year follow-up study (Thomsen, 1996), 209 children and adolescents initially diagnosed as having schizophrenia before age of 18 were deemed later to have personality disorders (primarily antisocial and borderline).

However, when probands are subjected to systematic sampling and independent best-estimate consensus diagnosis, there is greater diagnostic stability; in one such study, for example, only 1 out of 77 subjects received an adult diagnosis of a bipolar disorder (Maziade et al., 1996b). These differences in classification (including rates of misdiagnosis), sampling and duration of follow-up may explain some of the variations in reported outcome for those with early-onset schizophrenia. Outcomes reported have ranged from poor in several (Werry et al., 1991; McClellan et al., 1993; Schmidt et al., 1995; Maziade et al., 1996b) to those where the risk of chronicity is comparable with adult-onset schizophrenia (Eggers, 1978; Asarnow et al., 1994b; Eggers and Bunk, 1997).

Eggers (1978), in a 15-year follow-up of 71 schizophrenia patients aged 7–13 years, found that onset of illness before age of 10 was associated with a particularly poor outcome. Twenty per cent of the original sample was excluded from analysis as they did not exhibit adult schizophrenic symptoms. Furthermore, Eggers and Bunk (1997) reported a remarkable 42-year follow-up on the same population confirming the correlation of poor outcome with earlier age of onset, as well as noting an insidious type of onset that was more common with the early age. The small numbers precluded statistical assessment for causal predominance of these two factors in this sample.

Cawthorn and colleagues (1994), in their retrospective follow-up of 58 psychotic adolescents over a mean of 7.7 years, demonstrated the very poor outcome of those diagnosed initially with schizophrenia in comparison with those with bipolar and schizoaffective disorders. In an 11-year follow-up study looking specifically at adolescent-onset schizophrenia (ages 14 to 18), a high proportion (50%) developed a chronic course (Krausz and Muller-Thomsen, 1993).

In summary, outcome in early-onset and particularly childhood-onset schizophrenia is generally poorer over a range of indices than adult forms of the disorder and other childhood psychiatric disorders. Poor outcome appears also to be associated with premorbid dysfunction (Eggers, 1978; Werry et al., 1991; Werry, 1992; Schmidt et al., 1995; Maziade et al., 1996a) and with an insidious type of onset (Asarnow and Ben-Meir, 1988; Werry and McClellan, 1992) One potential confounder is that high familial loading for schizophrenia, which is associated with an early onset, is also associated with a poorer outcome (Suvisaari et al., 1998). At this stage, one cannot delineate the relative contribution to this poorer outcome of either the genetically determined factors of the illness, which may directly rift development of specific cerebral pathways (DeLisi, 1992), or the disruptive effects that an illness's early onset has on the social and psychological development (Häfner and Nowotny, 1995). It could well be that it is the dynamic, complex interaction of such factors during this dense maturational period that causes significant deviation from the expected developmental trajectory and also hampers the parallel development of protective factors, which in turn amplifies the pathoplastic effect.

Very-late-onset schizophrenia

With respect to very-late-onset patients, the longitudinal course of illness is one of the major pointers to such patients not merely having dementia. Indeed, Roth's (1955) landmark study showed a very much worse outcome, in terms of cognitive functioning and mortality, for dementia patients than for those with very-late-onset schizophrenia. However, some such patients do have a poor prognosis in this regard, suggestive of underlying 'organic' pathology. For example, the follow-up study of Holden (1987) found that a subgroup of patients with very-late-onset schizophrenia does have an 'organic' form of illness, with a relatively poor outcome.

Treatment issues

Early-onset schizophrenia

There is a paucity of controlled treatment trials in early-onset schizophrenia. Management should entail a multimodal approach that considers the judicious use of appropriate drug therapy, cognitive and psychotherapeutic strategies, behavioural modification procedures and family intervention (McClellan and Werry, 1994; Clark and Lewis, 1998). Furthermore, there may be comorbid learning and developmental problems that would need to be addressed through the implementation of a comprehensive educational programme. It is essential to consider issues of valid consent in relation to the developmental stage of the young patient (Clark and Lewis, 1998).

Antipsychotic drugs are a mainstay in the treatment of early-onset schizophrenia. The limited evidence available from controlled studies indicates the efficacy of typical neuroleptics (Pool et al., 1976; Realmuto et al., 1984; Spencer and Campbell, 1994). However, untoward effects are common, with high rates of EPS (extrapyramidal side effects) associated with the higher potency typical antipsychotics (haloperidol, loxapine) and sedation and postural hypotension with the lower potency antipsychotics (thioridazine).

There are data to support the clinical impression that an early age of onset is associated with both an increased sensitivity to EPS (Lewis, 1998) and a suboptimal response to typical antipsychotics (Meltzer et al., 1997). This has prompted the increasing use of atypical neuroleptics (Toren et al., 1998). However, further research is vital to investigate both the short- and the long-term safety and efficacy of these atypical drugs (Toren et al., 1998; Campbell et al., 1999) as well as to determine optimal dose ranges (Lewis, 1998). What is of interest is whether or not there is superior efficacy compared with typical neuroleptics and if there is a specific role for the various atypical antipsychotics such as risperidone and olanzapine in treatment-resistant early-onset schizophrenia. Clozapine has a demonstrated efficacy in this latter regard, but clinical application may be limited by a significant side effect burden, leading to a high dropout rate (Kumra et al., 1996).

Late-onset schizophrenia

With late-onset schizophrenia, it is imperative that adequate psychiatric and physical examinations be undertaken to exclude recognizable causes and to delineate comorbid physical illness. For example, the possibility of visual and auditory impairment should be investigated and appropriately remedied. Psychopharmacological therapy with antipsychotic medication forms the core approach in the treatment of very-late-onset schizophrenia. Available studies (mainly open studies) demonstrate efficacy in reducing both acute psychotic symptoms and relapse rates (Howard et al., 2000). Pearlson and colleagues (1989) reported complete or partial response of symptoms to traditional antipsychotics in 76% of 54 patients with very-late-onset schizophrenia. However, it would appear that in this population there is an increased sensitivity to side effects such as tardive dyskinesia (Jeste et al., 1999a). Age-related pharmacodynamic and pharmacokinetic changes require that drug treatment should commence at very low doses and increase with increments made gently and with caution. In view of their advantages in terms of side effects, the value of the atypical neuroleptics such as olanzapine, risperidone and possibly quetiapine as the mainstay initial drug treatment is being established (Jeste et al., 1999b; Howard et al., 2000), but further evaluation is required. The role and efficacy of nonpharmacological approaches, including psychological intervention, needs to be further investigated but is advocated as an essential component in the context of the wider therapeutic relationship (Aguera-Ortiz and Renes-Prieto, 1999).

Conclusions

Our main findings from the literature review are detailed in Tables 9.1 and 9.2. In terms of clinical manifestation of illness (Table 9.1), the similarities between the early and very-late-onset disorders are, in part at least, a reflection of case ascertainment itself, in that 'psychosis' is generally defined in terms of positive symptoms of delusions and hallucinations; therefore, the fact that both groups of patients tend to manifest such symptoms is hardly surprising. Of more interest, perhaps, are the differences between the two groups of patients in clinical manifestation of illness. For example, the rarity of negative and disorganization symptoms in very-late-onset schizophrenics is suggestive of a more benign form of disorder and/or might reflect rather different underlying aetiopathological processes from those in the early-onset group. Why so-called 'partition' delusions should be so much more common in the very-late-onset patients is again potentially instructive in this way.

Other clinical differences between the two onset groups might well reflect the life stage at which the disorder first manifests, rather than being reflective of true differences in disease process itself. For example, poor occupational and social outcomes in patients with the very-early-onset disease is hardly surprising given that the illness occurs before realisation of educational, vocational and social potential, and the disease process has a profound impact on those domains.

The aetiological parameters that tend to be more or less common at the extremes of life (Table 9.2) are of particular interest, though it must be acknowledged that many of the conclusions that can be drawn are tentative in that there are few methodologically sound comparison studies of such parameters across the ages. The fact that genetic risk appears to be higher in early-onset schizophrenia might either reflect a 'more genetic' subtype of illness or be a result of genes serving to influence age-at-onset itself. The excess of PBCs in the early-onset group might be interpreted in a similar way, or they might merely serve to 'bring forward' the onset of an illness that might otherwise only have manifested in late life (if at all). In the late-onset group, the coaggregation of a number of 'hits' (e.g. sensory deficits, social isolation, mild cerebral degeneration) might all be required to tip the less genetically prone individual into manifesting psychotic symptoms.

We believe that individuals who first manifest a schizophrenia-like illness at the extremes of life should not be dismissed as esoteric rarities. Indeed, detailed comparative studies of these groups of patients can enhance our understanding of schizophrenia at any age.

REFERENCES

Aguera-Ortiz L, Renes-Prieto B (1999) The place of non-biological treatments. In: Late Onset Schizophrenia, Howard R, Rabins P, Castle DJ, eds. Hampshire, UK: Wrightson Biomedical, pp. 233–260.

Alaghband RJ, McKenna K, Gordon CT et al. (1995) Childhood-onset schizophrenia: the severity of premorbid course. Journal of the American Academy of Child and Adolescent Psychiatry 34, 1273–1283.

Alaghband RJ, Hamburger SD, Giedd JN, Frazier JA, Rapoport JL (1997) Childhood-onset schizophrenia: biological markers in relation to clinical characteristics. American Journal of Psychiatry 154, 64–68.

Aleman A, Hijman R, de Haan EHF, Kahn RS (1999) Memory impairment in schizophrenia: a meta-analysis. American Journal of Psychiatry 156, 1358–1366.

Almeida OP, Howard RJ, Levy R, David AS, Morris RG, Sahakian BJ (1995) Cognitive features of psychotic states arising in late life (late paraphrenia). Psychological Medicine 25, 685–698.

American Psychiatric Association (1980) Diagnostic and Statistical Manual of Mental Disorders, 3rd edn. Washington, DC: American Psychiatric Press.

American Psychiatric Association (1987) Diagnostic and Statistical Manual of Mental Disorders III – Revised. Washington, DC: American Psychiatric Press.

Asarnow JR, Ben-Meir S (1988) Children with schizophrenia spectrum disorders: a comparative study of onset patterns, premorbid adjustment, and severity of dysfunction. Journal of Child Psychology and Psychiatry 29, 477–488.

Asarnow RF, Sherman T (1984) Studies of visual information processing in schizophrenic children. Child Development 55, 249–261.

Asarnow RF, Asamen J, Granholm E, Sherman T, Watkins JM, Williams ME (1994a) Cognitive/ neuropsychological studies of children with a schizophrenic disorder. Schizophrenia Bulletin 20, 647–669.

Asarnow RJ, Tomson MC, Goldstein MG (1994b) Childhood-onset schizophrenia: a follow-up study. Schizophrenia Bulletin 20, 599–617.

Barta PE, Powers RE, Aylward EH et al. (1997) Quantitative MRI volume changes in late onset schizophrenia and Alzheimer's disease patients compared to normal controls. Psychiatry Research 68, 65–75.

Bassett AS, Chow EWC (1999) 22q11 deletion syndrome: a genetic subtype of schizophrenia. Biological Psychiatry 46, 882–891.

Basso MR, Nasrallah HA, Olson SC, Bornstein RA (1997) Cognitive deficits distinguish patients with adolescent- and adult-onset schizophrenia. Neuropsychiatry, Neuropsychology, and Behavioural Neurology 10, 107–112.

Beitchman JH (1985) Childhood schizophrenia: a review and comparison with adult-onset schizophrenia. Psychiatric Clinics of North America 8, 793–814.

Burd L, Fisher W, Kerbeshian J (1987) A prevalence study of pervasive developmental disorders in North Dakota. Journal of the American Academy of Child and Adolescent Psychiatry 26, 704–710.

Campbell M, Rapoport JL, Simpson GM (1999) Antipsychotics in children and adolescents Journal of American Academic Child and Adolescent Psychiatry 38, 537–545.

Caplan R (1994) Communication deficits in childhood schizophrenia spectrum disorders. Schizophrenia Bulletin 20, 671–683.

Cardno AG, McGuffin P (1996) Aetiological theories of schizophrenia. Current Opinion of Psychiatry 9, 45–49.

Castle DJ (1999) Gender and age at onset in schizophrenia. In: Late Onset Schizophrenia, Howard R, Rabins P, Castle DJ, eds. Hampshire, UK: Wrightson Biomedical, pp. 147–164.

Castle DJ, Howard R (1992) What do we know about the aetiology of late-onset schizophrenia? European Psychiatry 7, 99–108.

Castle DJ, Murray RM (1993) The epidemiology of late-onset schizophrenia. Schizophrenia Bulletin 19, 691–699.

Castle DJ, Wessely S, Howard R, Murray RM (1997) Schizophrenia with onset at the extremes of adult life. International Journal of Geriatric Psychiatry 12, 712–717.

Castle DJ, Sham PC, Murray RM (1998) Differences in distribution of ages of onset in males and females with schizophrenia. Schizophrenia Research 33, 179–183.

Cawthorn P, James A, Dell J, Seagroatt V (1994) Adolescent onset psychosis. A clinical and outcome study. Journal of Child Psychology and Psychiatry 35, 1321–1332.

Clark AF, Lewis SW (1998) Practitioner review: treatment of schizophrenia in childhood and adolescence. Journal of Child Psychology and Psychiatry 39, 1071–1081.

DeLisi LE (1992) The significance of age of onset for schizophrenia. Schizophrenia Bulletin 2, 209–215.

Eggers C (1978) Course and prognosis of childhood schizophrenia. Journal of Autism and Childhood Schizophrenia 1, 21–35.

Eggers C, Bunk D (1997) The long-term course of childhood-onset schizophrenia: a 42-year followup. Schizophrenia Bulletin 23, 105–117.

Findling RL, Friedman L, Kenny JT, Swales TP, Cola DM, Schulz SC (1995) Adolescent schizophrenia: a methodologic review of the current neuroimaging and neuropsychologic literature. Journal of Autism and Developmental Disorders 25, 627–639.

Fish B (1977) Neurobiologic antecedents of schizophrenia in children: evidence for an inherited, congenital neurointegrative defect. Archives of General Psychiatry 34, 1297–1313.

Frangou S (1999) The Maudsley early onset schizophrenia study: abnormal genes, abnormal brains, abnormal families. Biological Psychiatry 45, 12S.

Frazier JA, Giedd JN, Hamburger SD et al. (1996) Brain anatomic magnetic resonance imaging in childhood-onset schizophrenia. Archives of General Psychiatry 53, 617–624.

Galdos P, van Os JJ, Murray RM (1993) Puberty and the onset of psychosis. Schizophrenia Research 10, 7–14.

Garralda ME (1985) Characteristics of the psychoses of late onset in children and adolescents (a comparative study of hallucinating children). Journal of Adolescence 8, 195–207.

Geddes JR, Lawrie SM (1995) Obstetric complications and schizophrenia: a meta-analysis. British Journal of Psychiatry 167, 786–793.

Giedd JN, Jeffries NO, Blumenthal J et al. (1999) Childhood-onset schizophrenia: progressive brain changes during adolescence. Biological Psychiatry 46, 892–898.

Gillberg C (1984) Infantile autism and other childhood psychoses in a Swedish urban region: epidemiological aspects. Journal of Child Psychology and Psychiatry 25, 35–43.

Gillberg C (2001) Epidemiology of early onset schizophrenia. In: Schizophrenia in Children and Adolescents, Remschmidt H, ed. Cambridge, UK: Cambridge University Press, pp. 43–59.

Goldberg TE, Gold JM (1995) Neurocognitive Deficits in Schizophrenia. In: Schizophrenia, Hirsch S, Weinberger D, eds. Oxford: Blackwell, pp. 146–162.

Goldberg TE, Karson CN, Leleszi JP, Weinberger DR (1988) Intellectual impairment in adolescent psychosis. A controlled psychometric study. Schizophrenia Research 1, 261–266.

Goldberg TE, Berman KF, Weinberger DR (1995) Neuropsychology and neurophysiology of schizophrenia. Current Opinion in Psychiatry 8, 34–40.

Gothelf D, Frisch A, Munitz H et al. (1999) Clinical characteristics of schizophrenia associated with velo-cardio-facial syndrome. Schizophrenia Research 35, 105–112.

Green WH, Padron-Gayol M, Hardesty AS (1992) Schizophrenia with childhood onset: a phenomenological study of 38 cases. Journal of American Academy of Child and Adolescent Psychiatry 31, 968–976.

Häfner H, Nowotny B (1995) Epidemiology of early-onset schizophrenia. European Archives of Psychiatry and Clinical Neuroscience 245, 80–92.

Häfner H, Hambrecht M, Loffler W, Munk-Jørgensen P, Riecher-Rossler A (1998) Is schizophrenia a disorder of all ages? A comparison of first episodes and early course across the life-cycle. Psychological Medicine 28, 351–365.

Harris MJ, Jeste DV (1988) Late-onset schizophrenia: an overview. Schizophrenia Bulletin 14, 39–55.

Hoff AL, Harris D, Faustman WO et al. (1996) A neuropsychological study of early onset schizophrenia. Schizophrenia Research 20, 21–28.

Holden NL (1987) Late paraphrenia or the paraphrenias? A descriptive study with 10-year follow-up. British Journal of Psychiatry 150, 635–639.

Hollis C (1995) Child and adolescent (juvenile onset) schizophrenia. British Journal of Psychiatry 166, 489–495.

Howard R, Castle DJ, O'Brien J, Almeida O, Levy R (1992) Permeable walls, floors, ceilings and doors. Partition delusions in late paraphrenia. International Journal of Geriatric Psychiatry 7, 719–724.

Howard R, Cox T, Almeida O, Mullen R, Levy R (1995) White matter signal hyperintensities in the brains of people with late paraphrenia and the normal community-living elderly. Biological Psychiatry 38, 86–91.

Howard R, Graham C, Sham P et al. (1997) A controlled family study of late-onset nonaffective psychosis (late paraphrenia). British Journal of Psychiatry 170, 511–514.

Howard R, Rabins PV, Seeman MV for the International Late-onset Schizophrenia Group (2000) Late-onset schizophrenia and very-late-onset schizophrenia-like psychosis: an international consensus. American Journal of Psychiatry 157, 172–178.

Hultman CM, Sparen P, Takei N, Murray RM, Cnattingius S (1999) Prenatal and perinatal risk factors for schizophrenia, affective psychosis, and reactive psychosis of early onset: case-control study. British Medical Journal 318, 421–426.

Jacobsen LK, Rapoport JL (1998) Research update: Childhood-onset schizophrenia, implications of clinical and neurobiological research. Journal of Child Psychology and Psychiatry 39, 101–113.

Jacobsen LK, Giedd JN, Castellanos FX et al. (1998) Progressive reduction of temporal lobe structures in childhood-onset schizophrenia. American Journal of Psychiatry 155, 678–685.

Jeste DV, Lacro JP, Palmer B, Rockwell E, Harris MJ, Caligiuri MP (1999a) Incidence of tardive dyskinesia in early stages of neuroleptic treatment for older patients. American Journal of Psychiatry 156, 309–311.

Jeste DV, Rockwell E, Harris MJ, Lohr JB, Lacro J (1999b) Conventional versus newer antipsychotics in elderly. American Journal of Geriatric Psychiatry 7, 70–76.

Jones PB, Bebbington P, Foerster A et al. (1993) Poor scholastic achievement and pre-psychotic social decline are specific to schizophrenia: results from the Camberwell Collaborative Psychosis Study. British Journal of Psychiatry 162, 65–71.

Jones P, Rodgers B, Murray R, Marmot M (1994) Child developmental risk factors for adult schizophrenia in the British 1946 birth cohort. Lancet 344, 1398–1402.

Kay DWK, Roth M (1961) Environmental and hereditary factors in the schizophrenias of old age ('late paraphrenia') and their bearing on the general problem of causation in schizophrenia. Journal of Mental Science 107, 649–686.

Kendler KS, Karkowski-Shuman L, Walsh D (1996) Age at onset in schizophrenia and risk of illness in relatives. Results from the Roscommon family study. British Journal of Psychiatry 169, 213–218.

Kirov G, Jones PB, Harvey I et al. (1996) Do obstetric complications cause the earlier age at onset in male than female schizophrenics? Schizophrenia Research 20, 117–124.

Kolvin I (1971) Studies in the childhood psychoses. Diagnostic criteria and classification. British Journal of Psychiatry 118, 381–384.

Kolvin I, Ounsted C, Richardson LM, Garside RF (1971a) Studies in the childhood psychoses. The family and social background in childhood psychoses. British Journal of Psychiatry 118, 396–402.

Kolvin I, Ounsted C, Humphrey M, McNay A (1971b) Studies in the childhood psychoses. The phenomenology of childhood psychoses. British Journal of Psychiatry 118, 385–395.

Kraepelin E (1919) Dementia Praecox and Paraphrenia. Edinburgh: E & S Livingstone.

Krausz M, Muller-Thomsen T (1993) Schizophrenia with onset in adolescence: an 11-year followup. Schizophrenia Bulletin 19, 831–841.

Kravariti J, Morris RG, Frangou S (1999) The Maudsley Early-onset Schizophrenia Study. Schizophrenia Research 36, 140.

Kumra S, Frazier JA, Jacobsen LK et al. (1996) Childhood-onset schizophrenia: a double-blind clozapine–haloperidol comparison. Archives of General Psychiatry 53, 1090–1097.

Kumra S, Wiggs E, Krasnewich D et al. (1998) Brief report: association of sex chromosome anomalies with childhood-onset psychotic disorders. Journal of American Academy of Child and Adolescent Psychiatry 37, 292–296.

Kumra S, Wiggs E, Bedwell J et al. (2000) Neuropsychological deficits in pediatric patients with childhood-onset schizophrenia and psychotic disorder not otherwise specified. Schizophrenia Research 42, 135–144.

Kydd RR, Werry JS (1982) Schizophrenia in children under 16 years. Journal of Autism and Developmental Disorders 12, 343–357.

Lewis R (1998) Typical and atypical antipsychotics in adolescent schizophrenia: efficacy, tolerability, and differential sensitivity to extrapyramidal symptoms. Canadian Journal of Psychiatry 43, 596–604.

Loranger AW (1984) Sex difference in age at onset of schizophrenia. Archives of General Psychiatry 41, 157–161.

Makowski D, Waternaux C, Lajonchere CM et al. (1997) Thought disorder in adolescent-onset schizophrenia. Schizophrenia Research 23, 147–165.

Matsumoto H, Takei N, Saito H, Kachi K, Mori N (1999) Childhood-onset schizophrenia and obstetric complications: a case-control study. Schizophrenia Research 38, 93–99.

Maziade M, Bouchard S, Gingras N et al. (1996a) Long-term stability of diagnosis and symptom dimensions in a systematic sample of patients with onset of schizophrenia in childhood and early adolescence. II: positive/negative distinction and childhood predictors of adult outcome. British Journal of Psychiatry 169, 371–378.

Maziade M, Gingras N, Rodrigue C et al. (1996b) Long-term stability of diagnosis and symptom dimensions in a systematic sample of patients with onset of schizophrenia in childhood and early adolescence. I: nosology, sex and age of onset. British Journal of Psychiatry 169, 361–370.

McClellan J, Werry J (1994) Practice parameters for the assessment and treatment of children and adolescents with schizophrenia. Journal of the American Academy of Child and Adolescent Psychiatry 33, 616–635.

McClellan J, Werry JS, Ham M (1993) A follow-up study of early onset psychosis: comparison between outcome diagnoses of schizophrenia, mood disorders, and personality disorders. Journal of Autism and Developmental Disorders 23, 243–262.

McGlashan TH, Fenton WS (1991) Classical subtypes for schizophrenia: Literature review for DSM-IV. Schizophrenia Bulletin 17, 609–623.

McGrath J, Murray R (1995) Risk factors for schizophrenia from conception to birth. In: Schizophrenia, Hirsch S, Weinberger D, eds. Oxford: Blackwell Scientific, pp. 187–205.

McGuffin P, Owen MJ, Farmer AE (1995) The genetic basis of schizophrenia. Lancet 346, 678–682.

Meltzer HY, Rabinowitz J, Lee MA et al. (1997) Age at onset and gender of schizophrenic patients in relation to neuroleptic resistance. American Journal of Psychiatry 154, 475–482.

Morice RD, Ingram JCL (1983) Language complexity and age of onset of schizophrenia. Psychiatry Research 9, 233–242.

Nicolson R, Rapoport JL (2000) Childhood-onset schizophrenia: what can it teach us? In: Childhood Onset of 'Adult' Psychopathology: Clinical and Research Advances, Rapoport JL, ed. Washington, DC: American Psychiatric Press, pp. 167–192.

Nicolson R, Giedd JN, Lenane M et al. (1999a) Clinical and neurobiological correlates of cytogenetic abnormalities in childhood-onset schizophrenia. American Journal of Psychiatry 156, 1575–1579.

Nicolson R, Malaspina D, Giedd JN et al. (1999b) Obstetrical complications and childhood-onset schizophrenia. American Journal of Psychiatry 156, 1650–1652.

O'Callaghan E, Gibson T, Colohan HA et al. (1992) Risk of schizophrenia in adults after obstetric complications and their association with early onset of illness: a controlled study. British Medical Journal 305, 1256–1259.

Parry-Jones WL (1991) Adolescent psychoses: treatment and service provisions. Archives of Disease in Childhood 66, 1459–1462.

Pearlson G (1999) Gender and age at onset in schizophrenia. In: Late Onset Schizophrenia, Howard R, Rabins P, Castle DJ, eds. Hampshire, UK: Wrightson Biomedical, pp. 191–204.

Pearlson GD, Kreger L, Rabins PV et al. (1989) A chart review study of late-onset and early-onset schizophrenia. American Journal of Psychiatry 146, 1568–1574.

Pearlson GD, Tune LE, Wong DF et al. (1993) Quantitative D_2 dopamine receptor PET and structural MRI changes in late onset schizophrenia: a preliminary report. Schizophrenia Bulletin 19, 783–795.

Pool D, Bloom W, Mielke D, Roniger JJ, Gallant DM (1976) A controlled evaluation of Loxitane in seventy-five adolescent schizophrenic patients. Current Therapeutic Research 19, 99–104.

Post F (1966) Persistent Persecutory States of the Elderly. Oxford: Pergamon.

Prager S, Jeste DV (1993) Sensory Impairment in Late-Life Schizophrenia. Schizophrenia Bulletin 19, 755–771.

Pulver AE, Brown CH, Wolyniec PS et al. (1990) Schizophrenia, age at onset, gender and familial risk. Acta Psychiatrica Scandinavica 81, 344–351.

Rapoport JL, Giedd J, Kumra S et al. (1997) Childhood-onset schizophrenia. Progressive ventricular change during adolescence. Archives of General Psychiatry 54, 897–903.

Realmuto GM, Erickson WD, Yellin AM, Hopwood JH, Greenberg LM (1984) Clinical comparison of thiothixene and thioridazine in schizophrenic adolescent patients. American Journal of Psychiatry 141, 440–442.

Remschmidt HE, Schulz E, Martin M, Warnke A, Trott G-E (1994) Childhood-onset schizophrenia: history of the concept and recent studies. Schizophrenia Bulletin 4, 727–745.

Retterstol N (1968) Paranoid psychoses. British Journal of Psychiatry 114, 553–562.

Rifkin L, Lewis S, Jones P, Toone B, Murray R (1994) Low birth weight and schizophrenia. British Journal of Psychiatry 165, 357–362.

Rosso IM, Cannon TD, Huttunen T, Huttunen MO, Lonnqvist J, Gasperoni TL (2000) Obstetric risk factors for early-onset schizophrenia in a Finnish birth cohort. American Journal of Psychiatry 157, 801–807.

Roth M (1955) The natural history of mental disorder in old age. Journal of Mental Science 101, 281–301.

Russell AT, Bott L, Sammons C (1989) The phenomenology of schizophrenia occurring in childhood. Journal of American Academic Child and Adolescent Psychiatry 28, 399–407.

Schmidt M, Blanz B, Dippe A, Koppe T, Lay B (1995) Course of patients diagnosed as having schizophrenia during first episode occurring under age 18 years. European Archives of Psychiatry and Clinical Neuroscience 245, 93–100.

Schultz SC, Koller MM, Kishore PR, Hamer RM, Gehl JJ, Friedel RO (1983) Ventricular enlargement in teenage patients with schizophrenia spectrum disorder. American Journal of
Psychiatry 140, 1592–1595.

Sham PC, Jones P, Russell A et al. (1994) Age at onset, sex, and familial psychiatric morbidity in
schizophrenia. British Journal of Psychiatry 165, 466–473.

Smith GN, Kopala LC, Lapointe JS et al. (1998) Obstetric complications, treatment response and
brain morphology in adult-onset and early-onset males with schizophrenia. Psychological
Medicine 28, 645–53.

Spencer EK, Campbell M (1994) Children with schizophrenia: diagnosis, phenomenology, and
pharmacotherapy. Schizophrenia Bulletin 20, 713–725.

Suvisaari JM, Haukka J, Tanskanen A, Lonnqvist JK (1998) Age at onset and outcome in schizophrenia are related to the degree of familial loading. British Journal of Psychiatry 173, 494–500.

Thomsen PH (1996) Schizophrenia with childhood and adolescent onset – a nationwide register-based study. Acta Psychiatrica Scandinavica 94, 187–193.

Toren P, Laor N, Weizman A (1998) Use of atypical neuroleptics in child and adolescent psychiatry. Journal of Clinical Psychiatry 59, 644–656.

Verdoux H, Geddes JR, Takei N et al. (1997) Obstetric complications and age at onset in schizophrenia, an international collaborative metaanalysis of individual patient data. American
Journal of Psychiatry 154, 1220–1227.

Volkmar FR, Cohen DJ, Hoshino Y, Rende RE, Paul R (1988) Phenomenology and classification
of the childhood psychoses. Psychological Medicine 18, 191–201.

Walker E, Savoie T, Davis D (1994) Neuromotor precursors of schizophrenia. Schizophrenia
Bulletin 20, 441–451.

Werry JS (1992) Child and adolescent (early onset) schizophrenia: a review in light of DSM-III-
R. Journal of Autism and Developmental Disorders 22, 601–624.

Werry JS, McClellan JM (1992) Predicting outcome in child and adolescent (early onset) schizophrenia and bipolar disorder. Journal of the American Academy of Child and Adolescent
Psychiatry 31, 147–150.

Werry JS, McClellan JM, Chard L (1991) Childhood and adolescent schizophrenic, bipolar, and
schizoaffective disorders: a clinical and outcome study. Journal of the American Academy of
Child and Adolescent Psychiatry 30, 457–465.

Werry JS, McClellan JM, Andrews LK, Ham M (1994) Clinical features and outcome of child and
adolescent schizophrenia. Schizophrenia Bulletin 20, 619–630.

Woody RC, Boylard K, Eisenhauer G, Altschuler L (1987) CT scan and MRI findings of a child
with schizophrenia. Journal of Child Neurology 2, 105–110.

World Health Organization (1967) International Classification of Diseases, 8th revision. Geneva:
World Health Organization.

Yang P-C, Liu C-Y, Chiang S-Q, Chen J-Y, Lin T-S (1995) Comparison of adult manifestations of
schizophrenia with onset before and after 15 years of age. Acta Psychiatrica Scandinavica 91,
209–212.

Part III

The genetic epidemiology of schizophrenia

Introduction

Genetic epidemiology is a relatively new discipline that seeks to elucidate the role of genetic factors and their interaction in the occurrence of disease in populations (Khoury et al., 1993). It is becoming more apparent that most diseases are not purely genetic or purely environmental in origin but depend on a complex interaction of the two. Even with 'infectious' or 'environmental' aetiology, differential genetic susceptibility may be involved in determining the ultimate clinical manifestation.

Historical observations that schizophrenia runs in families led to a number of family, twin and adoption studies, which provide strong evidence for a genetic component to the disorder. Cardno and Murray review these 'classical' genetic epidemiological studies in Chapter 10, with particular emphasis on the twin study approach. Although the size of the genetic contribution is still debated, even conservative estimates suggest heritabilities of greater than 60%. A polygenic model is most likely, but the question remains about what these individual genes might actually transmit. Cardno and Murray suggest that some families transmit a liability to traits for minor deviations that are relatively innocent in themselves but, in combination with other genetic or environmental risk factors, may propel an individual past a threshold for the expression of symptoms.

Zammit, Lewis and Owen take these issues further in Chapter 11 by discussing the methods that can be used to search for 'genes for schizophrenia' in the future. The authors point out that the first wave of molecular genetic studies of schizophrenia using linkage techniques 'effectively ignored the evidence for genetic complexity' and searched for genes of major effect segregating in large multiply affected pedigrees. As this approach has proved unsuccessful, the focus must now turn to the more epidemiological approaches such as association study designs. In addition, more work is needed to refine the phenotype and nosology of the schizophrenia syndrome. The identification of genetic risk factors will provide a new impetus to epidemiological studies of schizophrenia by allowing researchers to investigate ways in which genes and the enviroment interact. However Zammit and colleagues warn that 'the price of improved scientific rigor is likely to be considerably more expensive studies'.

Schizophrenia is a complex disorder that results from the action of both genetic and environmental factors. Many possible environmental risk factors were outlined in Sections I and II. In Chapter 12, van Os and Sham discuss gene–environment correlation and interaction and emphasize the importance of such concepts in furthering our understanding of schizophrenia. Four mechanisms by which genes and environment can co-influence disease outcome are outlined. The authors then examine how the (limited) current evidence for gene–environment interaction in schizophrenia can be viewed in the light of these models. In Chapter 13, van Erp and colleagues illustrate some novel approaches to the study of gene–environment interaction in schizophrenia by outlining a series of elegant studies that apply neuroimaging techniques to epidemiological twin, family and high-risk samples. The authors demonstrate that structural brain abnormalities are promising endophenotypic indicators for schizophrenia and further propose that a genetic factor in schizophrenia may render the fetal brain particularly susceptible to damage following hypoxia–ischaemia. This type of approach, which combine the use of imaging and molecular biological techniques with epidemiological study designs, will provide a powerful tool for solving complex disorders such as schizophrenia.

REFERENCE

Khoury M, Beaty TH, Cohen BH (1993) Fundamentals of Genetic Epidemiology. New York: Oxford University Press.

10

The 'classical' genetic epidemiology of schizophrenia

Alastair Cardno[1] and Robin M. Murray[2]
[1]University of Wales College of Medicine, Cardiff, UK
[2]Institute of Psychiatry, Kings College, London, UK

In the mid-1980s, it was widely predicted that family, twin and adoption studies of schizophrenia would be rendered obsolete by the application of molecular genetic techniques to this condition. However, the anticipated advances have yet to occur. Consequently, there has been a revival of interest in the classical genetic epidemiological approach to schizophrenia. Larger and better-designed investigations have been carried out, and new technologies such as brain imaging and neurophysiology have been incorporated into some of these. Family, twin and adoption studies have attempted to answer the following questions:

1 Do genetic factors contribute to the aetiology of schizophrenia?
If so,
2 What is the relative contribution of genetic and environmental factors?
3 What is the mode of inheritance?
4 What exactly is inherited?

Investigating whether a genetic effect is present

Since the studies that have addressed the first question have often been reviewed, we will only discuss the major findings and the main sources of bias.

Family studies

Family studies (reviewed by Gottesman and Shields, 1982; Kendler and Tsuang, 1988; Gottesman, 1991; Kendler and Diehl, 1993; McGuffin et al., 1994a, 1995) generally depend on the calculation of the lifetime expectation or morbid risk of schizophrenia in the relatives of probands. The lifetime morbid risk is basically the number of affected relatives divided by the total number of relatives, with an adjustment made for the fact that not all relatives will have passed through the period of risk at the time that they are studied. Various methods can be used to make this adjustment, including the Weinberg, the Strömgren and the

Kaplan–Meier methods (see Sham, 1998). Since the expected genetic covariance between parents and offspring differs from that between siblings if dominance or epistasis (gene–gene interaction) is present, and because schizophrenia is associated with a reduced rate of reproduction, it is best to calculate risks separately for parents, siblings and children.

The morbid risk of schizophrenia in relatives of probands is compared with the morbid risk in the general population or, preferably, in relatives of a demographically matched control sample. Control probands may be screened for psychiatric illness or may be unscreened. Using unscreened controls is a more conservative approach, since some of the control probands may have a psychiatric illness; unscreened controls sampled from the general population also allow estimates of population morbid risks to be made. Familial aggregation is indicated by a significantly higher morbid risk for schizophrenia in relatives of probands than in controls.

Results

Kendler and Diehl (1993) divided family studies into those from two periods: the first from 1917 to the early 1980s, and the second from the early 1980s onwards. Studies from the first period generally used a broad clinical definition of schizophrenia, and when Gottesman and Shields (1982) pooled the results they showed morbid risks of 6% for parents, 10% for siblings and 13% for children of probands with schizophrenia, compared with a population morbid risk of around 1%. The lower risks to parents than to other first-degree relatives are probably a consequence of the reduced rate of reproduction associated with schizophrenia (i.e. those with severe schizophrenia are less likely to have children).

However, these early studies were criticized for their methodological limitations (Pope et al., 1982; Abrams and Taylor, 1983), and a new generation of studies was initiated using structured interviews and operational diagnostic procedures. Kendler and Diehl (1993) have summarized these as showing a pooled morbid risk for first-degree relatives of probands with schizophrenia of 4.8%, versus 0.5% in first-degree relatives of controls. The lower risks for both relatives of probands and controls compared with the risks found in earlier studies is mainly the result of using relatively narrow definitions of schizophrenia in the more recent studies.

Even if systematically collected, a sample of probands ascertained via clinical services can be subject to ascertainment biases. Compared with the general population, such a sample will tend to be selected for (i) more severe forms of illness; (ii) comorbidity with other illnesses; and (iii) clinical profiles that are more likely to elicit treatment, for example suicidal thoughts or acts (Neale and Kendler, 1995). The ascertainment biases are probably smaller for schizophrenia than for studies of milder illnesses, because the vast majority of people with schizophrenia have contact with psychiatric services (Cooper et al., 1987; Castle et al., 1998). However, few family studies have examined all first-onset cases from a specific area.

To overcome the above potential biases, Kendler et al. (1993a) carried out an epidemiologically based family study in Roscommon County, Ireland. The morbid risks for DSM-III-R-defined schizophrenia (American Psychiatric Association, 1987) were 9.2% in siblings and 1.3% in parents of probands. Thus, methodologically rigorous studies have confirmed the results of earlier studies in showing substantial familial aggregation for schizophrenia, and higher morbid risks in siblings than in parents of probands.

High-risk studies

High-risk studies are variants of family studies that involve the longitudinal follow-up of children or young adults regarded as being at high risk of schizophrenia because they have one or more relatives (usually parents) affected by schizophrenia. There are ongoing studies in the USA (Nuechterlein, 1983; Erlenmeyer-Kimling et al., 1995), Denmark (Jørgensen et al., 1987; Parnas et al., 1993), Israel (Mirsky, 1995) and the UK (Byrne et al., 1999). As expected, such studies show high rates of schizophrenia of 11–16% in the high-risk offspring on follow-up (Parnas et al., 1993; Erlenmeyer-Kimling et al., 1995) However, the main focus has generally been on identifying premorbid predictors of schizophrenia (see Ch. 6).

Twin studies

The basic premise of twin studies is that if pairs of monozygotic (MZ) twins, who inherit all of their genes in common, are more similar for a phenotype than pairs of dizygotic (DZ) twins, who on average have 50% of their genes in common, a genetic contribution to the phenotype can be inferred. This premise is based on a number of assumptions.

The equal environments assumption

MZ and DZ twin pairs are assumed to share environmental risk factors for schizophrenia to the same degree. The assumption would be invalid if MZ twins shared environmental risk factors to a greater degree than DZ twins; in this case, a greater resemblance for liability to schizophrenia in MZ than DZ twins could not be attributed solely to genetic factors. MZ twins do show more general environmental sharing than DZ twins because they tend to socialize together more, and their parents emphasize their similarities more (Kendler and Gardner, 1998). However, concordance rates for schizophrenia are not predicted by the degree of environmental sharing, as inferred from the degree of physical resemblance or length of cohabitation of twins (Kendler, 1983; Cannon et al., 1998; Cardno et al., 1999a). To our knowledge, in twin studies of schizophrenia, the assumption has not been tested for more specific measures of environmental sharing, for example being dressed alike and having the same friends.

The effects of MZ twins having more similar environments can theoretically be avoided by studying MZ twins who have been reared apart. However, such twins are very rare, and those reported (see Gottesman and Shields, 1982) are probably not representative. It is also theoretically possible to adjust for such effects in biometrical modelling (see below), if they are found to be relevant.

The effects of environmental sharing in utero are unclear because they are difficult to measure. Such effects could potentially make MZ twins either more or less similar (Martin et al., 1997). About 65% of MZ twins share a common chorion, while DZ twins never do. A consequence of this shared blood supply could, on the one hand, be to increase the chances that a viral infection would affect both twins; on the other hand, competition for nutrition and sharing a crowded chorion could result in differences in growth rates, as in the twin transfusion syndrome. Comparison of monochorionic and dichorionic MZ twins could help to unravel these effects (Rose et al., 1981; Martin et al., 1997). Davis et al. (1995) attempted to do this using indirect indicators of chorionicity (such as mirroring of fingerprints) and reported much higher concordance rates in those MZ pairs that were categorized as monochorionic. However, this cannot be said to be a definitive study.

The risk of receiving the diagnosis is the same in monozygotic and dizygotic twins

This assumption would be invalid if MZ twins had a higher risk of receiving the diagnosis of schizophrenia than DZ twins. In this case, a higher concordance in MZ than DZ twin pairs would not be a result of MZ twins sharing a greater proportion of susceptibility genes, but they would resemble each other because of factors related to being a MZ twin. Most studies have found no significant differences in the rates of schizophrenia in MZ versus DZ twins (Rosenthal, 1960 (Luxenburger study); Kringlen, 1967; Fischer, 1973; Kendler and Robinette, 1983; Kendler et al., 1996b). Three studies of schizophrenia have shown notable differences, but their results have been inconsistent. The first study found a lower than expected rate in MZ twins (Rosenthal, 1960 (Essen-Möller study)); the second found a higher than expected rate (Tienari, 1963), and the third found a normal rate in MZ twins but a higher rate in DZ twins (Kläning, 1999).

The risk of receiving the diagnosis is the same in twins and singletons

If this assumption were shown to be invalid, the results of twin studies could not be extrapolated to the general population in a straightforward way. Most studies have not found an excess of schizophrenia in twins (Rosenthal, 1960; Allen et al., 1972; Fischer, 1973; Kendler et al., 1996b), but two studies have done so (Tienari, 1963; Kläning et al., 1996). The generalizability of twin studies can also be tested by extending studies to include other classes of relative and comparing these with the results of the twin data alone (Martin et al., 1997).

Monozygotic twins are genetically identical

A range of noninherited influences could potentially make MZ twins genetically discordant, for example differential trinucleotide repeat expansion or skewed X-inactivation (McGuffin et al., 1994a; Martin et al., 1997). Such factors would be labelled as nonshared environmental effects in the results of a standard twin study.

The same potential ascertainment biases apply to twin studies as we discussed above for family studies. In addition, there may be selection for (i) twin status; (ii) concordant pairs; and (iii) MZ pairs, by the rationale that such factors make twins stand out as being unusual and, therefore, more likely to be referred for specialist hospital treatment.

Twin pairs are usually counted probandwise (i.e. if both members of an affected twin pair are independently ascertained, they are counted as two pairs). This approach allows comparison between the general population morbid risk for the diagnosis and the rate of the diagnosis in co-twins of probands, which is a pre-requisite for calculating heritability estimates (see below). The alternative approach is to count pairwise (i.e. each pair is counted once but this rate cannot be directly compared with the population morbid risk). Thus, the resemblance for the diagnosis in twin pairs is initially expressed as the probandwise concordance rate, that is, the number of concordant probandwise pairs divided by the total number of probandwise pairs. A higher concordance rate in MZ than DZ pairs suggests a genetic contribution to the diagnosis. There is no standard adjustment for variable age of onset in twin studies; age correction is made problematic by the high correlation for age of onset in MZ pairs. However, in twin studies of other phenotypes, an adjustment has sometimes been made, for example using survival analysis (Meyer et al., 1991).

Results

Early studies carried out before the introduction of operational diagnoses showed pooled probandwise concordance rates of 46% for MZ and 14% for DZ pairs (Gottesman and Shields, 1982). Pooled probandwise concordance rates have now been calculated for studies that have employed operational diagnoses (Cardno and Gottesman, 2000). For the four studies that employed DSM-III-R criteria (Onstad et al., 1991a; Tsujita et al., 1992; Franzek and Beckmann, 1998; Cardno et al., 1999b), the pooled rates were 57/114 (50.0%) for MZ and 4/97 (4.1%) for DZ pairs. For the two studies that employed ICD-10 (World Health Organization, 1992) criteria (Kläning, 1996; Cardno et al., 1999b), the rates were 28/66 (42.4%) for MZ and 3/77 (3.9%) for DZ pairs. The results from the study of Cardno et al. (1999b)

Table 10.1. Results of a twin study based on the Maudsley twin psychosis series

Schizophrenia diagnosis	Probandwise concordance rate		Best-fitting model	Heritability estimate (% (95% CI))
	MZ (%)	DZ (%)		
RDC	20/49 (40.8)	3/57 (5.3)	AE	82 (71–90)
DSM-III-R[a]	20/47 (42.6)	0/50 (0.0)	ADE	84 (19–92)
ICD-10[a]	21/50 (42.0)	1/58 (1.7)	ADE	83 (7–91)

Notes:

MZ, monozygotic; DZ, dizygotic; CI, confidence interval; RDC, research diagnostic criteria (lifetime-ever diagnosis); DSM-III-R, Diagnostic and Statistical Manual III–Revised; IDC-10, International Classification of Disease 10th revision; AE, model comprising additive genetic and individual-specific environmental effects; ADE, model comprising additive genetic, genetic dominance and individual-specific environmental effects. (NB: best-fitting ADE models may be artifacts of low DZ concordance rates; see text for details.)

[a] Main-lifetime diagnosis based on OPCRIT system (McGuffin et al., 1991).

which employed both DSM-III-R and ICD-10 criteria, are shown in Table 10.1. Therefore, more recent twin studies have confirmed the earlier investigations in showing a pattern of results consistent with a genetic effect.

Adoption studies

There are three main types of adoption study.

1 Biological parent of adoptee as proband (adoptee study). Parents are ascertained who (i) have been given a diagnosis of schizophrenia and (ii) have had a child adopted away soon after birth. The risk of schizophrenia in their adopted children is compared with the risk in adoptees who had unaffected biological parents.

2 Adoptee as proband (adoptee's family study). Adoptees with schizophrenia are ascertained. The risk of schizophrenia is compared in their biological parents, their adoptive parents and in the biological and adoptive parents of unaffected control adoptees.

3 Cross-fostering design. The risk of schizophrenia is compared between adoptees who have affected biological parents but unaffected adopting parents, and adoptees with unaffected biological parents but affected adopting parents.

In each case, if the risk of schizophrenia is higher in biological relatives of probands (where genes but not environment are shared) than in the other control groups, a genetic contribution to the illness is suggested.

With the exception of the study of Heston (1966), adoption studies of schizophrenia have been carried out in Scandinavia, where systematic ascertainment can be achieved by linking population registers with adoption registers and registers of hospital treatment. There may be ascertainment biases relating to the identification of probands via hospital treatment, as with family studies. In addition, adoptees and their biological and adoptive parents may not be representative of the general population (e.g. adoptees frequently have a family history of psychiatric illness). Other potentially biasing factors include (i) rearing practices by adoptive parents (who have passed screening by the adoption agencies) may be biased towards health; (ii) correlations between the social classes of biological and adoptive parents (this may arise if adoption agencies have tried to match biological and adopting parents); and (iii) the partner of the psychotic parent whose child is sent for adoption may not be representative of partners of people who have schizophrenia in general (Gottesman and Shields, 1982).

Results

The early adoptee studies (Heston, 1966; Rosenthal et al., 1971), adoptee's family studies (Kety et al., 1994) and cross-fostering studies (Wender et al., 1974), which did not use operational diagnoses, all showed higher rates of schizophrenia and related disorders in the biological relatives of probands than in controls. The data of Kety et al. (1994) from Denmark have been re-analysed applying DSM-III criteria, with consistent results (Kendler et al., 1994a): 3 of 38 (7.9%) of first-degree biological relatives of proband adoptees had DSM-III schizophrenia (American Psychiatric Association, 1980), compared with 1 of 107 (0.9%) of first-degree relatives of control adoptees (not age corrected). Also, an ongoing Finnish study (Tienari et al., 1994) found a higher prevalence of DSM-III-R schizophrenia in the adopted-away offspring of mothers with schizophrenia or a related disorder, compared with control offspring (6/136 (4.4%) versus 1/186 (0.5%)).

Investigating the relative contribution of genetic and environmental factors

The consistent pattern of results across family, twin and adoption studies indicates the existence of a genetic contribution to the aetiology of schizophrenia. The next question is what size is this contribution?

The liability-threshold model

The relative contribution of genetic and environmental factors to the aetiology of schizophrenia has most commonly been investigated in twins, because of their genetic informativeness. The principles are derived from quantitative genetic approaches to continuous phenotypes, which generally involve investigating patterns of phenotypic variances and covariances or correlations (Neale and Cardon, 1992; Falconer and Mackay, 1996). Similar approaches can be applied to a dichotomous phenotype, such as the presence or absence of a diagnosis of schizophrenia, by assuming a liability-threshold model (Falconer, 1965). This postulates a hypothetical continuous liability distribution in the general population, contributed to by many genes of small effect and also environmental factors. Individuals below a particular threshold on this liability distribution are unaffected, while those above the threshold are affected.

Correlations in liability

Based on the liability-threshold model, correlations in respect of liability (or correlations in liability) (Falconer and Mackay, 1996) for schizophrenia can be calculated. These are tetrachoric correlations that make use of data on the population risk for schizophrenia, and the risk in a particular class of relative of probands. Correlations in liability can be calculated using computer programs (Jöreskog and Sörbom, 1988; Neale, 1999) and can be used to estimate the relative contribution of genetic and environmental factors to the aetiology or, more correctly, to the variance in liability to schizophrenia. This can be carried out with formulae that use, for example, correlations in MZ and DZ pairs to calculate variance in liability contributed by additive genetic effects (e.g. see McGuffin et al., 1994b); however, if the sample is of adequate size, it is preferable to employ biometrical model fitting.

Biometrical model fitting

Biometrical model fitting (Neale and Cardon, 1992) is a process by which one can formally test hypotheses concerning whether, and to what extent, various genetic and environmental effects contribute to variation in a phenotype. For the analysis of data on MZ and DZ twins this generally proceeds as follows:

1 A set of models is chosen that includes various combinations of genetic and environmental effects. Commonly, the models specify phenotypic variance contributed by

   a. nonshared environmental factors only (E model)
   b. shared (or common) and nonshared environmental factors (CE model)
   c. additive genetic and nonshared environmental factors (AE model)
   d. additive genetic, shared and nonshared environmental factors (ACE model)
   e. additive genetic, genetic dominance and nonshared environmental factors (ADE model).

   It is not possible to test a, d, c and e together using only data on twins reared together because in this case there are four parameters to estimate from only three statistics: the correlation in liability for MZ pairs, that for DZ pairs and the total variance in liability.

2 Equations are derived, for example from an approach such as path analysis (Neale and Cardon, 1992), showing the relationships between (a) correlations in liability for twins and (b) the parameters included in the model (e.g. a^2, c^2 and e^2 in the ACE model). This sets up a series of simultaneous equations to be solved. For example, under the ACE model, risk in MZ twins is $a^2 + c^2$, and risk in DZ twins is $1/2a^2 + c^2$.

3 The correlations in liability are inspected. Patterns of correlations that suggest particular effects are as follows:

a. additive genetic rMZ = 2rDZ
b. genetic dominance rMZ > 2rDZ
c. shared environment rMZ = rDZ
d. nonshared environment − degree to which rMZ < 1.0

If there are mixed effects (e.g. additive genetic and shared environment), the expected pattern is between (a) and (c), that is, the value of rMZ is between 1 and 2 times rDZ.

4 The fit of each model is formally calculated using a computer program, such as Mx (Neale, 1999) or LISREL (Jöreskog and Sörbom, 1989). This involves an iterative process in which the probability of obtaining the observed data is calculated for estimates of the parameters in the model (e.g. a^2, c^2 and e^2 for the ACE model), until convergence is reached (i.e. when the parameter estimates have been found that give the best agreement between the observed and expected correlations). This is usually done by maximizing a likelihood function or minimizing a goodness-of-fit χ^2. The degrees of freedom for the model-fitting statistic is given by the number of observed statistics minus the number of estimated parameters. For a study of MZ and DZ twin pairs ascertained probandwise, there are three observed statistics (MZ concordance, DZ concordance and total phenotypic variance). So there are two degrees of freedom for the E model $(3 - 1)$, one for the CE and AE models $(3 - 2)$, and none for the ACE and ADE models $(3 - 3)$. A good model has a fit with a high (nonsignificant) p value.

5 The fits of nested models are compared. Thus, models can be compared where one model is a submodel of the other, for example ACE can be compared with AE, CE and E. However, CE and AE, for example, cannot be compared. The fit of models is compared using a χ^2 difference test, with degrees of freedom equal to the difference between the degrees of freedom of the models being tested, for example one degree of freedom for ACE versus AE.

6 The best model is chosen on the grounds of goodness-of-fit and parsimony. Thus, if two models do not differ significantly in goodness-of-fit, the model with fewer parameters is chosen. Criteria such as the Akaike Information Criteria

(AIC), which is an index of the balance of goodness-of-fit and parsimony, can also be used.

7 The accuracy of the parameter estimates can be assessed by calculating, for example, 95% confidence intervals (CI).

Results

Two recent studies have employed these methods. First, Cannon et al. (1998) applied biometrical model fitting to a Finnish population-based sample with clinically diagnosed schizophrenia. The AE model fitted best and suggested that 83% of the variance in liability to schizophrenia was owing to additive genetic effects (i.e. there was a heritability of 83%), with the remaining 17% owing to individual-specific environmental effects.

Similarly, Cardno et al. (1999a) applied model fitting to a sample based on the Maudsley Hospital Twin Register, in London. Heritability estimates for three operational definitions of schizophrenia (RDC (Research Diagnostic Criteria; Spitzer et al., 1990), DSM-III-R and ICD-10) are shown in Table 10.1 and were very similar to those found by Cannon et al. (1998). The relatively wide CI values for DSM-III-R and ICD-10 schizophrenia were generated in the best-fitting model (ADE), suggesting that genetic dominance effects entirely accounted for the heritabilities. This appeared to be an artifact of the low DZ concordance rates: adding one concordant DZ pair to the analysis resulted, in both cases, in heritabilities accounted for by additive genetic effects (AE model: for DSM-III-R $a^2 = 83\%$ (95% CI 72–91); for ICD-10 $a^2 = 82\%$ (95% CI 71–90)). Patterns of inheritance in schizophrenia are compatible with the occurrence of some dominance or epistatic effects (Risch, 1990), but it is unlikely that a twin study of this size would be able to detect such effects reliably.

Therefore, model-fitting analyses suggest that schizophrenia is under a strong genetic influence, and that the heritability estimates do not differ greatly according to which diagnostic system is employed. However, it should be noted that the sample sizes were probably too small to exclude with confidence any common environmental effects as well as genetic dominance or epistasis. Also, it would be valuable to test the general representativeness of these results by performing further model fitting including data from family studies.

It is perhaps only fair to point out that not all researchers accept either the representativeness of the twin data or the model fitting. Some researchers who emphasize environmental effects dispute the assumptions made in heritability calculations and instead prefer to quote the population attributable risk. For example, Mortensen et al. (1999) estimated that the proportion of schizophrenia attributable to being born in an urban area was 34.6% compared with only 5.5% for having a parent or sibling with schizophrenia. However, it is important to note that determining the risk of schizophrenia in relatives is not the same as determining genetic risk, which will require information on risks associated with as-yet unidentified susceptibility genes.

What is the mode of inheritance?

Given the evidence for a substantial genetic contribution to the aetiology of schizophrenia, methods such as complex segregation analysis (Lalouel and Morton, 1981) have been used in an attempt to identify the most likely mode of inheritance. This is also a model-fitting approach, in this case based on the pattern of inheritance of schizophrenia shown by families. Commonly a mixed model (Morton and MacLean, 1974), in which there are both major gene and polygenic effects, is compared with the submodels of a single major locus and polygenic inheritance. Large sample sizes are required to distinguish between models, especially the polygenic and mixed models, which has limited the practical usefulness of segregation analysis as applied to schizophrenia to date.

Complex segregation analysis and related approaches have shown that the pattern of risks in family and twin studies is not compatible with a model in which a single locus accounts for all of the genetic liability to schizophrenia (O'Rourke et al., 1982; Risch and Baron, 1984; McGue et al., 1985). However, it has not been possible to distinguish between a polygenic and a mixed model as best fitting (Risch and Baron, 1984). The pattern of risks in family studies, in which the risk decreases rapidly as the degree of genetic relatedness decreases, is also compatible with a model of multiple loci with epistasis (i.e. interaction between genes) (Risch, 1990).

What exactly is transmitted?

Is the genetic liability to schizophrenia specific?

Quantitative genetic studies have found evidence that a number of other disorders probably share at least some genetic risk factors with schizophrenia. Relatives of probands with schizophrenia have elevated risks of schizoaffective disorder (Gershon et al., 1982; Kendler et al., 1986, 1993a; Maier et al., 1993) and schizotypal and paranoid personality disorders (Kendler et al., 1993b). In addition, there is some evidence for familial coaggregation between schizophrenia and schizophreniform disorder, and psychosis not otherwise specified (Kendler and Walsh, 1995), as well as evidence of familial aggregation with psychotic affective disorders (Kendler et al., 1986, 1993a), especially when the psychotic symptoms are mood incongruent (Maier et al., 1992). However, this last finding remains controversial, and two high-risk studies have not found an excess of psychotic affective disorders among offspring of parents with schizophrenia (Parnas et al., 1993; Erlenmeyer-Kimling et al., 1995).

The 'schizophrenia spectrum'

In the adoption studies of Kety et al. (1971), the term 'schizophrenia spectrum' was coined to encompass a broad range of disorders including chronic, acute, border-line, and possible schizophrenia. This group of disorders was found to have a higher prevalence in biological relatives than controls. Subsequently, in the reanalysis that applied DSM-III criteria (Kendler et al., 1994a), spectrum disorders were defined as schizophrenia, schizoaffective disorder mainly schizophrenic subtype, and schizotypal and paranoid personality disorders. The prevalence of spectrum disorders was 16 of 68 (23.5%) among first-degree biological relatives of adoptee pro-bands with spectrum disorders, compared with only 5 of 107 (4.7%) among first-degree relatives of controls. In the study of Tienari et al. (1994), who used DSM-III-R criteria, their 'soft spectrum' included schizophrenia, schizophreni-form disorder, delusional disorder and nonpsychotic personality disorders. The prevalence was 43 of 155 (27.7%) in offspring of mothers with spectrum disorders compared with 26 of 186 (14.0%) in control offspring.

In the Finnish twin sample we discussed above, Cannon et al. (1998) investigated whether clinically defined schizophrenia and other psychoses lie on a single contin-uum of liability. This analysis was based on a liability-threshold model with multi-ple thresholds (Reich et al., 1972) in which schizophrenia and other psychoses are assumed to share the same aetiological risk factors but a higher level of liability is required for schizophrenia to be expressed than for other psychotic disorders. The multiple-threshold model did not fit well, suggesting that schizophrenia and other psychoses do not lie on a single liability continuum. However, comparison with alternative models was not performed.

In the Maudsley twin sample, Cardno et al. (2002) performed a more general investigation of whether RDC schizophrenia, schizoaffective disorder and mania have genetic and environmental risk factors in common, when these disorders were defined on a nonhierarchical basis that allowed within-person comorbidity between disorders (i.e. a schizophrenic twin who had in the past met criteria for mania would be regarded as showing within-person comorbidity). They used a correlated liability model (Neale and Kendler, 1995) to test whether the three pos-sible pairings of these disorders had significant additive genetic and individual-specific environmental correlations in order to indicate the extent to which such effects were shared in common between the disorders. Significant additive genetic correlations were found for each pairing, but environmental correlations were non-significant. Analyses of all three disorders together under independent and common pathway models (Neale and Cardon, 1992) were consistent with schizo-phrenia and mania having both shared and diagnosis-specific genetic effects, while schizoaffective disorder had only genetic effects that were also shared with the other disorders. These results are consistent with those of Cannon et al. (1998) in suggesting that schizophrenia is genetically related to other psychoses but does not share all of its risk factors with them.

'Splitting' the schizophrenia syndrome
Subtypes of schizophrenia

The clinical variation among people suffering from schizophrenia has prompted numerous investigations to determine whether genetically distinct subtypes exist within the syndrome of schizophrenia. Most studies have investigated the degree of familial aggregation of classical schizophrenia subtypes (e.g. paranoid, hebephrenic) in pairs of affected siblings or twins. Since siblings selected on the basis that both have schizophrenia are likely to share most genetic risk factors in common, they would be expected to be highly concordant for schizophrenia subtype if the subtypes were genetically distinct.

In studies of affected sibling pairs, schizophrenia subtypes show only a modest degree of familial aggregation (Kendler and Adler, 1984; Kendler et al., 1997; Cardno et al., 1998), and a similar pattern of partial homotypia for subtype has been found in samples of concordant MZ twins (Gottesman and Shields, 1972; Farmer et al., 1984; McGuffin et al., 1987; Onstad et al., 1991b).

Nevertheless, twin studies have shown significantly higher MZ concordance rates for schizophrenia when probands had hebephrenic or nonparanoid subtypes than paranoid subtypes (Gottesman and Shields, 1972; Farmer et al., 1984; McGuffin et al., 1987; Onstad et al., 1991b). Also, most (reviewed by Kendler and Davis, 1981; McGuffin et al., 1987), but not all (Kendler et al., 1988, 1993c,d, 1994b; Kendler and Gardner, 1998), family studies (and a high-risk study: Jørgensen et al., 1987) have found higher familial risks for schizophrenia when probands had hebephrenic or nonparanoid subtypes, compared with paranoid subtypes.

Consequently, although classical schizophrenia subtypes are not totally genetically distinct from each other, they could differ quantitatively on a single liability continuum with multiple thresholds. Such a view postulates that the hebephrenic or nonparanoid subtype has a higher familial loading for schizophrenia than the paranoid subtype and represents a more extreme subtype than paranoid schizophrenia on the liability continuum. However, to our knowledge, this hypothesis has not been formally tested by model fitting on twin data.

Symptom dimensions

A similar pattern of only modest familial aggregation is seen when clinical variation within schizophrenia is subclassified in other ways, for example in terms of psychotic symptom dimensions derived from factor analysis (Burke et al., 1996; Kendler et al., 1997; Loftus et al., 1998; Cardno et al., 1999a), individual psychotic symptoms (Kendler et al., 1997; Cardno et al., 1998) or illness course (Kendler et al.,

1997; Cardno et al., 1998). Most studies have found no relationship between familial risk of psychoses and severity of positive symptoms in probands (Dworkin and Lenzenweger, 1984; Kendler et al., 1994c; Cardno et al., 1997; van Os et al., 1997). Some studies have found an increased familial risk associated with severity of negative symptoms (Dworkin and Lenzenweger, 1984; Verdoux et al., 1996), though others have not (Kendler et al., 1994c; Cardno et al., 1997). Finally, some studies have found increased familial risk associated with severity of disorganized symptoms (Cardno et al., 1997; van Os et al., 1997). In short, psychotic symptom dimensions consistently show only modest familial aggregation in affected sibling pairs, and rather weak and inconsistent relationships with familial risk of psychoses.

Age at onset

The pattern of results described above is similar to that found for age of onset in schizophrenia, which has been studied more extensively than other clinical variables to date. There is evidence of an important genetic contribution to age at onset of schizophrenia (Kendler et al., 1987; Cannon et al., 1998) with modest correlations in affected sibling and DZ twin pairs of around 0.3, and correlations in affected MZ twin pairs of around 0.7. A number of studies have shown higher familial risk to be associated with earlier age of onset (Kendler and MacLean, 1990; Pulver and Liang, 1991; Sham et al., 1994; Suvisaari et al., 1998). For example, Sham et al. (1994) showed that the morbid risk of schizophrenia is greater among the relatives of those probands who had an onset before rather than after age 21 years. The same group subsequently showed (Howard et al., 1997) that morbid risk in relatives was lowest for those with schizophrenia-like illnesses who presented for the first time in old age. However, other studies have found no significant relationship between familial risk and age of onset (Kendler et al., 1987, 1996a). This may be because the relationship is weak and, therefore, difficult to detect. Consistent with this, Neale et al. (1989) applied model fitting to a US veteran twin sample and found evidence that the genetic contribution to variation in age of onset in schizophrenia is predominantly caused by modifying genes, rather than susceptibility genes.

To the extent that susceptibility genes have some effect on clinical heterogeneity in schizophrenia, greater familial morbid risk tends to be associated with more severe illness (hebephrenic, negative, disorganized), earlier age of onset and also poor premorbid adjustment (Dworkin et al., 1991; Cardno and Gottesman, 2000). Therefore, some genes at least may be operating through a process of aberrant neurodevelopment.

Studies of endophenotypic abnormalities in twins and relatives
Studies of discordant twin pairs

Pairs of MZ twins where one has schizophrenia and the other does not offer important research opportunities. Two studies have shown that the risk of schizophrenia-like psychosis is similar in the offspring of both the affected and unaffected MZ twins (Gottesman and Bertelsen, 1989; Kringlen and Cramer, 1989). This implies that unaffected co-twins of affected MZ probands carry susceptibility genes for schizophrenia but have not expressed the phenotype. In view of this, studies of differences between the members of discordant MZ pairs offer the possibility of shedding light on noninherited or epigenetic mechanisms that contribute to the multifactorial aetiology of schizophrenia.

Following this logic, several groups have carried out brain imaging on MZ pairs discordant for schizophrenia. The first such study on twins from the Maudsley Register used computed tomographic (CT) scanning to demonstrate that the ill twins had larger ventricle to brain ratio (VBR) than their well co-twins, but nevertheless the well co-twins had greater VBR than normal control twin pairs (Reveley et al., 1982). This implies that both members of the discordant pair have inherited a tendency to increased cerebral ventricular size, and that this was then compounded by the operation on the affected twin of some additional environmental factor. Reveley and colleagues (1984) suggested that this additional factor might be pre- or perinatal hazards. These findings and speculations were supported by a series of magnetic resonance imaging (MRI) studies of MZ twins discordant for schizophrenia that had been collected by the US National Institute of Mental Health (Torrey et al., 1994). The affected twins had larger lateral ventricles and smaller hippocampal volume (Suddath et al., 1990), as well as smaller total brain volume (Noga et al., 1996), than their unaffected co-twins. Recently, McNeil et al. (2000) re-examined this sample and reported that the MZ twins with the largest lateral ventricles and smallest hippocampi compared with their well co-twins were those who had been subjected to the most severe perinatal complications.

Other studies of discordant pairs have investigated cognitive function (Goldberg et al., 1993, 1995), eye tracking (Litman et al., 1997), electroencephalogram (EEG) patterns (Stassen et al., 1999), obstetric complications (McNeil et al., 1994) and dermatoglyphic patterns suggestive of aberrant fetal development during the second trimester (Markow and Gottesman, 1989; Davis and Bracha, 1996). These findings have made important contributions to the hypothesis that aberrant neurodevelopment contributes to schizophrenia in at least a proportion of patients (Murray, 1994).

Phenotypic abnormalities in relatives

A number of investigators have asked whether the first-degree relatives of people with schizophrenia show any of the same abnormalities as their schizophrenic kin. One of these studies, the Maudsley Family Study, carried out MRI scans in patients and their well relatives from families with several schizophrenic members – these families were deliberately sampled on the basis that they were assumed to transmit a high genetic loading (Sharma et al., 1998). The study particularly focused on relatives who appeared to be transmitting liability to the disorder, for example a parent who, although well himself/herself, had a schizophrenic parent and child. These so-called 'obligate carriers' showed a similar increase in lateral ventricular volume to the patients themselves; other relatives were midway between patients and controls, as one might expect from a group where some, but not all, of whom are carrying susceptibility genes.

The Maudsley Family Study went on to contrast schizophrenic patients with a strong family history of the disorder and no obstetric complications with their counterparts who had no such family history but had been subject to obstetric complications (Stefanis et al., 1999): the latter but not the former group showed a decreased volume of the left hippocampus. This tends to confirm the work of McNeil et al. (2000), which suggested that decreased hippocampal volume in schizophrenia is a consequence of early environmental damage.

A variety of other abnormalities have been found in these well relatives. For example, the Maudsley Family Study reported that relatives show the same delay in the P300 event related potential that patients have (Frangou et al., 1997). Furthermore, some but not all families seem to transmit eye tracking abnormalities (Crawford et al., 1998) and relatives also show an excess of higher or integrative neurological signs (Griffiths et al., 1998). Neuropsychological deficits similar to those found in schizophrenic patients were also found in some of the relatives.

Gene–environment interaction

How are we to reconcile evidence that there is a major genetic component to schizophrenia and yet environmental factors appear to play an important role, for example in determining some of the structural abnormalities found in the brains of people with schizophrenia? (Models of gene–environment interaction are discussed in Ch. 12.) According to one model, individuals vary in their sensitivity to adverse environmental circumstances, and genetically sensitive individuals are more likely to develop psychiatric illness when exposed to certain environments than others. For example, Cannon et al. (1993) reported an association between exposure to obstetric complications and ventricular enlargement, and this association was especially pronounced among the offspring of mothers with psychosis. These findings led Cannon and his colleagues to conclude that part of the genetic susceptibility to schizophrenia may be a sensitivity to hypoxic-ischaemic damage at birth. These studies are outlined in detail in Chapter 13.

A similar gene–environment interaction was reported in the Finnish Adoptive Family Study, where the risk of developing schizophrenia spectrum disorders was higher in the adopted-away offspring of schizophrenic individuals but only in those who were exposed to a dysfunctional adoptive family rearing environment (Tienari et al., 1994).

Gene–environment interaction may also be the explanation for striking findings from two studies (Sugarman and Craufurd, 1994; Hutchinson et al., 1996) that examined the relatives of African-Caribbeans with schizophrenia living in England. This population is known to have a much increased incidence of schizophrenia, which is not shared by those living in the Caribbean (Wessely et al., 1991; van Os et al., 1996; see Ch. 4). While the risk for parents of African-Caribbeans with schizophrenia living in the UK was not examined in comparison with that for the parents of white schizophrenics, the risk of schizophrenia among siblings of the second generation (i.e. those born in England) was remarkably high, at up to six times higher than in siblings of white patients. These findings are compatible with the view that some environmental effect present in the UK but not the Caribbean is operating upon the second generation and increases risk in those who are genetically vulnerable.

Another question is whether individuals with certain genotypes may select environments that increase risk of the illness. For example, there is considerable evidence that abuse of certain drugs can increase the risk of schizophrenia. As noted in Chapter 16 of this volume, the first-degree relatives of individuals with cannabis-associated psychosis have an increased morbid risk of psychosis (McGuire et al., 1995). It may be that some individuals turn to the abuse of cannabis in an attempt to self-treat psychiatric symptoms to which they are genetically predisposed; it could equally be that among those individuals who abuse cannabis, it is those who have a genetic predisposition who are particularly likely to develop psychosis.

Conclusions and implications

There can be no doubt that schizophrenia is under a considerable genetic influence. The evidence of twin and family, as well as molecular genetic, studies indicates that this is not linked to the inheritance of a single major gene. Rather a number of such genes are likely to be involved. Some of these are shared with liability to other psychoses and to minor variants of the syndrome, termed schizophrenia spectrum disorders. One of the questions is whether the predisposition is actually to the syndrome per se or whether the so-called susceptibility genes are actually for traits found in the general population. There is some evidence, for example, that schizotypal characteristics in the general population are as heritable as schizophrenia itself (Linney et al., 2001).

If we accept the polygenic model, then the question is what do the individual genes transmit. Increasingly, studies are examining the relatives of schizophrenics to ascertain exactly what is transmitted. The evidence suggests that some families transmit a liability to traits for minor deviations that are relatively innocent in themselves, for example slightly decreased brain volume or a childhood intelligence quotient a few points lower than that of their siblings. However, when an individual is unlucky enough to inherit several of these, perhaps confounded by early environmental (e.g. perinatal hypoxia) or other hazards (e.g. cannabis abuse), then the cumulative effect of these risk factors may propel the individual past a threshold for the expression of symptoms.

An implication for molecular genetic studies is that defining the phenotype solely in terms of an operational diagnosis of schizophrenia may be inadequate. It may be more appropriate to adopt a fairly broad phenotype initially that includes the range of functional psychoses (and schizotypal and paranoid personality disorders, if feasible) and also to collect a wide range of good-quality phenotypic data including symptom profile, illness history and comorbidity variables, as well as making operational definitions. In addition, it would be valuable to obtain information on variables such as cognitive test performance, obstetric complications, neurophysiological measures and brain imaging in at least a representative subsample. Collecting this amount of phenotypic data is a major undertaking, but it would allow the relationship between genotypic and phenotypic variation to be explored in much more depth than has been possible so far.

REFERENCES

Abrams R, Taylor MA (1983) The genetics of schizophrenia: a reassessment using modern criteria. American Journal of Psychiatry 140, 171–175.

Allen MG, Cohen S, Pollin W (1972) Schizophrenia in veteran twins: a diagnostic review. American Journal of Psychiatry 128, 939–945.

American Psychiatric Association (1980) Diagnostic and Statistical Manual of Mental Disorders, 3rd edn. Washington, DC: American Psychiatric Press.

American Psychiatric Association (1987) Diagnostic and Statistical Manual III–Revised. Washington, DC: American Psychiatric Press.

Burke JG, Murphy BM, Bray JC, Walsh D, Kendler KS (1996) Clinical similarities in siblings with schizophrenia. American Journal of Medical Genetics (Neuropsychiatric Genetics) 67, 239–243.

Byrne M, Hodges A, Grant E, Owens DC, Johnstone EC (1999) Neuropsychological assessment of young people at high genetic risk for developing schizophrenia compared with controls: preliminary findings of the Edinburgh High Risk Study (EHRS). Psychological Medicine 29, 1161–1173.

Cannon TD; Mednick SA, Parnas J, Schulsinger F et al. (1993) Developmental brain abnormalities in the offspring of schizophrenic mothers: I. Contributions of genetic and perinatal factors. Archives of General Psychiatry 50, 551–564.

Cannon TD, Kaprio J, Lonnqvist J, Huttunen M, Koskenvuo M (1998) The genetic epidemiology of schizophrenia in a Finnish twin cohort: a population-based modeling study. Archives of General Psychiatry 55, 67–74.

Cardno AG, Gottesman II (2000) Twin studies of schizophrenia: from bow-and-arrow concordances to star wars Mx and functional genomics. American Journal of Medical Genetics (Seminars in Medical Genetics) 97, 00–00.

Cardno AG, Holmans PA, Harvey I, Williams MB, Owen MJ, McGuffin P (1997) Factor-derived subsyndromes of schizophrenia and familial morbid risks. Schizophrenia Research 23, 231–238.

Cardno AG, Jones LA, Murphy KC et al. (1998) Sibling pairs with schizophrenia or schizoaffective disorder: associations of subtypes, symptoms and demographic variables. Psychological Medicine 28, 815–823.

Cardno AG, Marshall EJ, Coid B et al. (1999a) Heritability estimates for psychotic disorders: the Maudsley twin psychosis series. Archives of General Psychiatry 56, 162–168.

Cardno AG, Jones LA, Murphy KC et al. (1999b) Dimensions of psychosis in affected sibling pairs. Schizophrenia Bulletin 25, 841–850.

Cardno AG, Rijsdijk FV, Sham PC, Murray RM, McGuffin P (2002) A twin study of genetic relationships between psychotic symptoms. American Journal of Psychiatry 159, 539–545.

Castle DJ, Wessely S, van Os J, Murray R (1998) Psychosis in the Inner City: The Camberwell First Episode Study. Hove: Psychology Press.

Cooper J, Goodhead D, Craig T, Harris M, Howards J, Korer J (1987) The incidence of schizophrenia in Nottingham. British Journal of Psychiatry 151, 619–626.

Crawford TJ, Sharma T, Puri BK, Murray RM, Berridge DM, Lewis SW (1998) Saccadic eye movements in families multiply affected with schizophrenia: the Maudsley Family Study. American Journal of Psychiatry 155, 1703–1710.

Davis JO, Bracha HS (1996) Prenatal growth markers in schizophrenia: a monozygotic co-twin control study. American Journal of Psychiatry 153, 1166–1172.

Davis JO, Phelps JA, Bracha HS (1995) Prenatal development of monozygotic twins and concordance for schizophrenia. Schizophrenia Bulletin 21, 357–366.

Dworkin RH, Lenzenweger MF (1984) Symptoms and the genetics of schizophrenia: implications for diagnosis. American Journal of Psychiatry 141, 1541–1546.

Dworkin RH, Bernstein G, Kaplansky LM et al. (1991) Social competence and positive and negative symptoms: a longitudinal study of children and adolescents at risk for schizophrenia and affective disorder. American Journal of Psychiatry 148, 1182–1188.

Erlenmeyer-Kimling L, Squires-Wheeler E, Hilldoff Adamo U et al. (1995) The New York High Risk Project: psychoses and cluster A personality disorders in offspring of schizophrenic parents at 23 years of follow-up. Archives of General Psychiatry 52, 857–865.

Falconer DS (1965) The inheritance of liability to certain diseases, estimated from the incidence among relatives. Annals of Human Genetics 29, 51–76.

Falconer DS, Mackay TFC (1996) Introduction to Quantitative Genetics, 4th edn. Harlow, UK: Longman.

Farmer AE, McGuffin P, Gottesman II (1984) Searching for the split in schizophrenia: a twin Farmer study perspective. Psychiatry Research 13, 109–118.

Fischer M (1973) Genetic and environmental factors in schizophrenia: a study of schizophrenic twins and their families. Acta Psychiatrica Scandinavica Suppl. 238.

Frangou S, Sharma T, Alarcon G et al. (1997) The Maudsley Family Study, II: endogenous event-related potentials in familial schizophrenia. Schizophrenia Research 23, 45–53.

Franzek E, Beckmann H (1998) Different genetic background of schizophrenia spectrum psychoses: a twin study. American Journal of Psychiatry 155, 76–83.

Gershon ES, Hamovit J, Guroff JJ et al. (1982) A family study of schizoaffective, bipolar I, bipolar II, unipolar, and normal control probands. Archives of General Psychiatry 39, 1157–1167.

Goldberg TE, Torrey EF, Gold JM, Ragland JD, Bigelow LB, Weinberger DR (1993) Learning and memory in monozygotic twins discordant for schizophrenia. Psychological Medicine 23, 71–85.

Goldberg TE, Torrey EF, Gold JM et al. (1995) Genetic risk of neuropsychological impairment in schizophrenia: a study of monozygotic twins discordant and concordant for the disorder. Schizophrenia Research 17, 77–84.

Gottesman II (1991) Schizophrenia Genesis: The Origins of Madness. New York: Freeman.

Gottesman II, Shields J (1972) Schizophrenia and Genetics: A Twin Vantage Point. New York: Academic Press.

Gottesman II, Shields J (1982) Schizophrenia: The Epigenetic Puzzle. Cambridge: Cambridge University Press.

Gottesman II, Bertelsen A (1989) Confirming unexpressed genotypes for schizophrenia: risks in the offspring of Fischer's Danish identical and fraternal discordant twins. Archives of General Psychiatry 46, 867–872.

Griffiths TD, Sigmundsson T, Takei N, Rowe D, Murray RM (1998) Neurological abnormalities in familial and sporadic schizophrenia. Brain 121, 191–203.

Heston LL (1966) Psychiatric disorders in foster home reared children of schizophrenic mothers. British Journal of Psychiatry 112, 819–825.

Howard RJ, Graham C, Sham P et al. (1997) A controlled family study of late-onset nonaffective psychosis (late paraphrenia). British Journal of Psychiatry 170, 511–514.

Hutchinson G, Takei N, Fahy T et al. (1996) Morbid risk of psychotic illness in first degree relatives of white and African-Caribbean patients with psychosis. British Journal of Psychiatry, 169, 776–780.

Jöreskog KG, Sörbom D (1988) PRELIS: A Program for Multivariate Data Screening and Data Summarization. A Preprocessor for LISREL, 2nd edn. Mooresville, Indiana: Scientific Software, Inc.

Jöreskog KG, Sörbom D (1989) LISREL 7: A Guide to the Program and Applications, 2nd edn. Chicago: SPSS Inc.

Jørgensen A, Teasdale TW, Parnas J, Schulsinger F, Schulsinger H, Mednick SA (1987) The Copenhagen High-Risk Project: the diagnosis of maternal schizophrenia and its relation to offspring diagnosis. British Journal of Psychiatry 151, 753–757.

Kendler KS (1983) Overview: a current perspective on twin studies of schizophrenia. American Journal of Psychiatry 140, 1413–1425.

Kendler KS, Adler D (1984) The pattern of illness in pairs of psychotic siblings. American Journal of Psychiatry 141, 509–513.

Kendler KS, Davis KL (1981) The genetics and biochemistry of paranoid schizophrenia and other paranoid psychoses. Schizophrenia Bulletin 7, 689–709.

Kendler KS, Diehl SR (1993) The genetics of schizophrenia: a current, genetic-epidemiologic perspective. Schizophrenia Bulletin 19, 261–285.

Kendler KS, Gardner CO Jr (1998) Twin studies of adult psychiatric and substance dependence disorders: are they biased by differences in the environmental experiences of monozygotic and dizygotic twins in childhood and adolescence? Psychological Medicine 28, 625–633.

Kendler KS, MacLean CJ (1990) Estimating familial effects on age at onset and liability to schizophrenia I: results of a large sample family study. Genetic Epidemiology 7, 409–417.

Kendler KS, Robinette CD (1983) Schizophrenia in the National Acadamy of Sciences National Research Council Twin Registry: a 16 year update. American Journal of Psychiatry 140, 1551–1563.

Kendler KS, Tsuang MT (1988) Outcome and familial psychopathology in schizophrenia. Archives of General Psychiatry 45, 338–346.

Kendler KS, Walsh D (1995) Schizophreniform disorder, delusional disorder and psychotic disorder not otherwise specified: clinical features, outcome and familial psychopathology. Acta Psychiatrica Scandinavica 91, 370–378.

Kendler KS, Gruenberg AM, Tsuang MT (1986) A DSM-III family study of the nonschizophrenic psychotic disorders. American Journal of Psychiatry 143, 1098–1105.

Kendler KS, Tsuang MT, Hays P (1987) Age at onset in schizophrenia: a familial perspective. Archives of General Psychiatry 44, 881–890.

Kendler KS, Gruenberg AM, Tsuang MT (1988) A family study of the subtypes of schizophrenia. American Journal of Psychiatry 145, 57–62.

Kendler KS, McGuire M, Gruenberg AM, O'Hare A, Spellman M, Walsh D (1993a) The Roscommon family study IV: affective illness, anxiety disorders, and alcoholism in relatives. Archives of General Psychiatry 50, 952–960.

Kendler KS, McGuire M, Gruenberg AM, O'Hare A, Spellman M, Walsh D (1993b) The Roscommon family study III: schizophrenia-related personality disorders in relatives. Archives of General Psychiatry 50, 781–788.

Kendler KS, McGuire M, Gruenberg AM, O'Hare A, Spellman M, Walsh D (1993c) The Roscommon family study I: methods, diagnosis of probands, and risk of schizophrenia in relatives. Archives of General Psychiatry 50, 527–540.

Kendler KS, McGuire M, Gruenberg AM, Spellman M, O'Hare A, Walsh D (1993d) The Roscommon family study II: the risk of nonschizophrenic nonaffective psychoses in relatives. Archives of General Psychiatry 50, 645–652.

Kendler KS, Gruenberg AM, Kinney DK (1994a) Independent diagnoses of adoptees and relatives as defined by DSM-III in the provincial and national samples of the Danish adoption study of schizophrenia. Archives of General Psychiatry 51, 456–468.

Kendler KS, McGuire M, Gruenberg AM, Walsh D (1994b) Outcome and family study of the subtypes of schizophrenia in the west of Ireland. American Journal of Psychiatry 151, 849–856.

Kendler KS, McGuire M, Gruenberg AM, Walsh D (1994c) Clinical heterogeneity in schizophrenia and the pattern of psychopathology in relatives: results from an epidemiologically based family study. Acta Psychiatrica Scandinavica 89, 294–300.

Kendler KS, Karkowski-Shuman L, Walsh D (1996a) Age at onset in schizophrenia and risk of illness in relatives: results from the Roscommon family study. British Journal of Psychiatry 169, 213–218.

Kendler KS, Pedersen NL, Farahmand BY, Persson P-G (1996b) The treated incidence of psychotic and affective illness in twins compared with population expectation: a study in the Swedish twin and psychiatric registries. Psychological Medicine 26, 1135–1144.

Kendler KS, Karkowski-Shuman L, O'Neill FA et al. (1997) Resemblance of psychotic symptoms and syndromes in affected sibling pairs from the Irish study of high-density schizophrenia families: evidence for possible etiologic heterogeneity. American Journal of Psychiatry 154, 191–198.

Kety SS, Rosenthal D, Wender PH, Schulsinger F (1971) Mental illness in the biological and adoptive families of adopted schizophrenics. American Journal of Psychiatry 128, 302–306.

Kety SS, Wender PH, Jacobsen B et al. (1994) Mental illness in the biological and adoptive relatives of schizophrenic adoptees: replication of the Copenhagen study in the rest of Denmark. Archives of General Psychiatry 51, 442–455.

Kläning U (1996) Schizophrenia in Twins: Incidence and Risk Factors. PhD thesis, University of Aarhus, Denmark.

Kläning U (1999) Greater occurrence of schizophrenia in dizygotic but not monozygotic twins: register-based study. British Journal of Psychiatry 175, 407–409.

Kläning U, Mortensen PB, Kyvik KO (1996) Increased occurrence of schizophrenia and other psychiatric illnesses among twins. British Journal of Psychiatry 168, 688–692.

Kringlen E (1967) Heredity and Environment in the Functional Psychoses: An Epidemiological–Clinical Twin Study. London: William Heinemann.

Kringlen E, Cramer G (1989) Offspring of monozygotic twins discordant for schizophrenia. Archives of General Psychiatry 46, 873–877.

Lalouel JM, Morton NE (1981) Complex segregation analysis with pointers. Human Heredity 31, 312–321.

Linney Y (2001) A Quantitative Genetic Analysis of Schizotypal Personality Traits and Neuropsychological Functioning. PhD thesis, University of London.

Litman RE, Torrey EF, Hommer DW, Radant AR, Pickar D, Weinberger DR (1997) A quantitative analysis of smooth pursuit eye tracking in monozygotic twins discordant for schizophrenia. Archives of General Psychiatry 54, 417–426.

Loftus J, DeLisi LE, Crow TJ (1998) Familial associations of subsyndromes of psychosis in affected sibling pairs with schizophrenia and schizoaffective disorder. Psychiatry Research 80, 101–111.

Maier W, Lichtermann D, Minges J, Heun R, Hallmayer J, Benkert O (1992) Schizoaffective disorder and affective disorders with mood-incongruent psychotic features: keep separate or combine? Evidence from a family study. American Journal of Psychiatry 149, 1666–1673.

Maier W, Lichtermann D, Minges J et al. (1993) Continuity and discontinuity of affective disorders and schizophrenia: results of a controlled family study. Archives of General Psychiatry 50, 871–883.

Markow TA, Gottesman II (1989) Fluctuating dermatoglyphic asymmetry in psychotic twins. Psychiatric Research 29, 37–44.

Martin N, Boomsma D, Machin G (1997) A twin-pronged attack on complex traits. Nature Genetics 17, 387–392.

McGue M, Gottesman II, Rao DC (1985) Resolving genetic models for the transmission of schizophrenia. Genetic Epidemiology 2, 99–110.

McGuffin P, Farmer A, Gottesman II (1987) Is there really a split in schizophrenia?: the genetic evidence. British Journal of Psychiatry 150, 581–592.

McGuffin P, Farmer A, Harvey J (1991) A polydiagnostic application of operational criteria in studies of psychotic illness: development and reliability of the OPCRIT system. Archives of General Psychiatry 48, 764–770.

McGuffin P, Asherson P, Owen M, Farmer A (1994a) The strength of the genetic effect: is there room for an environmental influence in the aetiology of schizophrenia? British Journal of Psychiatry 164, 593–599.

McGuffin P, Owen MJ, O'Donovan MC, Thapar A, Gottesman II (1994b) Seminars in Psychiatric Genetics. London: Gaskell.

McGuffin P, Owen MJ, Farmer AE (1995) The genetic basis of schizophrenia. Lancet 346, 78–682.

McGuire PK, Jones P, Harvey I, Williams M, McGuffin P, Murray RM (1995) Morbid risk of schizophrenia for relatives of patients with cannabis-associated psychosis. Schizophrenia Research 15, 277–281.

McNeil TF, Cantorgraae E, Torrey EF et al. (1994) Obstetric complications in histories of monozygotic twins discordant and concordant for schizophrenia. Acta Psychiatrica Scandinavica 89, 196–204.

McNeil TF, Cantor-Graae E, Weinberger DR (2000) Relationship of obstetric complications and differences in size of brain structures in monozygotic twin pairs discordant for schizophrenia. American Journal of Psychiatry 157, 203–212.

Meyer JM, Eaves LJ, Heath AC, Martin NG (1991) Estimating genetic influences on the age-at-menarche: a survival analysis approach. American Journal of Medical Genetics 39, 148–154.

Mirsky AF (1995) Israeli high-risk study: editor's introduction. Schizophrenia Bulletin 21, 179–204.

Mortensen PB, Pedersen CB, Westergaard T et al. (1999) Effects of family history and place and season of birth on the risk of schizophrenia. New England Journal of Medicine 340, 603–608.

Morton NE, MacLean CJ (1974) Analysis of family resemblance III: complex segregation analysis of quantitative traits. American Journal of Human Genetics 26, 89–503.

Murray RM (1994) Neurodevelopmental schizophrenia: the rediscovery of dementia praecox. British Journal of Psychiatry 165(Suppl. 25), 6–12.

Neale MC (1999) Mx: Statistical Modeling, 5th edn. Richmond, VA: Department of Psychiatry, Medical College of Virginia.

Neale MC, Cardon LR (1992) Methodology for Genetic Studies of Twins and Families. Dordrecht, the Netherlands: Kluwer Academic.

Neale MC, Kendler KS (1995) Models of comorbidity for multifactorial disorders. American Journal of Human Genetics 57, 935–953.

Neale MC, Eaves LJ, Hewitt JK, MacLean CJ, Meyer JM, Kendler KS (1989) Analysing the relationship between age at onset and risk to relatives. American Journal of Human Genetics 45, 226–239.

Noga JT, Bartley AJ, Jones DW, Torrey EF, Weinberger DR (1996) Cortical gyral anatomy and gross brain dimensions in monozygotic twins discordant for schizophrenia. Schizophrenia Research 22, 27–40.

Nuechterlein KH (1983) Signal detection in vigilance tasks and behavioral attributes among off-spring of schizophrenic mothers and among hyperactive children. Journal of Abnormal Psychology 92, 4–28.

Onstad S, Skre I, Torgersen S, Kringlen E (1991a) Twin concordance for DSM-III-R schizophrenia. Acta Psychiatrica Scandinavica 83, 395–401.

Onstad S, Skre I, Torgersen S, Kringlen E (1991b) Subtypes of schizophrenia: evidence from a twin-family study. Acta Psychiatrica Scandinavica 84, 203–206.

O'Rourke DH, Gottesman II, Suarez BK, Rice J, Reich T (1982) Refutation of the single locus model for the etiology of schizophrenia. American Journal of Human Genetics 34, 630–649.

Parnas J, Cannon TD, Jacobsen B, Schulsinger H, Schulsinger F, Mednick SA (1993) Lifetime DSM-III-R diagnostic outcomes in the offspring of schizophrenic mothers: results from the Copenhagen high-risk study. Archives of General Psychiatry 50, 707–714.

Pope HG, Jonas JM, Cohen BM, Lipinski JF (1982) Failure to find evidence of schizophrenia in first-degree relatives of schizophrenic probands. American Journal of Psychiatry 139, 826–828.

Pulver AE, Liang K-Y (1991) Estimating effects of proband characteristics on familial risk II: the association between age at onset and familial risk in the Maryland schizophrenia sample. Genetic Epidemiology 8, 339–350.

Reich T, James JW, Morris CA (1972) The use of multiple thresholds in determining the mode of transmission of semi-continuous traits. Annals of Human Genetics 36, 163–184.

Reveley AM, Reveley MA, Clifford CA, Murray RM (1982) Cerebral ventricular size in twins discordant for schizophrenia. Lancet 1, 540–541.

Reveley AM, Reveley MA, Murray RM (1984) Cerebral ventricular enlargement in non-genetic schizophrenia: a controlled study. British Journal of Psychiatry 144, 89–93.

Risch N (1990) Linkage strategies for genetically complex traits I: multilocus models. American Journal of Human Genetics 46, 222–228.

Risch N, Baron M (1984) Segregation analysis of schizophrenia and related disorders. American Journal of Human Genetics 36, 1039–1059.

Rose RJ, Uchida IA, Christian JC (1981) Placentation effects on cognitive resemblance of adult monozygotes. In: Twin Research 3: Intelligence, Personality, and Development. New York: Alan R Liss, pp. 5–41.

Rosenthal D (1960) Confusion of identity and the frequency of schizophrenia in twins. Archives of General Psychiatry 3, 297–304.

Rosenthal D, Wender PH, Kety SS, Welner J, Schulsinger F (1971) The adopted-away offspring of schizophrenics. American Journal of Psychiatry 128, 307–311.

Sham PC (1998) Statistics methods in psychiatric genetics. Statistical Methods in Medical Research 7, 279–300.

Sham PC, Jones P, Russell A et al. (1994) Age at onset, sex, and familial psychiatric morbidity in schizophrenia: Camberwell collaborative psychosis study. *British Journal of Psychiatry* 165, 466–473.

Sharma T, Lancaster E, Lee D et al. (1998) Brain changes in schizophrenia: volumetric MRI study of families multiply affected with schizophrenia – The Maudsley Family Study 5. *British Journal of Psychiatry* 173, 132–138.

Spitzer RL, Williams JBW, Gibbon M (1990) User's Guide for the Structured Clinical Interview for DSM-III-R (SCID). Washington, DC: American Psychiatric Press.

Stassen HH, Coppola R, Gottesman II et al. (1999) EEG differences in monozygotic twins discordant and concordant for schizophrenia. *Psychophysiology* 36, 109–117.

Stefanis N, Frangou S, Yakeley J et al. (1999) Hippocampal volume reduction in schizophrenia: effects of genetic risk and pregnancy and birth complications. *Biological Psychiatry* 46, 697–702.

Suddath RL, Christison GW, Torrey EF et al. (1990) Anatomical abnormalities in the brains of monozygotic twins discordant for schizophrenia. *New England Journal of Medicine* 322, 789–794.

Sugarman PA, Craufurd D (1994) Schizophrenia in the Afro-Caribbean community. *British Journal of Psychiatry* 164, 474–80.

Suvisaari JM, Haukka J, Tanskanen A, Lönnqvist JK (1998) Age at onset and outcome in schizophrenia are related to the degree of familial loading. *British Journal of Psychiatry* 173, 494–500.

Tienari P (1963) Psychiatric illnesses in identical twins. *Acta Psychiatrica Scandinavica* 39(Suppl.), 171.

Tienari P, Wynne LC, Moring J et al. (1994) The Finnish Adoptive Family Study of schizophrenia: implications for family research. *British Journal of Psychiatry* 164(Suppl.), 20–26.

Torrey EF, Bowler AE, Taylor EH, Gottesman II (1994) Schizophrenia and Manic Depressive Disorder: The Biological Roots of Mental Illness as Revealed by a Landmark Study of Identical Twins. New York: Basic Books.

Tsujita T, Okazaki Y, Fujimaru K et al. (1992) Twin concordance rate of DSM-III-R schizophrenia in a new Japanese sample. *Proceedings of the Seventh International Congress on Twin Studies*, Tokyo, abstract 152.

van Os J, Castle J, Takei N, Der G, Murray RM (1996) Psychotic illness in ethnic minorities: clarification from the 1991 census. *Psychological Medicine* 26, 203–208.

van Os J, Marcelis M, Sham P, Jones P, Gilvarry K, Murray R (1997) Psychopathological syndromes and familial morbid risk of psychosis. *British Journal of Psychiatry* 170, 241–246.

Verdoux H, van Os J, Sham P, Jones P, Gilvarry K, Murray R (1996) Does familiality predispose to both emergence and persistence of psychosis? A follow-up study. *British Journal of Psychiatry* 168, 620–626.

Wender PH, Rosenthal D, Kety SS, Schulsinger F, Welner J (1974) Crossfostering: a research strategy for clarifying the role of genetic and experiential factors in the etiology of schizophrenia. *Archives of General Psychiatry* 30, 121–128.

Wessely S, Castle D, Der G, Murray RM (1991) Schizophrenia and Afro-Caribbeans: a case control study. *British Journal of Psychiatry* 159, 795–801.

World Health Organization (1992) International Classification of Diseases, 10th draft. Geneva: World Health Organization.

11

Molecular genetics and epidemiology in schizophrenia: a necessary partnership

Stanley Zammit[1], Glyn Lewis[2] and Michael J. Owen[1]

[1]University of Wales College of Medicine, Cardiff, UK
[2]Division of Psychiatry, University of Bristol, UK

A genetic component to the aetiology of schizophrenia was established early in this century (Jablensky, 1999) but, apart from this, the aetiology still remains something of a mystery. In recent years, epidemiologists have tended to study environmental factors associated with disease (Ch. 5) whereas geneticists have focused on the application of model-fitting approaches to try to quantify the genetic component (Ch. 10) or on developing specialized methods to map and identify susceptibility genes. However, it is becoming increasingly clear that the identification of specific genes that increase risk factors will be greatly aided by the appropriate application of epidemiological principles. Moreover, geneticists and epidemiologists will need to work even more closely together once such genes are identified in order to establish the impact of specific genetic risk factors on populations and to study the interactions of these factors with each other and with environmental factors.

Schizophrenia is a complex, multifactorial condition that results from the influence of both genetic and environmental factors. Our understanding of other complex disorders has shown us that it is more productive to consider how these factors might be operating together to bring about disease rather than to classify them as distinct aetiological processes, since identified risk factors appear to be neither sufficient, nor always necessary, to cause disease. Additionally, the division between genetic and environmental causation is not always clear. For example, phenylketonuria may be considered as 100% genetic (eliminating all the disease genes from the population would eradicate the disease) or as 100% environmental (removing all phenylalanine from the environment would also eradicate the disease).

The diagnosis of schizophrenia covers patients with a variety of symptoms, courses, outcomes and responses to treatment, but despite considerable effort and ingenuity it has not been possible to delineate aetiologically distinct subgroups, or to establish clearly pathogenic mechanisms. In spite of these difficulties, the use of structured and semi-structured interviews together with explicit operational diagnostic criteria means that it is often possible to achieve high degrees of diagnostic reliability and to define a syndrome with high heritability. However, we have to accept that the disorder, as defined by current diagnostic criteria, may include a number of heterogeneous disease processes and that this will hinder any attempts at identifying aetiological factors.

The nature of the genetic effect

Historical observations that schizophrenia runs in families led to a number of family, twin and adoption studies, which, despite some variation in results, overall provide strong evidence for a genetic component to this disorder, with even conservative estimates suggesting a heritability of greater than 60% (McGuffin et al., 1994). These data are reviewed in detail in Chapter 10 of this volume.

While it is clear from these studies that there is a genetic contribution to schizophrenia, it is equally clear that what is inherited is not the certainty of disease accompanying a particular genotype but rather a predisposition or liability to develop the disorder. Moreover, twin and adoption studies have also shown that schizophrenia shares familial, and probably genetic, liability with a range of other psychotic illnesses (Kendler et al., 1993a) and personality disorders, such as schizotypal personality disorder (Kendler et al., 1993b), collectively known as the schizophrenia spectrum disorders.

Studies on the recurrence risk in various classes of relative allow us to exclude the possibility that schizophrenia is a single-gene disorder or a collection of single-gene disorders even when incomplete penetrance is taken into account (O'Rourke et al., 1982; McGue et al., 1985). Rather, the mode of transmission, like that of other complex disorders, is complex and nonmendelian (McGue and Gottesman, 1989). The commonest mode of transmission is probably oligogenic (a small number of genes of moderate effect), polygenic (many genes of small effect) or a mixture of the two (McGuffin et al., 1995). However, the number of susceptibility loci, the disease risk conferred by each locus and the degree of interaction between loci all remain unknown.

The contribution of individual genes to the familiality of a disorder can be expressed in terms of λ_s, which is the relative risk to siblings resulting from possession of the disease allele (Risch, 1990). Risch (1990) has calculated that the data for recurrence risks in the relatives of probands with schizophrenia are incompatible with the existence of a single locus of $\lambda_s > 3$ and, unless extreme epistasis (interaction between loci) exists, models with two or three loci of $\lambda_s \leq 2$ are more plausible. It should be emphasized that these calculations are based upon the assumption that the effects of genes are distributed equally across the whole population. It is quite possible that genes of larger effect are operating in a subset of patients.

Although the weight of evidence from genetic epidemiology suggests that genes play a substantial role in the aetiology of schizophrenia, it is equally clear from twin studies that environmental factors must also play a role. There are a number of genetic mechanisms, such as somatic mutation, genomic imprinting and mitochondrial inheritance, that could cause phenotypic differences, including discordance, between monozygotic twins and that would, therefore, contribute to the so-called 'environmental' effects observed in twin studies (McGuffin et al., 1995; Morgan et al., 1999), emphasizing that the distinction between genetic and environmental factors is not always as straightforward as at first appears. It is also possible that stochastic factors could play a role in mediating the effects of genotype on phenotype, particularly where a complex process such as brain development is concerned (McGuffin et al., 1995). These too would inflate the contribution of environmental effects estimated from twin and adoption studies. However, interactions between genes and environment tend to be included in the 'genetic' component of models; for example, phenylketonuria, as discussed above, is regarded very much as a genetic disorder. One way of describing the relationship between genes and environment, therefore, is to say that the disease occurs when one's genes are not adapted to one's environment. These issues are discussed further in Chapter 12.

Gene mapping strategies

Two main groups of strategies are used to identify genes in complex disorders: linkage and association. In linkage studies, the aim is to identify alleles that segregate with the disease in families with two or more affected individuals. This approach can detect the presence of genes over large chromosomal distances and, therefore, is readily applicable to genome-wide studies. It is ideally suited to detecting genes in monogenic disorders, but its power to detect genes of moderate-to-small effect is limited.

In association studies, the unit of study is a sample of unrelated people usually in the form of a case-control design. Here the aim is to detect alleles that are more (or less) common in cases than in controls. Association studies have considerable power to detect the genes of small effect that are most likely to be operating in complex disorders such as schizophrenia, but they depend upon the marker studied being either the pathogenic variant itself or so close to it as to be in linkage disequilibrium (LD) with it. LD refers to the nonrandom association in a population of alleles at two closely linked loci and can occur when most cases of a disease are caused by a mutation in a common ancestor, known as a founder mutation. The disequilibrium will be eroded by recombination during meioses, and, therefore, for LD to be maintained over many generations, marker alleles need to be much closer to susceptibility loci than they do for linkage-based studies. A systematic, genome-wide search for association would, therefore, require many thousands of markers.

Linkage studies

The first wave of molecular genetic studies of schizophrenia effectively ignored the evidence for genetic complexity by focusing on large multiply affected pedigrees on the assumption that aetiological heterogeneity exists and that such families, or at least a proportion of them, are segregating genes of major effect. This approach has been successful in other complex disorders, particularly Alzheimer's disease, where mutations in three genes, *APP*, *PS1* and *PS2*, are now known to cause rare forms of the disorder in which disease of unusually early onset is inherited in an autosomal dominant fashion (Goate et al., 1991; Levy-Lahad et al., 1995; Sherrington et al., 1995). Similar studies of large families segregating schizophrenia and related phenotypes also initially produced positive findings (Sherrington et al., 1989) but unfortunately these could not be replicated. The reasons for this have become clear as data from systematic genome scans have accumulated. It seems likely that highly penetrant mutations causing schizophrenia are at best extremely rare and quite possibly nonexistent (Craddock et al., 1995; McGuffin and Owen, 1996), with type I errors arising largely from a combination of multiple testing and the use of statistical methodology and significance levels derived from work on single-gene disorders.

In spite of the failure to identify genes of major effect in multiply affected families, moderately significant evidence for linkage has been found in more than one dataset in several chromosomal regions. Areas implicated include 6p24–22, 8p22–21 and 22q11–12 (reviewed by McGuffin and Owen, 1996; Moldin and Gottesman, 1997) for which supportive data have also been obtained from international collaborative studies (Schizophrenia Collaborative Linkage Group, 1996; Schizophrenia Collaborative Linkage Group for Chromosomes 3, 6 and 8, 1996). More recent findings include those on 13q14.1–q32 (Lin et al., 1995; Blouin et al., 1998; Brzustowicz et al., 1999), 5q21–q31, 18p 22–21 and 10p15–p11 (Schwab et al., 1997, 1988a,b; Straub et al., 1997, 1998; Faraone et al., 1998). However, in each case there are negative as well as positive findings, and in only one case, that of chromosome 13q, did any single study achieve genome-wide significance at $p=0.05$.

The pattern of findings from linkage studies of schizophrenia demonstrates several features that are to be expected in the search for genes involved in disorders that have a predisposition through the combined action of several genes of moderate effect (Lander and Schork, 1994; Suarez et al., 1994; Lander and Kruglyak, 1995). First, no finding replicates in all datasets; second, levels of statistical significance and estimated effect sizes are usually modest; and third, chromosomal regions of interest are typically broad (often >20–30 centimorgans). Unfortunately, it is debatable, at present, whether the statistical support for linkage associated with any of the regions is sufficiently strong to warrant large-scale and expensive efforts aimed at cloning putative linked loci, given that some or all of these findings could be type I errors.

Williams et al. (1999) conducted the largest systematic search for linkage in affected sibling pairs (ASPs) with schizophrenia published to date, with a power of >0.95 to detect a susceptibility locus of $\lambda_s = 3$ at a genome-wide significance of 0.05, and a power of 0.70 to detect a locus of $\lambda_s = 2$. However, none of the findings approached a genome-wide significance of 0.05, corresponding to Lander and Kruglyak's (1995) definition of 'significant' linkage. Under the assumption of no dominance variance, Williams and colleagues were able to exclude susceptibility genes with effects of $\lambda_s = 3$ and $\lambda_s = 2$ from 82.8% and 48.7% of the genome, respectively, while genes with an effect size of $\lambda_s = 1.5$ could only be excluded from 9.3% of the genome. Of course it remains possible that susceptibility alleles of larger effect may be more common in other samples owing to diagnostic, ethnic or geographical differences, or when families containing multiple affected members are studied. However, this search does demonstrate that, while progress has been made in pursuit of genes using linkage methods, so far linkage has largely enabled delineation of what is not the case rather than the unequivocal location of susceptibility genes.

Linkage methods can detect smaller-sized genetic effects of the magnitude likely to be operating in schizophrenia (λ_s 1.5–3) in sample sizes that are realistic (600–800 ASPs) (Hauser et al., 1996; Scott et al., 1997) but considerably larger than those used to date. Priority should now be given to collecting such samples using common and robust clinical methodology. However, if schizophrenia does just reflect the operation of many genes of small effect, then even these large-scale studies will be unsuccessful.

Association studies

Once genes of small effect are sought (i.e. those conferring a risk in siblings relative to the population of <1.5), the number of families that are required for linkage studies becomes prohibitively large (Hauser et al., 1996). Allelic association studies offer a powerful means of identifying such genes in realistically sized samples of unrelated cases. The requirement for markers to be themselves the susceptibility locus, or at least very close to it, means that this approach is ideally suited to the study of polymorphisms within candidate genes. The main problem with this approach is that we have such limited knowledge about the pathogenesis of schizophrenia that there are potentially thousands of genes that could be candidates for involvement with the disorder, most of which are yet to be identified/sequenced.

Given the difficulties and expense inherent in these types of study, some may question whether any priority should be given to finding such genes of small effect, though of course if a risk factor is common in the population then it can be associated with a high attributable risk, even though the relative risk may be low. For example, in schizophrenia, the population attributable fraction associated with possession of allele *C* of the T102C polymorphism in the 5-hydroxytryptamine type 2A receptor (5HT2A) is 0.35 (Williams et al., 1997). Furthermore, even associations of small effect provide evidence that a particular pathway is involved in a disease process, which is extremely important because, historically, it has been difficult to distinguish between biological measurements that are a consequence of a psychiatric disorder rather than a cause (cf amyloid precursor protein and Alzheimer's disease). Independent findings from genetics can, therefore, provide a firm foundation for further research efforts into these pathways and their modulators in the search for other aetiological factors, both genetic and environmental.

Some positive results for allelic association in schizophrenia have already been found (Williams et al., 1997, 1998), though once again conflicting results have been reported. Unfortunately, association studies are prone to type I errors, the most likely reasons being the low prior odds of association and the multiple testing involved (Owen et al., 1997; Risch and Teng, 1998), a problem that will be even more significant when genome-wide scans are undertaken. Additionally, association studies are heavily influenced by population structure, and confounding may occur owing to population stratification, resulting in different allele frequencies at the marker locus in the cases and controls. In fact, there are relatively few proven examples of population stratification causing false associations.

Family-based association studies

Family-based association methods can be used to avoid the effects of population stratification. In these studies, other family members, usually parents, are genotyped and the number of alleles transmitted to the affected proband is compared with the nontransmitted parental alleles, which thus make up a notional control group matched with the probands for parental origin (Ewens and Spielman, 1995; Schaid and Rowland, 1998). However, family members are difficult to sample in many instances and especially in adult disorders. These studies also lack power in many situations (Risch and Teng, 1998) and offer less potential for future studies of interaction between genetic and environmental risk factors than traditional case-control designs.

Spurious associations may also arise from confounding caused by recent admixture and selection or drift between unlinked loci (Khoury and Beaty, 1994; Lander and Schork, 1994; Weeks and Lathrop, 1995). Confounding can be controlled for through various analytic strategies, with stratification and logistic regression being the methods most commonly used for case-control studies.

The most successful application of the association approach in psychiatric genetics has been the identification of the *e4* allele of the gene encoding apolipoprotein

E (APOE) as a risk factor for Alzheimer's disease (Corder et al., 1993). It has usually been assumed that the lack of replicated findings in schizophrenia reflect the tendency of association studies to produce type I errors. However, we should not discount the possibility of type II errors since, where small effects (odds ratios of approximately 1.2–1.5) are concerned, larger samples than those used in many studies may be required to have adequate power to achieve replication. For example, an association between schizophrenia and allele C of the T102C polymorphism in the gene for 5HT2A was recently observed in a large collaborative study (Williams et al., 1996). A number of small 'failures to replicate' have been published, but a meta-analysis of all published data, which included over 3000 subjects, supported the original finding with an odds ratio of 1.2 and suggested that publication bias was unlikely (Williams et al., 1997).

Consequently, it is with some urgency that association studies which aim to test putative associations should be based upon large enough samples (usually several hundred to a thousand cases with as many, if not more, controls) to provide meaningful tests of association hypotheses. Nevertheless, LD may still not be found if mutational events at either the marker locus or the disease locus are common, even when markers are very close to a disease locus.

Methodological problems

A further problem is that samples are often ascertained in widely differing and unsystematic ways, and any associations reported might, therefore, be with other confounding variables such as comorbidity or with modifying factors such as those influencing disease severity or age at onset. For example, genes involved in the monoamine system implicated in the aetiology of schizophrenia may help to determine drug response rather than contribute to the aetiology in any way. The design of studies using only incident cases may be required before explanations of this sort can be excluded. Selection bias can occur in case-control studies if the cases and controls are not drawn from the same population and, to date, no-one has done a population-based case-control study for genetic association in schizophrenia that would meet epidemiology study design criteria.

There are also problems in interpreting discrepancies between association studies that cannot simply be addressed by study design. For example, if there are differences in the contribution of a given allele in different ethnic groups (arising from different allele frequencies or different allele frequencies at interacting loci), aetiological heterogeneity can always provide a convenient but untested explanation for the discrepancies. Further potential for heterogeneity occurs if the association with the marker is a result of tight linkage with the true susceptibility allele. Similarly, in the face of aetiological heterogeneity in diseases for which there are no biologically meaningful diagnostic tests, it is possible that conflicting studies contain different balances of subtypes, known or unknown, of the disease, which might again dramatically alter the power for excluding association. At present, there are no simple ways to take such possibilities into account other than to recognize their potential existence.

It will be apparent, therefore, that basing future studies on sound epidemiological principles will be essential to avoid some of the problems inherent in studies to date and to maximize the potential for finding true associations.

The future

Refining phenotypes

The effectiveness of molecular genetic studies will depend upon the genetic validity of the phenotypes. It might be possible to improve genetic validity by focusing upon aspects of clinical variation or by identifying biological markers that define more homogeneous subgroups, though, despite much work, it has not been possible to identify genetically distinct subtypes to date. Indeed, clinical variation is likely to reflect, in part at least, a combination of quantitative variation in genetic risk for the disorder and the effect of modifying genes that influence illness expression, rather than the risk of illness per se.

The search for trait markers aims to move genetic studies beyond the clinical syndrome by identifying indices of genetic risk that can be measured in asymptomatic individuals. Indeed, it may be that there are no genes 'for' schizophrenia as such, but only those for other factors such as personality and intelligence, which increase risk of the disorder. Candidate trait markers for schizophrenia include schizotypal personality traits, measures of cognitive processing, brain evoked potentials and abnormalities in eye movements (DeLisi, 1999), though ensuring that the traits identified are highly heritable will itself require a return to classic twin studies and model fitting.

Efforts to improve the selection of phenotypes are also concerned with enhancing the traditional categorical approach to defining psychiatric disorders by identifying genetically valid phenotypes that can be measured quantitatively. These can be used in quantitative trait locus (QTL) approaches to gene mapping. QTL linkage (Kruglyak and Lander, 1995) is generally carried out in sibling pairs and is based on the principle that, at a locus influencing a trait or at a linked marker locus, siblings with more similar phenotypic scores should share more alleles identical-by-descent (ibd). QTL association (Page and Amos, 1999) is based on samples of unrelated individuals and seeks evidence of differences in phenotypic values according to allelic differences at a locus.

Genome-wide association studies

In recent years, there has been increasing interest in the possibility of systematic, genome-wide association studies (Owen, 1992; Risch and Merikangas, 1996; Collins et al., 1997; Owen et al., 1997, 2000). These have the potential of allowing systematic searches for genes of small effect in polygenic disorders. Optimism has been fuelled by the fact that the most abundant form of genetic variation, the single nucleotide polymorphism (SNP), is usually biallelic and potentially amenable to binary, high-throughput genotyping assays, the most promising of which are at present microarrays (so-called DNA chips). Moreover, as the amount of sequence data accumulates through the work of the Human Genome Project, it has become possible to contemplate the construction and application of very dense maps of hundreds of thousands of SNPs (Wang et al., 1998).

Essentially, two types of genome-wide association study have been proposed: direct and indirect. In the former, association is sought between the disease and a comprehensive catalogue of every variant that can alter the structure, function or expression of every single gene. In contrast, indirect studies seek associations between markers and disease that are caused by LD between the markers and susceptibility variants. The hope is that, if dense enough marker maps can be applied, the whole genome can be systematically screened for evidence of LD without the requirement of actually screening every single functional SNP in the genome. However, a number of uncertainties and difficulties remain. These include, in particular, the difficulty in identifying functional SNPs in regulatory, rather than coding, regions of the genome; uncertainty as to the distances over which LD is maintained; and the lack at the present time of a rapid, accurate and cheap method for SNP genotyping (Owen et al., 2000).

Another important unknown is the extent to which susceptibility to psychiatric disorders results from relatively common variants conferring small relative risks, such as *APOE e4*, or from rarer variants with larger effect sizes. The safest assumption is that both sorts of variant play a role, but there are important differences in the optimum strategies to detect the two types. Thus, to achieve power of 0.8 for detecting relatively common alleles present at a frequency of 0.3 in the general population, only three unselected individuals need be screened, whereas the corresponding figure for a rare variant with an allele frequency of 0.01 is 80 subjects (Owen et al., 2000). Common variants are, therefore, likely to be detected by generic SNP harvesting approaches, whereas rarer ones will most readily be detected in those with the disease in question and, preferably, those with a strong family history. However, both will require large samples to detect and confirm association. Rarer variants of larger effect will be more readily detected if the samples can be stratified on the basis of genetically valid variables such as family history, age at onset, severity and symptom profile, though the last three might reflect modifying loci rather than being an index of loading at a specific susceptibility locus.

Given the above considerations, it seems clear that the era of genome-wide association studies, direct or indirect, is not yet at hand. Instead, studies in the next few years should probably focus mainly upon the direct approach, utilizing SNPs from the coding sequence that actually alter protein structure in a wide range of functional and positional candidate genes. Preferably, complete functional systems should be dissected by a combination of sensitive methods for mutation detection followed by association studies in appropriately sized samples. We should also use our knowledge of functional pathways to make predictions about likely epistatic interactions between genes. However, given our ignorance of pathophysiology, the expectation should be that most reported associations will be false, and this will only be resolved by replication in large well-characterized samples. At present, although the indirect approach is not widely applicable at a genome-wide level, smaller-scale studies focusing upon specific regions indicated by the results of linkage studies may allow loci to be mapped and will have the added benefit of generating the type of information concerning patterns of LD in typical 'association samples' that will be required in order to determine whether genome-wide studies are likely to be feasible and what density of map will be required.

Functional studies

The most important, and the most obvious, implication of identifying genetic risk factors for schizophrenia is that it will inspire a new wave of neurobiological studies from which new and more effective therapies will hopefully emerge. However, while the unequivocal identification of associated genetic variants will represent a great advance, many years of work will still be required before this is likely to translate to bedside treatment. An early problem will be to determine exactly which genetic variation amongst several in LD in a given gene is actually responsible for the functional variation. Even where a specific variant within a gene can be identified as the one of functional importance, functional analysis, in terms of effect at the level of the organism, is likely to be particularly difficult for behavioural phenotypes in the absence of animal models. An extra level of complexity is that we will need to be able to produce model systems, both in vivo and in vitro, that allow gene–gene and gene–environment interactions to be studied.

Nosology

While the development of new therapies will take time, it is likely that the identification of susceptibility genes will have an earlier impact on psychiatric nosology. By correlating genetic risk factors with clinical symptoms and syndromes, it should be possible to study heterogeneity and comorbidity in order to improve the diagnosis and classification of psychosis, which will clearly facilitate all avenues of research into these disorders. Improvements in diagnosis and classification should enhance our ability to detect further genetic and environmental risk factors; thus, a positive feedback between nosology, epidemiology and molecular genetics can be envisaged.

Molecular epidemiology

The identification of genetic risk factors can be expected to provide a new impetus to epidemiological studies of schizophrenia by allowing researchers to investigate the ways in which genes and environment interact. Studies of this kind will require large epidemiologically based samples, together with the collection of relevant environmental data. This work could start now with DNA being banked for future use, although in schizophrenia the identification of plausible environmental measures might require clues from the nature of the genetic risk factors yet to be identified. A requirement of this approach will be to bring together methodologies from genetics and epidemiology, which have traditionally adopted somewhat differing analytical approaches (Sham, 1998). Treating susceptibility alleles as risk factors in an epidemiological context will allow estimates of effect sizes within a population to be made. Accounting for specific genetic effects will also facilitate the search for independent environmental factors, and the investigation of potential gene–environment interactions. Scientific validity is likely to be enhanced by ensuring as far as possible that control samples are drawn from the same base population as the cases. In addition, the use of incident cases should guard against the risk of identifying loci related to confounds such as chronicity of illness rather than susceptibility. Phenotypic assessment is likely to benefit from a prospective element to studies, to counteract the tendency of patients to forget historical details and the difficulty of making observed ratings retrospectively from case records. However, the price of improved scientific rigour is likely to be a requirement for considerably more expensive studies, as a result of the longer period and larger number of investigators that will be needed to ascertain the detailed data on the thousands of subjects that will probably be required.

Genetic testing

Finally, one other implication of genetic epidemiology studies concerns genetic testing. Given that susceptibility to schizophrenia almost certainly depends upon the combined effects of predisposing and protective alleles at a number of loci, as well as interactions with various environmental factors, the predictive value of genetic tests is likely to be low (Owen et al., 2000). Although determining exact risk may be impossible, investigation of gene–environment interactions may allow for the introduction of lifestyle changes to reduce risk in individuals identified as having increased susceptibility to the disorder. It may also encourage closer medical supervision for early diagnosis, repeatedly shown to be an important prognostic factor in schizophrenia. Genetic testing could also help to optimize treatment choices by testing genes that are found to influence treatment responses in schizophrenia, leading to a greater individualization of treatment.

Conclusion

It is clear that, over the next few decades, the completion of the Human Genome Project and the identification of polymorphisms that affect disease risk will have a significant impact on our understanding of pathogenic mechanisms and encourage the development of more specific treatments for many diseases, including schizophrenia. Only by studying genes in the environment to which the organism is exposed will we be able to understand the pathophysiology and psychopathology of this disorder. The study of how genes interact with each other and with non-genetic environmental factors is likely to be a fascinating and productive one, with the reduction of the population impact of schizophrenia likely to be an attainable result from the interaction of molecular genetics and epidemiology.

REFERENCES

Blouin JL, Dombroski BA, Nath SK et al. (1998) Schizophrenia susceptibility loci on chromosomes 13q32 and 8p21. Nature Genetics 20, 1061–4036.

Brzustowicz LM, Honer WG, Chow EWC et al. (1999) Linkage of familial schizophrenia to chromosome 13q32. American Journal of Human Genetics 65, 1096–1103.

Collins FS, Guyer MS, Chakravarti A (1997) Variation on a theme: cataloguing human DNA sequence variation. Science 278, 1580–1581.

Corder EH, Saunders AM, Strittmatter WJ et al. (1993) Gene dose of apolipoprotein E type-4 allele and the risk of Alzheimer's disease in late-onset families. Science 261, 921–3.

Craddock N, Khodel V, Van Eerdewegh P, Reich T (1995) Mathematical limits of multilocus models: the genetic transmission of bipolar disorder. American Journal of Human Genetics 57, 690–702.

DeLisi LE (1999) A critical overview of recent investigations into the genetics of schizophrenia. Current Opinion in Psychiatry 12, 29–39.

Ewens WJ, Spielman RS (1995) The transmission disequilibrium test: history, subdivision and admixture. American Journal of Human Genetics 57, 455–464.

Faraone SV, Matise T, Svrakic D et al. (1998) Genome scan of European-American schizophrenia pedigrees. Results of the NIMH Genetics Initiative and Millenium Consortium. American Journal of Medical Genetics 81, 290–295.

Goate A, Chartier-Harlin MC, Mullan ME (1991) Segregation of a missense mutation in the amyloid precursor protein gene with familial Alzheimer's disease. Nature 349, 704–706.

Hauser ER, Boehnke M, Guo SW, Risch N (1996) Affected-sib-pair interval mapping and exclusion for complex genetic traits – sampling considerations. Genetic Epidemiology 13, 117–137.

Jablensky A (1999) The 100-year epidemiology of schizophrenia. In: Search for the Causes of Schizophrenia, Vol. 4, Balance of the Century, Gattaz WF, Häfner H, eds. London: Springer, pp. 3–20.

Kendler KS, McGuire M, Gruenberg AM (1993a) The Roscommon Family Study II. The risk of nonschizophrenic nonaffective psychoses in relatives. Archives of General Psychiatry 50, 645–652.

Kendler KS, McGuire M and Gruenberg AM (1993b) The Roscommon Family Study III. Schizophrenia-related personality disorders in relatives. Archives of General Psychiatry 50, 781–788.

Khoury MJ, Beaty TH (1994) Applications of the case-control method in genetic epidemiology. Epidemiology Reviews 16, 134–150.

Kruglyak L, Lander ES (1995) Complete multipoint sib-pair analysis of qualitative and quantitative traits. American Journal of Human Genetics 57, 439–454.

Lander E, Kruglyak L (1995) Genetic dissection of complex traits: guidelines for interpreting and reporting linkage results. Nature Genetics 11, 241–247.

Lander ES, Schork NJ (1994) Genetic dissection of complex traits. Science 265, 2037–2048.

Levy-Lahad E, Wasco W, Poorkaj P et al. (1995) Candidate gene for the chromosome-1 familial Alzheimers-disease locus. Science 269, 973–977.

Lin MW, Curtis D, Williams N et al. (1995) Suggestive evidence for linkage of schizophrenia to markers on chromosome 13q14.1–q22. Psychiatric Genetics 5, 117–126.

McGue M, Gottesman II (1989) Genetic linkage and schizophrenia, perspectives from genetic epidemiology. Schizophrenia Bulletin 15, 453–464.

McGue M, Gottesman II, Rao DC (1985) Resolving genetic models for the transmission of schizophrenia. Genetic Epidemiology 2, 99–110.

McGuffin P, Owen MJ (1996) Molecular genetic studies of schizophrenia. Cold Spring Harbor Symposia on Quantitative Biology 61, 815–822.

McGuffin P, Owen MJ, O'Donovan MC, Thapar A, Gottesman I (1994) Seminars in Psychiatric Genetics. London: Gaskell.

McGuffin P, Owen MJ, Farmer AE (1995) The genetic basis of schizophrenia. Lancet 346, 678–682.

Moldin SO, Gottesman II (1997) At issue: genes, experience, and chance in schizophrenia – positioning for the 21st century. Schizophrenia Bulletin 23, 547–561.

Morgan HD, Sutherland HE, Martin DIK, Whitelaw E (1999) Epigenetic inheritance at the agouti locus in the mouse [letter]. Nature Genetics 23, 314–318.

O'Rourke DH, Gottesman II, Suarez BK et al. (1982) Refutation of the single locus model in the aetiology of schizophrenia. American Journal of Human Genetics 33, 630–649.

Owen MJ (1992) Will schizophrenia become a graveyard for molecular geneticists? Psychological Medicine 22, 289–293.

Owen MJ, Holmans P, McGuffin P (1997) Association studies in psychiatric genetics. Molecular Psychiatry 2, 270–273.

Owen MJ, Cardno AG, O'Donovan MC (2000) Psychiatric genetics: Back to the future. Molecular Psychiatry 5, 28–31.

Page GP, Amos CI (1999) Comparison of linkage-disequilibrium methods for localization of genes influencing quantitative traits in humans. American Journal of Human Genetics 64, 1194–1205.

Risch N (1990) Linkage strategies for genetically complex traits (1) multilocus models. American Journal of Human Genetics 46, 222–228.

Risch N, Merikangas K (1996) The future of genetic studies of complex human diseases. Science 273, 1516–1517.

Risch N, Teng J (1998) The relative power of family-based and case-control designs for linkage disequilibrium studies of complex human diseases: I. DNA pooling. Genome Research 8, 1273–1288.

Schaid DJ, Rowland C (1998) Use of parents, sibs and unrelated controls for detection of associations between genetic markers and disease. American Journal of Human Genetics 63, 1492–1506.

Schizophrenia Collaborative Linkage Group (1996) A combined analysis of D22S278 marker alleles in affected sib-pairs: support for a susceptibility locus for schizophrenia at chromosome 22q12. American Journal of Medical Genetics: Neuropsychiatric Genetics 67, 40–45.

Schizophrenia Linkage Collaborative Group for Chromosomes 3, 6, and 8 (1996) Additional support for schizophrenia linkage on chromosomes 6 and 8. A multicentre study. American Journal of Medical Genetics 67, 580–594.

Schwab SG, Eckstein SG, Hallmayer J et al. (1997) Evidence suggestive of a locus on chromosome 5q31 contributing to susceptibility for schizophrenia in German and Israeli families by multipoint affected sib-pair linkage analysis. Molecular Psychiatry 2, 156–160.

Schwab SG, Hallmayer J, Albus M et al. (1998a) A potential susceptibility locus on chromosome 10p14–p11 in 72 families with schizophrenia. American Journal of Medical Genetics 81, 528–529.

Schwab SG, Hallmayer J, Lerer B et al. (1998b) Support for a chromosome 18p locus conferring susceptibility to functional psychoses in families with schizophrenia, by association and linkage analysis. American Journal of Human Genetics 63, 1139–1152.

Scott WK, Pericak-Vance MA, Haines J (1997) Genetic analysis of complex diseases. Science 275, 1327.

Sherrington R, Brynjolfsson J, Petursson et al. (1989) Localization of a susceptiblity locus for schizophrenia on chromosome 5. Nature 336, 164–167.

Sherrington R, Rogaev EI, Liang Y et al. (1995) Cloning of a gene bearing missense mutations in early-onset familial Alzheimer's disease. Nature 375, 754–760.

Sham PC (1998) Statistical methods in psychiatric genetics. Statistical Methods in Medical Research 7, 279–300.

Straub RE, Maclean CJ, O'Neill FA, Walsh D, Kendler KS (1997) Support for a possible schizophrenia vulnerability locus in region 5q22–31 in Irish families. Molecular Psychiatry 2, 148–155.

Straub RE, Maclean CJ, Martin RB et al. (1998) A schizophrenia locus may be located in region 10p15–p11. American Journal of Medical Genetics 81, 296–301.

Suarez BK, Hampe CL, van Eerdewegh P (1994) Problems of replicating linkage claims in psychiatry. In: Genetic Approaches to Mental Disorders, Gershon ES, Cloninger CR, eds. Washington, DC: American Psychiatric Press, pp. 23–46.

Wang DG, Fan JB, Siao CJ et al. (1998) Large-scale identification, mapping, and genotyping of single-nucleotide polymorphisms in the human genome. Science 280, 1077–1082.

Weeks DE, Lathrop GM (1995) Polygenic disease: methods for mapping complex disease traits. Trends in Genetics 11, 513–519.

Williams J, Spurlock G, McGuffin P et al. (1996) Association between schizophrenia and the T102C polymorphism of 5-hydroxytryptamine type 2A receptor gene. Lancet 347, 1294–1296.

Williams J, McGuffin P, Nothen M, Owen MJ, EMASS Collaborative Group (1997) Meta-analysis of association between the 5HT2a receptor T102C polymorphism and schizophrenia. Lancet 349, 1221.

Williams J, Spurlock G, Holmans P et al. (1998) A meta-analysis and transmission disequilibrium study of association between the dopamine D_3 receptor gene and schizophrenia. Molecular Psychiatry 3, 141–149.

Williams NM, Rees MI, Holmans P et al. (1999) A teo-stage genome scan for schizophrenia susceptibility genes in 196 affected sibling pairs. Human Molecular Genetics 8, 1729–1739.

12

Gene–environment correlation and interaction in schizophrenia

Jim van Os[1,2] and Pak Sham[2]

[1]Department of Psychiatry and Neuropsychology, Maastricht University, the Netherlands
[2]Institute of Psychiatry, King's College London, UK

Mental health practitioners used to think in terms of 'visible' environmental risks in relation to onset and persistence of psychiatric disorders. Stressful life events, obstetric complications and dysfunctional parental interactions are but a few examples. Traditional psychiatric epidemiology was concerned mainly with such environmental risks. Conversely, clinical genetics was until recently almost exclusively concerned with Mendelian syndromes, for which single-gene defects could be mapped by positional cloning. Over the past decades, however, there has been increasing awareness that, for common psychiatric disorders, 'hidden' genetic factors can have a substantial influence on the effect of environmental exposures or even pose as risk factors. As genes can be considered as a conventional epidemiological risk factor in association studies (Sham, 1996), and epidemiological theory can be readily applied to genetically sensitive datasets (Susser and Susser, 1989; Ottman, 1990), epidemiologists and human geneticists have been gradually integrating their respective fields of research into a new discipline called genetic epidemiology (Khoury et al., 1993). Within genetic epidemiology, the term ecogenetics refers to the study of specific gene–environment relationships, the application of which to schizophrenia is relevant though still in the initial stages (van Os and Marcelis, 1998; Malaspina et al., 1999).

The interplay of genes and environment

The models of gene–environment relationships presented below all assume that genetic and environmental factors increase the risk for schizophrenia rather than reducing it. However, the underlying principles are the same for protective effects, although some extensions may be necessary. Interaction between genes and environment means more than simply stating that both are involved in disease aetiology. There are several biological plausible mechanisms by which genes and environment can coinfluence disease outcome (Plomin et al., 1977; Kendler and Eaves, 1986; Khoury et al., 1993; Ottman, 1996; van Os and Marcelis, 1998).

Correlation: genes influence environmental exposure

A gene may increase the likelihood that a person becomes exposed to an environmental risk factor, which in turn increases the risk for schizophrenia. For example, liability to the use of cannabis is influenced by genetic factors, especially heavy use (Kendler and Prescott, 1998). Therefore, as far as heavy cannabis use is a risk factor for schizophrenia (Andreasson et al., 1987), part of the apparently environmental risk may be of genetic origin. Conversely, it can be envisaged that an environmental factor influences whether or not a genotype is present, for example by affecting the rate of germline or somatic mutations in a population. These first two mechanisms are examples of genotype–environment correlation, so called because if in the population the occurrence of E (the environmental risk factor) depends on the occurrence of G (the genetic risk factor) their prevalences will be correlated.

Synergism: genes and environment coparticipate in the same cause

In genotype–environment synergism, the biological effects of G and E are dependent on each other in such a way that exposure to neither or either one alone does not result in disease, whereas exposure to both does. For example, a gene could influence the sensitivity to or, conversely, could influence the effect of G by controlling the degree of gene expression (Agid et al., 1999) or affecting epigenetic mechanisms such as DNA methylation (Petronis et al., 1999). It is also possible that other nongenetic, stochastic factors affect gene expression (McGuffin et al., 1994; Woolf, 1997).

Models describing gene–environment synergism

Describing a theory of synergism between genes and environment in nature is one thing, devising a statistical model that will aid us in quantifying such mechanisms in collected data is another. Let us assume that there are two risk factors for schizophrenia; one is E, and one is a single-gene risk factor G in the population. Risk is the proportion of individuals who get schizophrenia. If there are two risk factors G and E, there are four possible exposure states according to whether each factor is present or absent, and each of these four exposure states carries a specific risk. Therefore, the risk for schizophrenia in the population exposed to E only is R(E) and the risk in the population exposed to G only is R(G). The risk of schizophrenia in the population exposed to neither E or G is R, whereas the risk in the population exposed to both G and E is R(GE). On the additive scale, the effect of a risk factor is expressed as a risk difference. For example, if R(G) is 0.25 and R is 0.10, the effect of G is $0.25 - 0.10 = 0.15$. We can, therefore, express the effect of G as

$R(G) - R$, the effect associated with E as $R(E) - R$, and the effect associated with the GE-exposure as $R(GE) - R$. Table 12.1 shows the effects associated with the four different exposure states.

Table 12.1. Effects, measured on the additive scale, of the four exposure states occasioned by a genetic (G) and an environmental (E) risk factor for schizophrenia

Risk factor	G absent	G present
E absent	R	$R(G) - R$
E present	$R(E) - R$	$R(GE) - R$

As the combined effect of G and E is $R(GE) - R$, the excess of this over the sum of the solitary effects of G and E is:

$$[R(GE) - R] - [R(G) - R] - [R(E) - R] = [R(GE) - R(G) - R(E) + R] \tag{1}$$

If $[R(GE) - R(G) - R(E) + R] > 0$, G and E are said to interact on the additive scale. We will hereafter refer to $[R(GE) - R(G) - R(E) + R]$ as the statistical additive interaction.

How can we quantify the extent to which G and E act synergistically, that is in some way depend on each other, or coparticipate in disease causation? Let us consider the proportion of individuals in the population who developed schizophrenia after exposure to both G and E, or have risk $R(GE)$. It is possible that some of these individuals would also have contracted the disorder after exposure to either G or E alone. The degree to which some individuals would have also contracted the disorder after exposure to either G or E alone is referred to as the degree of parallelism. If there is parallelism, G and E 'compete' to cause schizophrenia, and the more they compete, the smaller the proportion of individuals that contracted the disease because of the coparticipation of G and E. Therefore, parallelism can be thought of as the opposite of synergism. For example, in the extreme case of 100% parallelism where all individuals exposed to G and E had developed the disease because of the causal action of either G or E alone, no individual could have contracted schizophrenia because of the coparticipation of G and E. In this case, the amount of synergism would be zero. In practice, it is impossible to assess the amount of parallelism and the amount of synergy in individuals exposed to both G and E. However, it can be shown that the amount by which synergism exceeds parallelism equals the excess of $R(GE)$ over the sum of the solitary effects of G and E (i.e. the statistical additive interaction as shown above) (Darroch, 1997). In other words:

$$|synergism| - |parallelism| = [R(GE) - R(G) - R(E) + R] \tag{2}$$

Previous models of synergy tended to ignore parallelism and assumed that synergy was equal to the additive interaction (Rothman, 1986). However, assuming that parallelism does not exist may underestimate synergism. In practice, therefore, the amount of synergy has to be approximated using Table 12.2 (Darroch, 1997).

Table 12.2. Approximation of synergy

|synergism| |$x1$|	|$x2$| |parallelism|	$R(GE) - R(G)$ $R(G) - R$
$R(GE) - R(E)$	$R(E) - R$	

The variables $x1$ and $x2$ are two unknowns that sum with synergism and parallelism to $[R(GE) - R(E)]$ and $[R(E) - R]$, respectively. For example, in the Finnish Adoption Study, G was measured by diagnosis of schizophrenia in the mother, E by the level of communication deviance and thought disorder in the adopting family, and the outcome variable consisted of broadly defined schizophrenia spectrum disorder (Tienari et al., 1994). The risks associated with the schizophrenia spectrum outcome were around 4% for the group exposed to neither G nor E, and, for the group exposed to G only. R(E) was 34%, and R(GE) was 62%. Filling in these risks in Table 12.2 results in the following estimates (Table 12.3).

Table 12.3. Approximation in the Finnish Adoption Study

|synergism| |$x1$|	|$x2$| |parallelism|	0.58 0.0
0.28	0.30	0.58

It can be seen that \|$x2$\| must be between 0 and 0.30. Therefore \|synergism\| must be between 0.28 and 0.58. In other words, between 45% (0.28/0.62) and 94% (0.58/0.62) of patients with schizophrenia spectrum disorder exposed to both communication deviance and a mother with schizophrenia were attributable to the synergistic action of these two factors. In another publication of the Finnish Adoption Study, the outcome was not schizophrenia, but a measure of schizophrenia thought disorder (Wahlberg et al., 1997). The baseline risk of having a high score on an index of primitive thought disorder was 64%, and this risk was approximately the same in individuals exposed to genetic risk of schizophrenia and individuals exposed to adoptive parents' communication deviance. However, the risk associated with exposure to both communication deviance and genetic risk was around 77%. Filling in these risks in Table 12.2 shows that only around 19–22% of those with schizophrenic thought disorder exposed to both communication deviance and a mother with schizophrenia can be attributed to the synergistic action of these two factors.

It is useful to estimate the fraction of cases attributable to the synergistic action of G and E. If the greatest proportion of patients with schizophrenia exposed to G and E is the result of the synergistic, codependent, action of G and E, the incidence of schizophrenia could be reduced by targeting either G or E. However, if a population is exposed to G and E, the degree of synergism is small and parallelism is dominant, schizophrenia incidence could be reduced most effectively by targeting both G and E.

Additive: genes and environment add to each other's effect

Some models of disease causation imply that there is no synergism. For example, an individual may get schizophrenia only if in possession of a certain type of vulnerability conferred by either genetic or environmental factors. An environmental factor could disrupt early brain development in the same fashion as a genetic mutation. If synergism is zero, the effect of genes and environment is said to be additive. As we have seen that

|synergism| – |parallelism| = statistical additive interaction,

it follows that, if synergism is zero, the statistical additive interaction equals − |parallelism| and is less than or equal to zero. Therefore, if genetic and environmental risk factors act additively to cause disease, their joint effect equals the sum of their individual risks, after taking into account the negative effect of parallelism. It follows that G and E cannot act additively to cause schizophrenia if the data show that the statistical additive interaction is positive, and some other model of disease causation involving synergism must apply. However, if the statistical additive interaction is zero, there may still be synergism if parallelism is not zero.

Multiplicative: genes and environment multiply each other's effects

Other disease models imply that there is no parallelism. For example, schizophrenia may be caused by genes and environment in multiple stages. Under a two-stage model, the clinical manifestation of schizophrenia is the result of a second stage of disease, which can only be reached via a first stage. Genetic factors may influence risk for the first stage of disease, and the first stage only, whereas an environmental factor may influence risk for the second stage of disease, and the second stage only. Transition from stage one to schizophrenia can only take place after passing first from stage one to stage two, and stage two will only result in schizophrenia if it was first preceded by stage one. Under this model, G and E cannot 'compete' to cause disease, and, therefore, parallelism will be zero. If parallelism is zero, the additive statistical interaction will equal |synergism| and will always be non-negative. In other words, if the additive interaction is negative, the multistage model cannot hold.

The multistage model is associated with a multiplicative model of disease causation. On the multiplicative scale, the effect of a risk factor is expressed as a risk ratio. Thus, the effect of G would be expressed as R(G)/R. For example, if R(G) is 0.25 and R is 0.10, the effect of G is 0.25/0.10 = 2.5. Under the hypothesis of a multistage model, it can be shown that the magnitude of the combined effect of G and E will be equal to the product of their individual effects. Thus, if the effect of G on schizophrenia is 10, and the effect of E is 2, the effect of their combined exposure will be 20. The importance of the multiplicative interaction lies not only in the possible underlying validity of the model of disease causation but also in the fact that many of our standard statistical procedures (such as logistic regression analysis) are carried out on the multiplicative scale. Researchers presenting their results in terms of multiplicative risks should be aware of the underlying assumptions of disease causation and, for example in the case of the multistage model, their (bold) assumption that there is no parallelism.

Research findings on GE interaction and correlation

Gene–environment correlation

There is evidence that many of the factors thought to represent environmental risks for schizophrenia are partly under the control of genetic factors. These include, apart from the cannabis use mentioned above, exposure to certain pregnancy complications (Marcelis et al., 1998), life events (Kendler et al., 1993a) and head injury resulting from trauma and accidents (Lyons et al., 1993; Matheny et al., 1997). In the study of obstetric complications by Marcelis et al. (1998), it was found that familial clustering for affective disorder increased the risk for exposure to an obstetric complication at birth. This would be a mechanism whereby the risk for environmental exposure leading to the schizophrenia phenotype may be influenced by the affective disorder genotype. As environmental factors cannot be directly influenced by DNA, genetic control of exposure to such factors must be mediated by some characteristic of the person (Plomin, 1994). For example, the genetic influence on exposure to life events was shown to be mediated by personality traits such as neuroticism, extraversion and openness to experience (Saudino et al., 1997). Genetic control of exposure to obstetric complications could be mediated by liability to depression (Marcelis et al., 1998), and accident-proneness may be associated with genetic factors through the personality trait sensation-seeking (Koopmans et al., 1995; Jonah, 1997). As discussed in Chapter 10, it is possible that part of the genetic liability to schizophrenia is expressed in the form of personality vulnerability traits, such as a high degree of social anxiety (Jones et al., 1994). A high level of social anxiety could give rise to a low level of exposure to social interaction with other individuals, which, in turn, through lack of correction of early abnormal mental states could facilitate the development of psychotic symptoms. Consequently, it can easily be envisaged that genotype–environment correlations play a significant role in the cascade of events leading to the development of psychosis.

Gene–environment interaction

As no genes that increase the risk for schizophrenia have been unequivocally identified, gene–environment interaction studies necessarily have to do with proxy variables, each of which has its particular problems (Table 12.4). While some studies suggest the possibility of gene–environment interaction, it is clear that more new research and more replication research is needed. Unfortunately, the published twin, adoption and high-risk studies that have yielded the most convincing evidence so far (Gottesman and Bertelsen, 1989; Cannon et al., 1993; Tienari et al., 1994; see also Ch. 10) cannot be replicated easily. Once genes that increase the risk for schizophrenia have been identified, it will be possible to investigate interaction between genotype and environmental risk factors directly.

Consequences for risk studies

Gene–environment interaction and gene–environment correlation are likely to play a role in schizophrenia but the precise mechanisms remain to be elucidated. As epidemiological studies are rarely, if ever, able to model specific gene–environment relationships, the question arises of how such underlying mechanisms distort our estimates of epidemiological parameters such as relative risk and the amounts of synergism and parallelism in individuals exposed to both G and E. An example can readily demonstrate these issues. In a given population of 1 million, let the prevalence of schizophrenia be 0.6%, and the prevalence of the single-gene G and E be 1% each. There is some degree of gene–environment correlation so the population proportion exposed to both E and G (GE) is 0.1% (instead of $1\% \times 1\% = 0.01\%$ if their prevalences had not been correlated). The risk of schizophrenia in individuals with exposure to E or G is increased by around a factor 5 (0.03), compared with the risk of 0.006 in the population as a whole. An investigator, unaware of any underlying genotype–environment relationship, separately calculates relative risks for G and E. We consider four different scenarios, depending on whether parallelism or synergism is the dominant class in those exposed to both G and E and on whether there is additional gene–environment correlation (Table 12.5).

Under the first scenario, the effects of G and E are independent of each other and

Table 12.4. Studies of gene–environment interaction in schizophrenia

Proxy genetic variable	Proxy environmental variable	Findings	Remarks
Positive family history (FH)	Ethnic group	Familial morbid risk for schizophrenia higher in siblings of African-Caribbean probands than in siblings of white probands (Sugarman and Crauford, 1994; Hutchinson et al., 1996)	Unlikely to be informative unless both environmental exposure status and clinical status is measured in both cases *and* all first-degree relatives and analyses are adjusted for age, sex and number of relatives
	Urban birth	No association between urban birth and a positive family history for schizophrenia (Mortensen et al., 1999)	Even then, however, the level of misclassification is likely to be very high because many unaffected relatives may carry the high-risk genotype
	Obstetric complications	Mostly inconclusive findings with regard to family history (Nimgaonkar et al., 1988; O'Callaghan et al., 1992; Kunugi et al., 1996)	Also not informative because *absence* of an association between positive family history and environmental exposure does *not* rule out gene–environment interaction, and *presence* of an association does not rule out *lack* of gene–environment interaction (Marcelis et al., 1998)
	Birth in winter/spring	Positive, negative and inconclusive associations with family history (Shur, 1982; Baron and Gruen, 1988; Pulver et al., 1992; Dassa et al., 1996)	
	Stressful life events	Positive association with family history (van Os et al., 1994)	
Having an identical twin with schizophrenia	Being discordant for schizophrenia	Children of both affected and nonaffected twin in discordant pair have higher rate of schizophrenia (Fischer, 1971; Gottesman and Bertelsen, 1989; Kringlen and Cramer, 1989)	Suggests environmental factor is necessary for expression of high-risk genotype in affected twin or inhibition of protective genotype in unaffected twin

Biological parent with schizophrenia	Growing up in dysfunctional adoptive family environment	Risk of schizophrenia spectrum disorder or schizophrenia-associated thought disorder higher in high-risk adoptees who had been brought up in dysfunctional adoptive family environment (Tienari et al., 1994; Wahlberg et al., 1997)	Risk of schizophrenia spectrum disorder 3% in absence of environmental risk, and 62% in presence of environmental risk; this difference seems extremely high. Children destined to develop schizophrenia may have contributed to dysfunctional family environment rather than the other way round
Having neither, one or two parents with schizophrenia	Obstetric complications	The greater the proxy genetic risk, the greater the effect of obstetric complications on ventricular enlargement (the schizophrenia endophenotype) (Cannon et al., 1993)	Genetic risk may increase risk of obstetric complication. Genetic risk may increase risk of heavy alcohol consumption or head injury resulting in greater obstetric complication effect sizes
Having a parent with schizophrenia and additionally having an electrodermal abnormality as a child	Paternal absence	Higher rate of paternal absence in children who subsequently developed schizophrenia (Walker, 1981)	Status of electrodermal abnormality as a marker of genetic risk for schizophrenia unclear
Having a monozygotic (MZ) twin with schizophrenia	Sharing the same chorion with the co-twin	Concordance rate was higher for MZ twins whose marker suggested they were monochorionic, than those whose marker indicated they were dichorionic (Davis et al., 1995)	These results are compatible with a factor in the prenatal environment facilitating expression of genetic risk for schizophrenia

Table 12.5. Standard epidemiological parameters under different gene–environment relationships[a]

Parameter	Scenario			
	No correlation;[b] no synergism; 100% parallelism	No correlation;[b] no synergism; 50% parallelism	GE correlation; no synergism; 50% parallelism	No GE correlation; 50% synergism; 50% parallelism
Prevalence GE (%)	0.1	0.1	0.4	0.1
Observed RR (GE)[c]	5.0 (3.5–7.2)	7.6 (5.7–10.1)	7.7 (6.7–8.9)	15.2 (12.5–18.6)
Observed RR(G) = RR(E)[c]	5.7 (5.2–6.4)	6.0 (5.4–6.7)	8.6 (7.9–9.4)	6.9 (6.2–7.6)
Dominant class in those exposed to both G and E (estimation of class size, %)	Parallelism (90–100)	Parallelism (40–60)	Parallelism (94–100)	Synergism (20–57)

Notes:
G, genetic risk factor; E, environmental risk factor; GE, joint G and E exposure; RR, relative risk.
[a] Prevalence schizophrenia 0.6%; prevalence G, 1%; prevalence E, 1%; true risk G and E 3%.
[b] Not in addition to that already present (see p. 243).
[c] Relative risk given with 95% confidence interval in parentheses.

there is 100% parallelism because individuals exposed to both G and E will only develop disease because of exposure to either G or E (G and E do not coparticipate in causation). The risk associated with GE is, therefore, the same as with either G or E alone. The second scenario is the same, but we assume that there is 50% parallelism in those exposed to both G and E and that there is no synergism (i.e. the risks are additive in the other 50% exposed to both G and E). The number of cases produced by joint GE exposure is, therefore, 50% higher than under the previous scenario. The third scenario is like the second but there is additional genotype–environment correlation, such that the risk of exposure to E is increased by a factor of four in individuals with genotype G. The fourth scenario is also like the second, but in the other 50% of those exposed to both G and E there is synergism such that joint exposure results in a fivefold increased risk.

If an investigator were to examine the population under the first scenario with 100% parallelism, he/she would find that R(GE), R(G) and R(E) were all around 5 and that 90–100% of schizophrenics exposed to both G and E were caused by G and E competing for individuals (parallelism). Under the second scenario with 50% parallelism and no synergism, all risks are increased, but R(GE) increases more than R(E) and R(G), and parallelism would still be the dominant class, although now only between 40 and 63%. Under the third scenario, the additional gene–environment correlation would increase all risks, but R(G) and R(E) more than R(GE). Parallelism is again the dominant class but the estimate is much higher at 94–100%.

The effect of gene–environment synergism in addition to parallelism under scenario four would only slightly increase R(G) and R(E) but dramatically increase R(GE). Synergism now becomes the dominant class.

In practice, of course, we remain ignorant about the underlying genotype–environment relationships. The examples shown here demonstrate that current estimates of relative risk are the result of many complex underlying relationships, and also that estimates of parallelism and synergism may be affected by underlying gene–environment correlation. At present, therefore, it is extremely difficult to interpret relative risk estimates from studies. It is perhaps best to calculate the risks under different assumptions of gene–environment relationships so that at least an idea is formed about the likely extremes between which the true estimates lie.

Consequences for twin studies

Twin studies are frequently used to calculate the heritability of a disease (Ch. 10). In this type of analysis, statistical model fitting is used to establish how much of the variation in liability to a disorder can be ascribed to the effects of additive genes (A), environment shared with family members (C), environment that is not shared with family members (E) and genetic dominance effects (D). By means of statistical comparison of nested models, for example a model comprising the influences of additive genes, shared and nonshared environment (ACE model) versus a model comprising the influences of additive genes and nonshared environment only (AE model), the statistical significance of a source of variation can be tested. However, because of the need also to compare non-nested models and the sensitivity of significance tests to sample size, the preferred model is often identified using a criterion that balances goodness-of-fit and parsimony, according to the Akaike Information Content (AIC) (Sham, 1998). For example, a model comprising the effect of additive genes and nonshared environment (AE model) was the preferred model with the smallest AIC in a recent study of RDC-defined (Research Diagnostic Criteria; Spitzer et al., 1990) schizophrenia (Cardno et al., 1999). Model-fitting studies of psychiatric disorders such as schizophrenia rarely consider the role of gene–environment interaction and correlation, although it can be readily shown that the failure to consider these mechanisms may lead to erroneous inferences concerning the role of genes in the aetiology of mental disorders.

The consequences of gene–environment interaction in family and twin studies have been examined recently by Guo (2000a,b,c). It was concluded that commonly used measures of genetic effects such as recurrence risk ratios for relative pairs, concordance rates for twins and heritability coefficients are functions not only of genetic effects and gene frequency but also of environmental effects and the distribution of environmental factors, in the presence of gene–environment interaction.

To illustrate the potential impact of gene–environment interaction and correlation on heritability estimates from twin studies, we consider three scenarios. We assume that there is a single gene G that is a necessary, but not sufficient, cause of schizotypy (i.e. risk in individuals exposed to G only is zero), that this gene has a 10% prevalence in nonaffected individuals and that the gene interacts synergistically (see above) with various environmental factors. A (fictitious) large and fully representative sample of twins in a given population was collected in order to establish the heritability of schizotypy. Schizotypy was dichotomously defined using a standard clinical interview. According to this definition, the prevalence of schizotypy was around 12.5%. The co-twin affection status contingency tables were constructed separately for monozygotic (MZ) and dizygotic (DZ) twin pairs (Table 12.6). According to these tables, the probandwise concordance rates (2x concordant affected pairs divided by 2× concordant affected pairs + discordant pairs) were 29% and 21% for MZ and DZ twins, respectively.

Table 12.6. Schizotypy affection status in monozygotic and dizygotic twins under hypothesized baseline circumstances

(*a*) *Monozygotic twins*

Twin 1	Twin 2	
	Noncase	Case
Noncase	1000	110
Case	110	45

Notes:
Probandwise concordance: 29%.

(*b*) *Dizygotic twins*

Twin 1	Twin 2	
	Noncase	Case
Noncase	1000	130
Case	130	35

Notes:
Probandwise concordance: 21%.

We now assume that 20% of an exact copy of this twin sample had been additionally exposed to an environmental risk factor (E). This factor does not in itself increase the risk for schizotypy (i.e. risk in individuals exposed to E only is zero), but it interacts with the genetic risk factor such that 100% of individuals who are exposed to both E and G will develop the disease (i.e. risk in individuals exposed to both is unity). If the environmental exposure is completely random and if we assume that twin pairs are always exposed together, the consequences for the contingency tables are predictable (Table 12.7). The probandwise concordance rates have changed, and are now 39% and 28% for MZ and DZ twins, respectively.

Table 12.7. Schizotypy affection status in monozygotic and dizygotic twins assuming gene–environment interaction

(*a*) *Monozygotic twins*

Twin 1	Twin 2	
	Noncase	Case
Noncase	980	107.8
Case	107.8	69.4

Notes:
Probandwise concordance: 39%.

(*b*) *Dizygotic twins*

Twin 1	Twin 2	
	Noncase	Case
Noncase	980	132.4
Case	132.4	50.2

Notes:
Probandwise concordance: 28%.

Apart from the occurrence of gene–environment interaction described above, we could now assume additionally that the risk of environmental exposure is influenced by the genetic risk factor, such that individuals with G have a threefold increased risk of exposure to E. Because of the additional gene–environment correlation, environmental exposure is now nonrandom, individuals with the genotype having a 60% exposure rate instead of 20%. If we again assume that twin pairs are always exposed together, the contingency tables will change, as displayed in Table 12.8. The probandwise concordance rates are now 47% and 33%, respectively, for MZ and DZ twin pairs.

We will now calculate the heritability of the liability to schizotypy under the three different circumstances (baseline, GE interaction only, GE interaction plus GE correlation) by fitting liability-threshold models to the respective contingency tables using the program Mx (Neale et al., 1999). The program calculates how much of

Table 12.8. Schizotypy affection status in monozygotic and dizygotic twins assuming gene–environment interaction and gene–environment correlation

(*a*) *Monozygotic twins*

Twin 1	Twin 2	
	Non-case	Case
Noncase	960	105.6
Case	105.6	93.8

Notes:
Probandwise concordance: 47%.

(*b*) *Dizygotic twins*

Twin 1	Twin 2	
	Noncase	Case
Noncase	960	134.8
Case	134.8	65.4

Notes:
Probandwise concordance: 33%.

the differences in liability to a disorder in a population can be ascribed to the effects of additive genes (A), dominance genetic effects (D), environment shared with family members (C) and environment that is not shared with family members (E). The most parsimonious model according to AIC was identified for each situation (Table 12.9). The AE model proved to be the most parsimonious under all three circumstances. However, the parameter estimates were different, such that the proportion of the liability owing to additive genes increased from the baseline to the GE interaction scenario, and again further from the GE interaction to the correlation scenario. This suggests that model-fitting procedures are quite sensitive to gene–environment interactions, and that reported estimates of separate contribution of genes and environment may be heavily contaminated by these interactions and correlations.

Another important point is that under the scenario of gene–environment correlation, the use of the twin design may be invalidated because of transgression of the so-called equal-environment assumption (EEA). The argument that MZ and DZ twins can be used to separate out genetic from environmental influences is based on the assumption that MZ and DZ twins experience the same degree of similarity in their environments, with respect to factors having an effect on the trait being

Table 12.9. Heritability model fitting outcomes assuming different gene–environment relationships

	Baseline	GE interaction	GE interaction and correlation
Most parsimonious model[a]	AE	AE	AE
F of model fit (degrees of freedom)	0.32 (2)	0.67 (2)	1.89 (2)
Akaike information criterion	4.32	4.67	5.89
Liability explained by effect additive genes	0.40	0.54	0.64
Liability explained by effect common environment	(0)	(0)	(0)
Liability explained by nonshared environment	0.60	0.46	0.36
Liability explained by effect of genetic dominance	(0)	(0)	(0)

Notes:

[a] For description of models, see the text.

considered (e.g. schizophrenia or schizotypy). The fact that MZ twins tend to be treated more similar by their parents than DZ twins would appear to be a violation of this assumption, but research suggests that the influence of perceived zygosity is small (Kendler et al., 1993b). However, if exposure to E is influenced by genes, then MZ twins will always share this influence, whereas DZ twins will only share it in 50% of cases. This would constitute a violation of the EEA and wrongly ascribe the greater degree of MZ resemblance to genetic instead of environmental factors. The fact that gene–environment correlation has been demonstrated for a number of environmental factors, including possible risk factors for schizophrenia such as the use of illicit drugs and stressful life events, suggests that current heritability estimates may be exaggerated at the expense of the environmental contribution to liability.

Consequences for gene-mapping studies

The discovery of polymorphic DNA markers throughout the genome and the development of efficient methods of genotyping have enabled the application of linkage and association analysis to the mapping of disease loci. This approach is called *positional cloning* because it is based on the estimation of genetic distances from the cotransmissions or cooccurrences of alleles and not on knowledge of gene function. Positional cloning has been successful in mapping the genes responsible for hundreds of simple Mendelian diseases. However, application of this approach to complex disorders has so far been less successful; most initial reports of linkage have been weak and subsequently replicated in only a proportion of studies. The usual explanation for the lack of strong and consistent linkage findings is the limited power of linkage analysis to detect genes of small or modest effect.

Table 12.10. A model of gene–environment interaction for exploring effect on linkage analysis

Genotype	Unexposed	Exposed	Marginal penetrance
DD	0.1000	0.3500	0.1250
Dd	0.0010	0.2000	0.0209
dd	0.0001	0.2000	0.0201
Marginal risk	0.0044	0.2060	0.0246

Notes:
Allele frequency of D 0.2; frequency of exposure 0.1; sibling correlation in exposure 0.7.

Although it is possible that gene effect is uniformly low in all populations, it is more likely that there are variations in gene effect according to the environment. In the presence of gene–environment interaction, the average effect of a gene may be small, but the actual effect may be quite high under certain environmental conditions. Guo has examined the impact of gene–environment interaction on the power of an affected sibling pair design to detect a gene, under a simplified model of a single gene and a single environmental factor (Guo, 2000c). As an example, consider the model given in Table 12.10. This model is one where penetrances are greater under the exposed condition than the unexposed condition, but the ratios of penetrances are greater under the unexposed condition. Under this model, Guo evaluated the number of sibling pairs necessary for 80% power and a type 1 error rate of 0.000022 for various designs (Guo, 2000c). It turns out that a random sample of affected sibling pairs regardless of exposure status is very uninformative, with a required sample size of 11 714 pairs. In contrast, if only affected sibling pairs who are also concordant for being unexposed are sampled, then the required sample size is only 28 pairs! The reason for the superior power of concordant unexposed affected sibling pairs is that the ratios of penetrances are far greater under the unexposed than the exposed condition. Under other underlying models, a different design might be more appropriate (e.g. affected sibling pairs who are discordant for exposure status); what is certain is that ignoring exposure status in the study design and data analysis can result in drastic reduction in power.

Gene–environment interactions will also have an impact on the optimal design of allelic association studies. It is clearly advantageous to study individuals exposed to an environment that maximizes the adverse effect of the susceptibility gene. Family and twin studies that incorporate environmental risk factors may provide valuable information regarding the heritability of the disease in different environments. Such information would be very useful in optimizing the design of studies to identify susceptibility genes.

Conclusion

Although research findings on gene–environment interactions and correlations remain scarce, the examples described in this chapter suggest that they may have a profound influence on commonly used epidemiological and genetic parameters. More intensive use of research designs that can elucidate these interactions will enhance our understanding of the pathways of risk leading to onset and persistence of psychiatric illness in the general population.

REFERENCES

Agid O, Shapira B, Zislin J et al. (1999) Environment and vulnerability to major psychiatric illness: a case control study of early parental loss in major depression, bipolar disorder and schizophrenia [see comments]. Molecular Psychiatry 4, 163–172.

Andreasson S, Allebeck P, Engstrom A, Rydberg U (1987) Cannabis and schizophrenia. A longitudinal study of Swedish conscripts. Lancet ii, 1483–1486.

Baron M, Gruen R (1988) Risk factors in schizophrenia: season of birth and family history [see comments]. British Journal of Psychiatry 152, 460–465.

Cannon TD, Mednick SA, Parnas J, Schulsinger F, Praestholm J, Vestergaard A (1993) Developmental brain abnormalities in the offspring of schizophrenic mothers. I. Contributions of genetic and perinatal factors [see comments]. Archives of General Psychiatry 50, 551–564.

Cardno AG, Marshall EJ, Coid B et al. (1999) Heritability estimates for psychotic disorders: the Maudsley Twin Psychosis Series. Archives of General Psychiatry 56, 162–168.

Darroch J (1997) Biologic synergism and parallelism [see comments]. American Journal of Epidemiology 145, 661–668.

Dassa D, Sham PC, van Os J, Abel K, Jones P, Murray RM (1996) Relationship of birth season to clinical features, family history, and obstetric complication in schizophrenia. Psychiatry Research 64, 11–17.

Davis JO, Phelps JA (1995) Twins with schizophrenia: genes or germs? Schizophrenia Bulletin 21, 13–18.

Fischer M (1971) Psychoses in the offspring of schizophrenic monozygotic twins and their normal co-twins. British Journal of Psychiatry 118, 43–52.

Gottesman, II, Bertelsen A (1989) Confirming unexpressed genotypes for schizophrenia. Risks in the offspring of Fischer's Danish identical and fraternal discordant twins [see comments]. Archives of General Psychiatry 46, 867–872.

Guo SW (2000a) Familial aggregation of environmental risk factors and familial aggregation of disease. American Journal of Epidemiology 151, 1121–1131.

Guo SW (2000b) Gene–environment interaction and the mapping of complex traits: some statistical models and their implications. Human Heredity 50, 286–303.

Guo SW (2000c) Gene–environment interactions and the affected-sib-pair designs. Human Heredity 50, 271–285.

Hutchinson G, Takei N, Fahy TA et al. (1996) Morbid risk of schizophrenia in first-degree relatives of white and African-Caribbean patients with psychosis. British Journal of Psychiatry 169, 776–780.

Jonah BA (1997) Sensation seeking and risky driving: a review and synthesis of the literature. Accident Analysis and Prevention 29, 651–665.

Jones P, Rodgers B, Murray R, Marmot M (1994) Child developmental risk factors for adult schizophrenia in the British 1946 birth cohort. Lancet 344, 1398–1402.

Kendler KS, Eaves LJ (1986) Models for the joint effect of genotype and environment on liability to psychiatric illness. American Journal of Psychiatry 143, 279–289.

Kendler KS, Prescott CA (1998) Cannabis use, abuse, and dependence in a population-based sample of female twins. American Journal of Psychiatry 155, 1016–1022.

Kendler KS, Neale M, Kessler R, Heath A, Eaves L (1993a) A twin study of recent life events and difficulties. Archives of General Psychiatry 50, 789–796.

Kendler KS, Neale MC, Kessler RC, Heath AC, Eaves LJ (1993b) A test of the equal-environment assumption in twin studies of psychiatric illness. Behavior Genetics 23, 21–27.

Khoury MJ, Beaty TH, Cohen BH (1993) Genetic Epidemiology. Oxford: Oxford University Press.

Koopmans JR, Boomsma DI, Heath AC, van Doornen LJ (1995) A multivariate genetic analysis of sensation seeking. Behavior Genetics 25, 349–356.

Kringlen E, Cramer G (1989) Offspring of monozygotic twins discordant for schizophrenia. Archives of General Psychiatry 46, 873–877.

Kunugi H, Nanko S, Takei N, Saito K, Murray RM, Hirose T (1996) Perinatal complications and schizophrenia. Data from the Maternal and Child Health Handbook in Japan. Journal of Nervous and Mental Disease 184, 542–546.

Lyons MJ, Goldberg J, Eisen SA et al. (1993) Do genes influence exposure to trauma? A twin study of combat. American Journal of Medical Genetics 48, 22–27.

Malaspina D, Sohler N, Susser ES (1999) Interaction of genes and prenatal exposures in schizophrenia. In: Prenatal Exposures in Schizophrenia, Susser ES, Brown AS, Gorman JM, eds. Washington, DC: American Psychiatric Press, pp. 47–68.

Marcelis M, van Os J, Sham P et al. (1998) Obstetric complications and familial morbid risk of psychiatric disorders. American Journal of Medical Genetics 81, 29–36.

Matheny AP, Jr, Brown AM, Wilson RS (1997) Behavioral antecedents of accidental injuries in early childhood: a study of twins. Injury Prevention 3, 144–145.

McGuffin P, Asherson P, Owen M, Farmer A (1994) The strength of the genetic effect. Is there room for an environmental influence in the aetiology of schizophrenia? British Journal of Psychiatry 164, 593–599.

Mortensen PB, Pedersen CB, Westergaard T et al. (1999) Effects of family history and place and season of birth on the risk of schizophrenia [see comments]. New England Journal of Medicine 340, 603–608.

Motulsky AG (1977) Ecogenetics: genetic variation in susceptibility to environmental agents. In: Human Genetics, Armendares S, Lisker R, eds. Amsterdam: Excerpta Medica, pp. 375–385.

Neale MC, Boker SM, Maes HH (1999) Mx: Statistical Modeling. Richmond, VA: Department of Psychiatry.

Nimgaonkar VL, Wessely S, Murray RM (1988) Prevalence of familiality, obstetric complications, and structural brain damage in schizophrenic patients. British Journal of Psychiatry 153, 191–197.

O'Callaghan E, Gibson T, Colohan HA et al. (1992) Risk of schizophrenia in adults born after obstetric complications and their association with early onset of illness: a controlled study [see comments]. British Medical Journal 305, 1256–1259.

Ottman R (1990) An epidemiologic approach to gene–environment interaction. Genetic Epidemiology 7, 177–185.

Ottman R (1996) Gene–environment interaction: definitions and study designs. Preventive Medicine 25, 764–770.

Petronis A, Paterson AD, Kennedy JL (1999) Schizophrenia: an epigenetic puzzle? Schizophrenia Bulletin 25, 639–655.

Plomin R (1994) Genetics and Experience. London: Sage.

Plomin R, de Fries JC, Loehlin JC (1977) Genotype–environment interaction and correlation in the analysis of human behavior. Psychological Bulletin 84, 309–322.

Pulver AE, Liang KY, Brown CH et al. (1992) Risk factors in schizophrenia. Season of birth, gender, and familial risk [see comments]. British Journal of Psychiatry 160, 65–71.

Rothman KJ (1986) Modern Epidemiology. Boston, MA: Little, Brown.

Saudino KJ, Pedersen NL, Lichtenstein P, McClearn GE, Plomin R (1997) Can personality explain genetic influences on life events? Journal of Personality and Social Psychology 72, 196–206.

Sham P (1996) Genetic epidemiology. British Medical Bulletin 52, 408–433.

Sham P (1998) Statistics in Human Genetics. London: Arnold.

Shur E (1982) Season of birth in high and low genetic risk schizophrenics. British Journal of Psychiatry 140, 410–415.

Spitzer RL, Williams JBW, Gibbon M (1990) User's Guide for the Structured Clinical Interview for DSM-III-R (SCID). Washington, DC: American Psychiatric Press.

Sugarman PA, Craufurd D (1994) Schizophrenia in the Afro-Caribbean community. British Journal of Psychiatry 164, 474–480.

Susser E, Susser M (1989) Familial aggregation studies. A note on their epidemiologic properties. American Journal of Epidemiology 129, 23–30.

Tienari P, Wynne LC, Moring J et al. (1994) The Finnish adoptive family study of schizophrenia. Implications for family research [see comments]. British Journal of Psychiatry Suppl. 20–26.

van Os J, Marcelis M (1998) The ecogenetics of schizophrenia: a review. Schizophrenia Research 32, 127–135.

van Os J, Fahy TA, Bebbington P et al. (1994) The influence of life events on the subsequent course of psychotic illness. A prospective follow-up of the Camberwell Collaborative Psychosis Study. Psychological Medicine 24, 503–513.

Wahlberg KE, Wynne LC, Oja H et al. (1997) Gene–environment interaction in vulnerability to schizophrenia: findings from the Finnish Adoptive Family Study of Schizophrenia. American Journal of Psychiatry 154, 355–362.

Walker E (1981) Attentional and neuromotor functions of schizophrenics, schizoaffectives, and patients with other affective disorders. Archives of General Psychiatry 38, 1355–1358.

Woolf CM (1997) Does the genotype for schizophrenia often remain unexpressed because of canalization and stochastic events during development? Psychological Medicine 27, 659–668.

13

Investigating gene–environment interaction in schizophrenia using neuroimaging

Theo G. M. van Erp, Timothy L. Gasperoni, Isabelle M. Rosso and Tyrone D. Cannon

Department of Psychology, University of California at Los Angeles, USA

Applications of classical epidemiological methods have led to general acceptance of a multifactorial threshold model of schizophrenia, whereby multiple genetic influences and environmental factors aggregate together, additively and/or interactively, to form a continuum of disease liability. Studies that make use of clinical diagnostic categories are limited in what they can tell us about the precise nature of the aetiological factors involved in schizophrenia because of the inherent limitations of categorical measures in reflecting a continuous liability scale. We propose that new methodologies that can represent this liability continuum on a quantitative scale are needed to aid in the search for schizophrenia susceptibility genes and in elucidating the pathophysiological mechanisms by which these genes and environmental factors act. Here we review evidence concerning structural brain abnormalities as markers of aetiological influences in schizophrenia, concluding that use of quantitative neuroanatomical measures will facilitate the detection of predisposing gene loci and help to clarify whether nongenetic influences contribute independently of or interactively with genetic factors in influencing disease liability. The eventual discovery of such genes will spawn a new era of epidemiological research, in which the effects of specific predisposing genotypes and specific environmental factors on schizophrenia phenomenology and pathophysiology can be studied.

Investigating gene–environment interaction in schizophrenia

Family, twin, and adoption studies have demonstrated that schizophrenia is a substantially heritable disorder. These studies are reviewed in Chapter 10. Still, attempts at isolating specific genes that confer vulnerability to schizophrenia have so far been only moderately successful (Moldin, 1997). These efforts have been complicated by an inability to detect nonclinically penetrant carriers of the predisposing genes and by uncertainties concerning the nature of nongenetic influences and their potential interaction with genetic factors. The pattern of affection with schizophrenia in families is not consistent with simple Mendelian transmission of a single major gene influencing disease liability. Rather, genetic epidemiological studies point strongly to a polygenic mode of inheritance in schizophrenia, whereby multiple genes of small effect contribute to increasing risk for the disorder but only result in its overt expression if their combined effects cross a hypothetical 'threshold of liability' (Gottesman & Shields, 1982; Ch. 11). Because genetic liability to schizophrenia is likely to vary on a continuous rather than categorical scale, our chances of isolating particular susceptibility genes are likely to be greatly improved by employing quantitative rather than qualitative measures of phenotypic affection. Quantitative symptom-based measures of affection represent one such approach but are sensitive to variation only above a certain threshold on the liability continuum. Quantitative indicators of pathological processes mediating between causative genetic factors and symptomatic phenotypic expression ('endophenotypes') are likely to represent more sensitive markers of underlying liability status than symptom-based measures of affection, whether quantitative or qualitative in nature. Such endophenotypic indicators are likely to be closer to the mechanism of simple gene action than clinical symptomologic status and, as such, should be more sensitive to variation in underlying disease liability among both affected and nonaffected members of high-density pedigrees (Cannon and Marco, 1994; Cannon, 1996). Their use should, therefore, greatly facilitate the isolation of susceptibility genes in linkage studies.

Obstetric complications

Of the various environmental factors proposed to be involved in schizophrenia, obstetric complications (OCs), particularly those associated with fetal hypoxia, have shown the most robust association (for reviews see Ch. 5; Cannon, 1997; McNeil and Kaij, 1988). Because no study using objective birth records has found that hypoxic OCs are more frequent in the first-degree relatives of schizophrenic patients than in the general population (Mirdal et al., 1974; Hanson et al., 1976; Rieder et al., 1977; Marcus et al., 1981; Fish et al., 1992; Gunther-Genta et al., 1994; Cannon et al., 2000a; Rosso et al., 2000a), these complications do not appear to be consequences of genetic liability to schizophrenia. While not impossible, it is also unlikely that these early influences cause schizophrenia on their own, since over 90% of individuals exposed to fetal hypoxia, even in severe form, do not develop schizophrenia (Done et al., 1991; Buka et al., 1993; Cannon et al., 2000a; Rosso et al., 2000a). Hypoxic OCs must, therefore, act additively or interactively with genetic factors in influencing disease liability. An extension of the endophenotype model developed above is to use quantitative liability indicators in epidemiological studies of individuals with and without a genetic background for schizophrenia, and with and without a history of OCs, to determine whether genetic factors and OCs contribute independently or interactively to variation in liability. In this chapter we review work conducted within this framework using structural brain abnormalities as quantitative endophenotypic indicators of liability.

Detecting causes of brain morphological changes in schizophrenia

Structural brain abnormalities are robust correlates of schizophrenia, but their roles in the aetiology and pathophysiology of the disorder have not been conclusively established. Evidence of neuromotor and cognitive deficits in preschizophrenic children (Walker et al., 1994; Rosso et al., 2000b; Cannon et al., 2000b) and of heterotopic neuronal displacements in frontal and temporal lobe regions in patients at postmortem (Arnold et al., 1991; Benes et al., 1991; Akbarian et al., 1993a,b), suggest that at least some of the anatomical changes in schizophrenia are neurodevelopmental in origin, reflecting factors intrinsic to disease causation (Cannon, 1998). Our hypotheses concerning the differential contributions of genetic and nongenetic influences to the neuroanatomical changes in schizophrenia grew out of a series of structural imaging studies in schizophrenic patients and their relatives. These studies employed either a vertical (parent–offspring) or horizontal (sibling–sibling or twin–twin) high-risk design format. In the vertical high-risk design, offspring of parents with schizophrenia are chosen prior to knowledge of their own diagnostic outcomes and compared with offspring of healthy controls. In the horizontal high-risk design, patients with schizophrenia and their non-ill siblings or co-twins are compared with healthy controls without a family history of schizophrenia. In both types of study, the influences of putative environmental aetiological factors on brain morphology can be examined at two or more clearly separable levels of genotypic risk for schizophrenia. Both approaches offer a distinct advantage in this respect over studies that compare schizophrenic patients with and without affected first-degree relative(s). That is, because many unaffected relatives of schizophrenic patients are expected to carry one or more genes in a predisposing configuration but nevertheless remain clinically unaffected, it is not valid to infer that schizophrenic patients without an affected first-degree relative lack a predisposing genotype. Further, because the mode of genetic transmission of schizophrenia is complex, and potentially heterogeneous, it is not clear whether there is a qualitatively or quantitatively meaningful difference in genotypic loading among schizophrenic patients with and without affected first-degree relatives.

Most neuroimaging studies of schizophrenia have utilized samples of convenience (e.g. patients being treated in a particular clinical setting). However, probands and relatives ascertained in this way may not adequately represent the distribution of liability to schizophrenia (and hence its causes) in the general population. Another advantage of our approach is the use of population-based sampling methods, which result in excellent correspondence between studied and nonstudied probands in terms of demographic and clinical history variables. (See Rössler & Rössler (1998) for a review of the advantages of epidemiological ascertainment methods.)

Below we describe two such studies, one involving the offspring of schizophrenic and normal parents in Denmark and the other involving patients with schizophrenia, their unaffected siblings and matched controls from a Helsinki birth cohort.

Danish High-Risk Project: pilot study

In 1962, Mednick and Schulsinger (1965, 1968) started a prospective high-risk study including 207 Danish children with schizophrenic mothers and 104 demographically matched controls without a family history of psychiatric illness. These children were selected by cross-referencing the Danish National Psychiatric Register, which maintains a central file on every psychiatric hospitalization in Denmark, with the Danish Folkeregister, which maintains a lifelong and up-to-date register of the address of every resident of Denmark. These and other population registries are a valuable resource for the selection of experimental and control groups because they allow for the potential for random sampling of probands and precise matching of control subjects on relevant demographic variables. Additionally, the demographic characteristics of a selected sample can easily be compared with the rest of the population to ensure representativeness. Another virtue of population registries is that the attrition rate during follow-up is reduced enormously because the participants can be relocated at follow-up.

At the time of the first assessment, the mean age of the children was 15.1 years, and none was diagnosed with any psychiatric illness. Between 1972 and 1974, these subjects underwent clinical assessments, and the clinical information was later used to make diagnoses according to DSM-III criteria (American Psychiatric Association, 1980). Among the offspring of schizophrenic mothers, 15 were diagnosed with schizophrenia, 29 with schizotypal personality disorder (SPD), 108 with a number of other diagnoses and 23 with no mental illness. Following up on several early imaging studies that suggested involvement of both genetic (Weinberger et al., 1981; Reveley et al., 1982; DeLisi et al., 1986) and environmental factors (Schulsinger et al., 1984; Silverton et al., 1985; DeLisi et al., 1988; Suddath et al., 1990) in the structural abnormalities seen in schizophrenia, we conducted a pilot computed tomography (CT) study on a subsample of 34 high-risk subjects, including 7 subjects with schizophrenia, 12 with schizotypal personality disorder, and 15 with no mental illness.

Results

In this sample, we examined the independence of structural abnormalities in schizophrenia based on their aetiological antecedents (i.e. genetic risk and OCs) by comparing subjects at two levels of genetic risk for developing schizophrenia: high risk (offspring with a schizophrenic mother) and super high risk (offspring with a schizophrenic mother and a schizophrenia spectrum father). Information on pregnancy and delivery complications, as well as birthweight, was collected prospectively from original birth records. A factor analysis of six CT scan measures yielded two factors that differed in their relationships with the aetiological precursors (Cannon et al., 1989). The first factor, labelled 'multisite neural deficits,' comprised of widening of the Sylvian and interhemispheric fissures and cortical sulci and of cerebellar vermis abnormalities; it was related to genetic risk status but not to any of the OCs examined. The second factor, labelled 'periventricular damage,' was reflected by increased ventricular cerebrospinal fluid (CSF) to brain ratio (VBR) and increased third ventricular size; this was highly correlated with delivery complications and low birthweight – and more highly so among super-high-risk than high-risk offspring. This study was the first to suggest that two types of structural brain abnormality may reflect independent aetiological processes in schizophrenia, based on differential contributions of genetic and obstetric influences. In addition, we interpreted these results as consistent with a gene–OC interaction model of schizophrenia, in which genetic liability confers a heightened vulnerability to fetal brain injury, perhaps specific to regions surrounding the ventricular system.

This study had several noteworthy unique advantages. First, the obstetric data were gathered prospectively from the records of the original midwives who attended the births, rather than retrospectively by an interview of the mother about the pregnancy and labour periods. Second, the obstetric, genetic and CT measurements were all obtained independently of each other and blindly with respect to diagnosis, eliminating any possible confound in any of these measures from prior knowledge of adult psychiatric diagnosis. Third, the sample is known to be representative in terms of the proportion of hospitalized and nonhospitalized cases, neuroleptic usage and other psychiatric treatments (Parnas and Teasdale, 1987).

However, this study also had several limitations that merit explicit mention. The small sample size ($n = 34$) did not allow us to examine the potential contribution of specific types of OC to morphological variation. In addition, we did not statistically control for possible confounding factors such as age, sex, substance abuse, organic brain syndromes and head injuries. Also, because we did not exclude from the analyses individuals who had developed schizophrenia, we could not rule out the possibility that the association between genetic and perinatal factors and structural brain deficits was an artifact of the increase in brain deviance associated with the disease process and/or its treatment. Finally, because there was not a nongenetically predisposed control group, we could not address the possibility that the contributions of OCs and low birthweight to ventricular abnormalities were caused by a covariation between level of genetic risk and these obstetric variables. The lack of a control group at low risk for schizophrenia also made it impossible to determine whether the genetic contribution to cortical and cerebellar abnormalities (and vulnerability to OCs) represented a stepwise increase from low risk (neither parent with schizophrenia) to high risk (one parent with schizophrenia) to super high risk (both parents with a schizophrenia spectrum disorder).

Danish High-Risk Project: follow-up study

In order to address these limitations, we performed a follow-up study with CT on 60 low-risk, 72 high-risk, and 25 super-high-risk offspring. Analyses of the CT data replicated and extended results of the initial pilot study. Increasing levels of genetic risk for schizophrenia (low to high to super high) were related to stepwise linear increases in both cortical, CSF to brain ratio and VBR, after controlling for the effects of age, sex, substance abuse and history of organic brain syndromes and head injuries (Fig. 13.1; Cannon et al., 1993). Genetic risk also interacted with OCs in predicting increased VBR but not cortical CSF to brain ratios. That is, the effect of delivery complications on VBR was greater among those with two affected parents compared with those with one affected parent, and greater among those with one affected compared with those with healthy parents. The exclusion of the schizophrenic patients from the analyses did not alter these results. In addition, we found that neither low birthweight nor any of the other OCs systematically varied with the level of genetic risk for schizophrenia, rejecting the gene–environment covariation model, which predicts that pre- and perinatal complications are a mere consequence of the predisposition to the disorder, rather than a cause. We concluded that the type and degree of brain abnormality shown by adult offspring of schizophrenic and healthy parents are strongly predicted by the independent and interacting influences of genetic risk for schizophrenia and OCs (Cannon et al., 1993).

We further examined the differences in VBR and sulcal CSF to brain ratio as a function of lifetime psychiatric diagnosis in this sample (Cannon et al., 1994). Based on substantial evidence of a genetic relationship between SPD and schizophrenia and our finding that cortical sulcal enlargement is specifically related to genetic risk for schizophrenia, we hypothesized that schizophrenic patients and individuals with SPD would both show cortical sulcal enlargement compared with that in low-risk offspring. Further, in view of our findings that OCs were related to an increased risk for schizophrenia but not to SPD in the high-risk children and that ventricular enlargement reflects an interaction between genetic risk and OCs, we hypothesized that schizophrenics would evidence larger ventricles than individuals with SPD and low-risk offspring. We found that high-risk individuals with

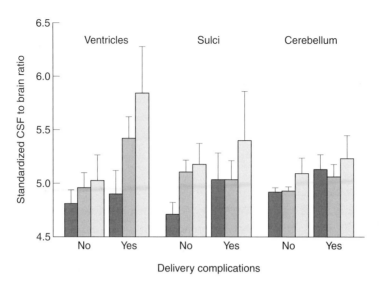

Fig. 13.1.   Mean (±SEM) ventricular, sulcal, and cerebellar cerebrospinal fluid (CSF) to brain ratios
by delivery complications and level of genetic risk for schizophrenia. The interaction of
delivery complications and risk for schizophrenia was significant only for the ventricular
measure ($p < 0.01$). The effect of delivery complications on ventricular enlargement was
significant in the super-high-risk (shaded bars) and high-risk (open bars) groups $p < 0.01$
and $p < 0.01$, respectively) but not in the low-risk (solid bars) group. Adapted from
Cannon et al., 1993.)

schizophrenia and SPD had an equivalent degree of cortical sulcal enlargement,
and that both groups had significantly larger sulci to brain ratios than the high-risk
offspring with nonschizophrenia spectrum disorders and those with no psychiatric disorders, and than the low-risk individuals with and without psychiatric diagnoses. However, only high-risk individuals with schizophrenia evidenced
significantly enlarged VBR compared with each of the other groups, including the
SPDs. These data suggest that in the offspring of schizophrenic parents, cortical
abnormalities are expressed equally across the range of syndromes in the schizophrenia spectrum and that they are, therefore, likely to be reflective of the genetic
predisposition to the disorder. In contrast, subcortical abnormalities (measured by
VBRs) are more pronounced in the more severe syndrome (i.e. schizophrenia) and
are reflective of a more severe, environmentally complicated form of the disorder
(Cannon et al., 1994; Zorrilla et al., 1997).

The Danish High-Risk Study thus provided suggestive preliminary evidence for
the influence of genetic and environmental risk factors on structural brain abnormalities in schizophrenia. However, these studies relied on CSF to brain ratios to
quantify measures of cortical and subcortical volumes. This method confounds two

potentially dissociable anatomical features, namely, increased sulcal or ventricular CSF volumes and reduced brain parenchymal volumes. CT methodology also does not have the spatial or contrast resolution required to measure specific brain structures and distinguish between grey and white matter. Another shortcoming of this study is that the possibility of a specific pathogenic mechanism underlying the effects of OCs was not explicitly tested.

Helsinki Cohort Study

To overcome these limitations, we examined the magnetic resonance images (MRI) of 75 psychotic probands, 60 of their nonpsychotic full siblings, and 56 demographically matched control subjects without a personal or family history of treated psychiatric morbidity. The participants were drawn from the total population of individuals born in Helsinki, Finland in 1955 ($n = 7840$) and all their full siblings ($n = 12796$), who (along with their parents) were screened in national case registries for psychiatric morbidity (Fig. 13.2).

A total of 267 (1.3%) members of this population had a register diagnosis of schizophrenia, schizoaffective disorder, or schizophreniform disorder, according to the ICD-8 (World Health Organization, 1967) numbering scheme. Probands were randomly selected from this total pool and approached initially via their treating psychiatrists. Those who expressed interest in participating were contacted by project staff, who evaluated and obtained informed consent from 80 patients. An attempt was made to recruit at least one nonschizophrenic sibling of each studied proband, but this was possible for only 62 of the 80 cases. In addition, 56 nonschizophrenic control subjects (28 sibling pairs from 28 independent families) were randomly selected from the same study population after excluding any individual with a personal or family history of treated psychiatric morbidity. Studied probands were equivalent to the remainder of the proband population in terms of year of birth, nuclear family size (i.e. parents and siblings), sex, history of inpatient admission, age at first inpatient admission, history of comorbid substance abuse disorder and work disability, but the studied group had more hospital admissions than the non-studied group (Cannon et al., 1998). MRI scans were not usable for five patients and two siblings because of movement artifact or other technical problems.

Of the 75 probands with usable MRI data, 63 had lifetime diagnoses of schizophrenia and 12 of schizoaffective disorder. The proband, sibling and control groups were balanced in terms of age, sex, handedness, social class, nuclear family size (i.e. parents and siblings), history of any DSM-III-R-defined (American Psychiatric Association, 1987) substance use or dependence disorder (primarily alcohol-related disorders), total intracranial volume, birthweight, exposure to infection during gestation, and history of perinatal hypoxia. The sibling and control groups were also balanced in terms of percentage of group with a DSM-III-R diagnosis of

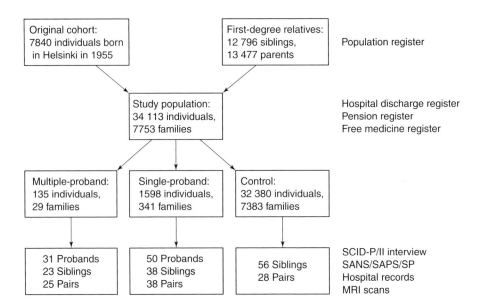

Fig. 13.2.   Selection of the population-based sample of individuals born in Helsinki, Finland, in 1955, using the national case registries. See text for the assessment methods.

depression or anxiety disorder. A standard form was used to code information on maternal health, fetal monitoring, prenatal and perinatal complications and neonatal conditions from the original antenatal clinic and obstetric hospital records by a worker blind to diagnosis and imaging results.

Brain changes

In an initial analysis of the scans, we reliably measured the left and right frontal, temporal, posterior and ventricular brain regions classified into grey matter, white matter and CSF. Both schizophrenic patients and their full siblings exhibited significant reductions in frontal and temporal grey matter volumes and significant increases in frontal and temporal sulcal CSF volumes, compared with controls, after controlling for the effects of age, sex and whole brain volume (Fig. 13.3). However, ventricular CSF volume increase and white matter volume reduction were found in schizophrenics but not their siblings (Cannon et al., 1998). These results suggest that frontal and temporal lobe grey matter reductions in schizophrenia may be caused by genetic (or shared environmental) factors. In contrast, ventricular enlargement and white matter deficits were specific to the clinical phenotype and may, therefore, reflect the influences of unique environmental factors or factors secondary to illness expression.

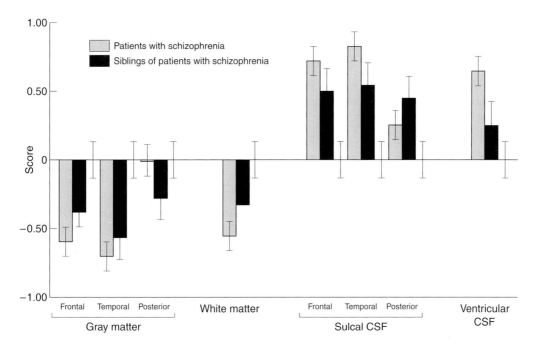

Fig. 13.3   Mean (±SEM) *z* scores for ratio measures of regional gray matter, overall white matter, regional sulcal cerebrospinal fluid (CSF), and overall ventricular CSF in patients (*n* = 75), siblings (*n* = 60), and control subjects (error bars; *n* = 56). The data shown are corrected for total intracranial volume, age, sex and history of substance abuse and are collapsed across any nonsignificant within-subject dimensions (hemisphere or region). Asterisks above and below error bars indicate statistically significant differences from controls. (Adapted from Cannon et al., 1998.)

Perinatal hypoxia

Subsequent analyses examined perinatal hypoxia as a possible environmental mechanism underlying some of these brain abnormalities (Cannon et al., 2002). In our earlier study, we had found evidence supporting the genotype–environment interaction model in that the contribution of OCs to subcortical pathology scaled with an increase in genetic risk, i.e. the contribution of OCs to subcortical pathology was larger in super-high-risk offspring compared with high-risk offspring, and larger in high-risk offspring compared with low-risk offspring (Cannon et al., 1993). Furthermore, Suddath and colleagues (1990) have demonstrated that the affected twins of discordant monozygotic twin pairs evidence enlarged ventricular volumes and reduced temporal lobe, but not frontal lobe, volumes compared with their nonschizophrenic co-twins, and McNeil and colleagues (2000) have found that intrapair differences in ventricular and hippocampal volumes may relate to higher rates of OCs in the affected co-twins. Based on these findings, we hypothesized that the ventricular and temporal lobe volumes of individuals at high genetic risk for schizophrenia (i.e. the patients and their full siblings) but not those of low genetic risk (i.e. healthy volunteers without a personal or family history of treated psychiatric morbidity) may be modulated by perinatal hypoxia.

To test this hypothesis, we devised a scale based on hypoxia-associated OCs. Hypoxia was scored as present if the subject was coded as blue at birth or neonatally or had two or more complications that were significantly related to birth or neonatal asphyxia in the overall sample: cord knotted or wrapped tightly around neck, placental infarcts, third trimester bleeding, pre-eclampsia, anaemia during pregnancy, anorexia/malnutrition during pregnancy, fetal distress and breech presentation. We found that grey matter in the frontal lobe, temporal lobe and posterior region of patients and their full siblings exposed to perinatal oxygen deprivation were smaller and the sulcal CSF volumes were larger than of those who were not. There was also a group by hypoxia by region interaction in that the temporal lobes of both the patients and their siblings showed the largest grey matter reduction and sulcal CSF increase. That cortical sulcal enlargement did not vary by obstetric history among those at genetic risk for schizophrenia in the Danish study (Cannon et al., 1993), as it did in the Helsinki study, most likely reflects a greater reduction in signal at the cortical surface (owing to partial volume artifacts) associated with CT compared with MRI. Hypoxia also appeared to be differentially related to increased ventricular CSF in the patients only. In contrast, there were no differences in any of the volumetric measurements of low-risk control subjects with and without hypoxia-associated OCs, and there were no associations of white matter with hypoxia in any of the groups (Cannon et al., 2002).

Genotype–perinatal hypoxia interaction

We interpreted these results as consistent with a genotype–environment interaction of perinatal influences, especially those that provoke hypoxia, in schizophrenia. That is, a genetic factor in schizophrenia may create a heightened susceptibility to the neurally disruptive effects of fetal oxygen deprivation. It could be argued that the results suggest an influence other than fetal hypoxia since some of the macroscopic sequelae of hypoxia-ischaemia – in particular periventricular white matter damage – were not observed. However, the neural sequelae of hypoxia are numerous and vary in severity from alterations in neurite outgrowth to neuronal cell death (Nyakas et al., 1996). In the latter, loss of both grey and white matter would be expected. In the former, immature neurons may survive the hypoxic insult but still have a compromised elaboration of synaptic interconnections (Nyakas et al., 1996). Studies in fetal sheep have shown that hypoxia secondary to chronic mild or subacute placental insufficiency results in a reduction in cortical thickness and an increase in cortical neuronal density, without any observable neuronal loss or white matter damage (Rees et al., 1998). These reductions in neuropil volume, in the absence of neuronal cell loss and associated gliosis, would be expected to manifest as reductions in grey but not white matter volume at the macroscopic level (i.e. on MRI). Nevertheless, the findings reviewed above are based on clinical indicators of hypoxia rather than molecular markers of fetal blood oxygenation. Further work is needed to determine whether hypoxia as confirmed via blood gas analysis alters brain morphology differentially among infants at genetic risk for schizophrenia and whether other consequences of fetal distress, such as the induction of proinflammatory cytokines, play a role in this association.

Other studies

Several other structural brain imaging studies in schizophrenia have indicated genetic load effects on hippocampal and amygdaloid (Seidman et al., 1997, 1999) as well as thalamic (Staal et al., 1998) volumes. On the basis of these findings, one could conclude that these volumetric measurements may be likely endophenotypic indicators – that is, markers of a predisposing genotype. However, apart from the study of McNeil and colleagues (2000), none of these studies have factored in measures of OCs, which, in view of our findings, may interact with genetic risk in determining at least some of the neuromorphological abnormalities in schizophrenia. Therefore, these subcortical brain measures may not be pure genetic markers (i.e. endophenotypes) that can be used in quantitative trait loci analyses without covarying for the level of hypoxia exposure. It will be important, however, to examine more regionally specific brain measures. The cingulate gyrus, for instance, has a relatively high density of N-methyl-D-aspartate (NMDA) receptors (Tamminga, 1999), and it is, therefore, possible that a more fine-grained parcelation of the frontal lobes will reveal that some subregions are susceptible to the effects of perinatal oxygen deprivation while others are more purely related to genetic risk. Whether or not the amygdaloid, thalamic and cingulate morphological changes in schizophrenics are under the influence of hypoxia-related OCs remains to be determined.

Conclusions and future directions

In complex diseases such as schizophrenia, quantitative measures of liability are likely to provide a more sensitive basis for elucidating aetiological factors and determining their mechanisms of influence than more traditional approaches based on clinical diagnostic categories. The work reviewed in this chapter suggests that structural brain abnormalities are promising endophenotypic indicators for schizophrenia. Some of these abnormalities (e.g. frontal and temporal cortical grey matter reductions) are shared by schizophrenic patients and their non-ill family members, while other abnormalities (e.g. ventricular enlargement, cortical white matter reduction) are unique to schizophrenic patients. Further, a history of fetal hypoxia was associated with reductions of cortical grey matter and increases of sulcal CSF in schizophrenic patients and their non-ill family members, but not in control subjects at low genetic risk for schizophrenia. It appears, therefore, that a genetic factor in schizophrenia may render the fetal brain particularly susceptible to damage following hypoxia–ischaemia.

The imaging studies reviewed above suggest two directions that may aid in the search for schizophrenia susceptibility genes. First, they suggest that we should continue to evaluate structural brain abnormalities in the search for more purely genetically mediated neuroendophenotypic indicators of schizophrenia. Such measures should facilitate the identification of specific susceptibility loci by encouraging a search for genes that contribute to quantitative variation in discrete aspects of disease liability and by making nonclinically penetrant gene carriers informative for linkage. Second, these results encourage search for genes that predispose to the disorder by creating heightened susceptibility to the neurally disruptive effects of hypoxia. In this approach, linkage analyses would be performed that make use of obstetric and genetic variation as predictors of variation in regional brain volumes. These two suggestions, which both combine the use of neuroimaging and molecular biological techniques with epidemiological study designs, may provide us with more powerful approaches to solving complex disorders such as schizophrenia (Susser & Susser, 1996; Ambrosone and Kadlubar, 1997).

REFERENCES

Akbarian S, Bunney WE Jr, Potkin SG et al. (1993a) Altered distribution of nicotinamide-adenine dinucleotide phosphate–diaphorase cells in frontal lobe of schizophrenics implies disturbances in cortical development. Archives of General Psychiatry 50, 169–177.

Akbarian S, Vinuela A, Kim JJ, Potkin SG, Bunney WE, Jr, Jones EG (1993b) Distorted distribution of nicotinamide-adenine dinucleotide phosphate–diaphorase neurons in temporal lobe of schizophrenics implies anomalous cortical development. Archives of General Psychiatry 50, 178–187.

Ambrosone CB, Kadlubar FF (1997) Toward an integrated approach to molecular epidemiology. American Journal of Epidemiology 146, 912–918.

American Psychiatric Association (1980) Diagnostic and Statistical Manual of Mental Disorders, 3rd edn. Washington, DC: American Psychiatric Press.

American Psychiatric Association (1987) Diagnostic and Statistical III–Revised. Washington, DC: American Psychiatric Press.

Arnold SE, Hyman BT, van Hoesen GW, Damasio AR (1991) Some cytoarchitectural abnormalities of the entorhinal cortex in schizophrenia. Archives of General Psychiatry 48, 625–632.

Benes FM, McSparren J, Bird ED, San Giovanni JP, Vincent SL (1991) Deficits in small interneurons in prefrontal cingulate cortices of schizophrenic and schizoaffective patients. Archives of General Psychiatry 48, 996–1001.

Buka SL, Tsuang MT, Lipsitt LP (1993) Pregnancy/delivery complications and psychiatric diagnosis: a prospective study. Archives of General Psychiatry 50, 151–156.

Cannon TD (1996) Abnormalities of brain structure and function in schizophrenia: implications for aetiology and pathophysiology. Annals of Medicine 28, 533–539.

Cannon TD (1997) On the nature and mechanisms of obstetric influences in schizophrenia: a review and synthesis of epidemiologic studies. International Review of Psychiatry 9, 387–397.

Cannon TD (1998) Neurodevelopmental influences in the genesis and epigenesis of schizophrenia: an overview. Applied and Preventive Psychology 7, 47–62.

Cannon TD, Marco E (1994) Structural brain abnormalities as indicators of vulnerability to schizophrenia. Schizophrenia Bulletin 20, 89–102.

Cannon TD, Mednick SA, Parnas J (1989) Genetic and perinatal determinants of structural brain deficits in schizophrenia. Archives of General Psychiatry 46, 883–889.

Cannon TD, Mednick S, Parnas J, Schulsinger F, Praestholm J, Vestergaard A (1993) Developmental brain abnormalities in the offspring of schizophrenic mothers: I. Contributions of genetic and perinatal factors. Archives of General Psychiatry 50, 551–564.

Cannon TD, Mednick S, Parnas J, Schulsinger F, Praestholm J, Vestergaard A (1994) Developmental brain abnormalities in the offspring of schizophrenic mothers: II. Structural brain characteristics of schizophrenia and schizotypal personality disorder. Archives of General Psychiatry 51, 955–962.

Cannon TD, van Erp TGM, Huttunen M et al. (1998) Regional grey matter, white matter, and cerebrospinal fluid distributions in schizophrenic patients, their siblings, and controls. Archives of General Psychiatry 55, 1084–1091.

Cannon TD, Rosso IM, Hollister JM, Bearden CE, Sanchez LE, Hadley T (2000a) A prospective cohort study of genetic and perinatal influences in the aetiology of schizophrenia. Schizophrenia Bulletin 26, 351–366.

Cannon TD, Bearden CE, Hollister JM, Rosso IM, Sanchez LE, Hadley F (2000b) Childhood cognitive functioning in schizophrenia patients and their unaffected siblings: a prospective cohort study. Schizophrenia Bulletin 26, 370–393.

Cannon TD, van Erp TGM, Rosso IM et al. (2002) Fetal hypoxia and structural brain pathology in schizophrenic patients, their siblings, and controls. Archives of General Psychiatry 59, 34–35.

DeLisi LE, Goldin LR, Hamovit, JR, Maxwell E, Kurtz D, Gershon ES (1986) A family study of the association of increased ventricular size with schizophrenia. Archives of General Psychiatry 43, 148–153.

DeLisi LE, Dauphinais ID, Gershon ES (1988) Perinatal complications and reduced size of brain limbic structures in familial schizophrenia. Schizophrenia Bulletin 14, 185–191.

Done DJ, Johnstone EC, Frith CD, Godling J, Shepherd PM, Crow RJ (1991) Complications of pregnancy and delivery in relation to psychosis in adult life: data from the British perinatal mortality survey sample. British Medical Journal 302, 1576–1580.

Fish B, Marcus J, Hans SL, Auerbach JG, Perdue S (1992) Infants at risk for schizophrenia: sequelae of a genetic neurointegrative defect. A review and replication analysis of pandysmaturation in the Jerusalem Infant Development Study. Archives of General Psychiatry 49, 221–235.

Gottesman II, Shields J (1982) Schizophrenia: the Epigenetic Puzzle. New York: Cambridge University Press.

Gunther-Genta F, Bovet P, Hohlfeld P (1994) Obstetric complication and schizophrenia: A case control study. British Journal of Psychiatry 64, 165–170.

Hanson DR, Gottesman II, Heston LL (1976) Some possible childhood indicators of adult schizophrenia inferred from children of schizophrenics. British Journal of Psychiatry 129, 142–154.

Marcus J, Auerback J, Wilkinson L, Burack CM (1981) Infants at risk for schizophrenia: the Jerusalem Infant Development Study. Archives of General Psychiatry 38, 703–713.

McNeil TF, Kaij L (1988) Obstetric factors and perinatal injuries. In: Handbook of Schizophrenia, Vol. 3. Nosology, Epidemiology and Genetics, Tsuang MR, Simpson JC, eds. New York: Elsevier Science, pp. 319–344.

McNeil MF, Cantor-Graae EC, Weinberger DR (2000) Relationship of obstetric complications and differences in size of brain structures in monozygotic twin pairs discordant for schizophrenia. American Journal of Psychiatry 157, 203–212.

Mednick SA, Schulsinger F (1965) A longitudinal study of children with a high risk for schizophrenia: a preliminary report. In: Methods and Goals in Human Behavior Genetics, Vandenberg S, ed. Orlando: Academic Pres, pp. 255–296.

Mednick SA, Schulsinger F (1968) Some premorbid characteristics related to breakdown in children with schizophrenic mothers. Journal of Psychiatric Research 6, 267–291.

Mirdal GKM, Mednick, SA, Schulsinger F, Fuchs F (1974) Perinatal complications in children of schizophrenic mothers. Acta Psychiatrica Scandinavica 50, 553–568.

Moldin SO (1997) The maddening hunt for madness genes. Nature Genetics 17, 127–129.

Nyakas C, Buwalda B, Luiten PGM (1996) Hypoxia and brain development. Progress in Neurobiology 49, 1–51.

Parnas J, Teasdale TW (1987) Treated versus untreated schizophrenia spectrum cases: a matched paired high risk population study. Acta. Psychiatrica Scandinavica 75, 44–50.

Rees S, Mallard C, Breen S, Stringer M, Cock M, Harding R (1998) Foetal brain injury following prolonged hypoxemia and placental insufficiency: a review. Comparative Biochemistry and Physiology 119, 653–660.

Reveley, AM, Reveley, MA, Clifford, CA, Murray, MA (1982) Cereberal ventricular size in twins discordant for schizophrenia. Lancet i, 540–541.

Rieder RO, Broman SH, Rosenthal D (1977) The offspring of schizophrenics: II. Perinatal factors and IQ. Archives of General Psychiatry 34, 789–799.

Rössler, AR, Rössler, W (1998) The course of schizophrenia psychoses: what do we really know? A selective review from an epidemiological perspective. European Archives of Psychiatry and Clinical Neuroscience 248, 189–202.

Rosso IM, Cannon TD, Huttunen MO, Huttunen T, Lonnqvist J, Gasperoni TL (2000a) Obstetric risk factors for early-onset schizophrenia in a Finnish birth cohort. American Journal of Psychiatry 157, 801–807.

Rosso IM, Bearden CE, Hollister JM et al. (2000b) Childhood neuromotor dysfunction in schizophrenia patients and their unaffected siblings: a prospective cohort study. Schizophrenia Bulletin 26, 367–378.

Schulsinger FJ, Parnas J, Petersen ET et al. (1984) Cerebral ventricular size in the offspring of schizophrenic mothers: a preliminary study. Archives of General Psychiatry 41, 602–606.

Seidman LJS, Faraone V, Goldstein JM et al. (1997) Reduced subcortical brain volumes in non-psychotic siblings of schizophrenic patients: a pilot magnetic resonance imaging study. American Journal of Medical Genetics 74, 507–514.

Seidman LJS, Faraone V, Goldstein JM et al. (1999) Thalamic and amygdala-hippocampal volume reductions in first-degree relatives of patients with schizophrenia: an MRI-based morphometric analysis. Biological Psychiatry 46, 941–954.

Silverton L, Finello KM, Schulsinger F, Mednick SA (1985) Low birth weight and ventricular enlargement in a high-risk sample. Journal of Abnormal Psychology 94, 405–409.

Staal WG, Hulshoff-Pol HE, Schnack H, van der Schot A, Kahn RS (1998) Partial volume decrease of the thalamus in relatives of patients with schizophrenia. American Journal of Psychiatry 155, 1784–1786.

Suddath RL, Christison GW, Torrey EF, Casanova MF, Weinberger DR (1990) Anatomical abnormalities in the brains of monozygotic twins discordant for schizophrenia. New England Journal of Medicine 322, 789–794.

Susser M, Susser E (1996) Choosing a future for epidemiology: I. Eras and paradigms. American Journal of Public Health 85, 668–673.

Tamminga C (1999) Glutamatergic aspects of schizophrenia. British Journal of Psychiatry 37(Suppl.), 12–15.

Walker EF (1994) Developmentally moderated expressions of the neuropathology underlying schizophrenia. Schizophrenia Bulletin 20, 453–480.

Weinberger DR, DeLisi LE, Neophytides AN, Wyatt RJ (1981) Familial aspects of CT scan abnormalities in chronic schizophrenic patients. Psychiatry Research 4, 65–71.

World Health Organization (1967) Manual of the International Statistical Classification of Diseases, Injuries, and Causes of Death, 8th edn. Geneva: World Health Organization.

Zorrilla LTE, Cannon TD, Kronenberg S et al. (1997) Structural brain abnormalities in schizophrenia: a family study. Biological Psychiatry 42, 1080–1086.

Part IV

Special issues in the epidemiology of schizophrenia

Introduction

It has long been known that people with schizophrenia have higher mortality rates from a number of causes, particularly suicide, than the general population. Higher than expected rates of comorbid substance abuse and violent behaviour have also been noted. The chapters in this section examine the epidemiological evidence for these associations, which have important implications for treatment and management.

Mortensen in Chapter 14 finds strong evidence that individuals with schizophrenia have elevated mortality rates from natural causes, thus leading to the expectation that individuals with schizophrenia have higher rates of a range of physical disorders. However, the epidemiological investigations of this issue have not been systematic. Investigators have tended to focus on certain diseases such as rheumatoid arthritis, diabetes mellitus or multiple sclerosis among schizophrenic patients in an effort to support an autoimmune aetiological hypothesis. Mortensen emphasizes the logistic difficulties inherent in such enterprises: 'the study of one relatively uncommon disorder among patients with another relatively uncommon disorder requires very large study populations to be followed up for a long time'. Some studies have found a reduced rate of cancer in schizophrenia, while others have found higher rates. Few studies have examined rates and risk factors for cardiovascular disease, although this is one of the major causes of the excess mortality. Mortensen argues that studies of 'the distribution of common risk factors for common diseases among patients with schizophrenia' and preventive programmes aimed at reducing known risk factors such as smoking and alcohol abuse are the types of research most likely to improve the life expectancy of individuals with schizophrenia.

Suicide is the largest cause of premature death in schizophrenia and rates appear to be increasing at present. In Chapter 15, Heilä and Lönnqvist review the literature on prevalence and risk factors for suicide in schizophrenia from an epidemiological perspective. They point out the methodological difficulties inherent in this field of study, such as the definition of suicide and the reliance on retrospective information. The authors urge that treatment-related factors related to suicide in schizophrenia should be urgently explored, in particular the effect of deinstitution-alization on suicide rates, the inadequate treatment of psychosis or comorbid depression, and the possible role of some atypical antipsychotic medication in suicide prevention.

Murray and colleagues in Chapter 16 examine the relationship between sub-stance abuse and schizophrenia. Having reviewed the international literature, they conclude that there is, indeed, evidence that individuals with schizophrenia are more likely to abuse substances than the general population, although there is no particular pattern of abuse associated with the disorder. The authors then proceed to investigate the reasons underlying this association. Does substance abuse cause schizophrenia? Do factors associated with the established illness increase the risk of substance abuse? Or does some common factor predispose individuals both to sub-stance abuse and schizophrenia?

Up until the early 1980s, the general consensus was that individuals with schizo-phrenia were no more likely to be violent than the general population. However, new epidemiological evidence has emerged in recent years to challenge this view. In Chapter 17, Walsh and Buchanan provide a critique of the studies that have influenced current thinking about this issue. They estimate that a diagnosis of schizophrenia is associated with a two- to sevenfold increased risk of violent beha-viour, but only a small proportion of violence in society can be attributable to people with this disorder.

14

Mortality and physical illness in schizophrenia

Preben Bo Mortensen

National Centre for Register-based Research, Aarhus University, Denmark

Mortality among psychiatric patients has been studied for almost as long as mental hospitals have existed (Farr, 1841), and studies of mortality and physical illness among schizophrenic patients have also been conducted for almost as long as the concept of schizophrenia has been in clinical use (Hahnemann, 1931; Alström, 1942). However, mortality studies on the one hand and studies of physical illness in schizophrenia on the other have traditionally been conducted with very different perspectives. Mortality studies have generally been conducted as part of long-term outcome studies of schizophrenia and the finding has generally been excess risk from some cause of death. Studies of physical illness have focused on the identification of illnesses occurring particularly uncommonly among schizophrenic patients, thus implying some biological antagonism that might give clues to aetiology. However, these fields of research are closely related and share many of the same methodological problems.

Studies of mortality

Mortality studies in schizophrenia have been reviewed by Simpson (1988) and Allebeck (1989). Harris and Barraclough (1998) have reviewed papers on schizophrenia mortality published in English during the period 1966–1995 together with weighted SMR (standardized mortality ratio) estimates for individual causes of death. The very large literature on suicide in schizophrenia has been reviewed by Drake et al. (1985) and Caldwell and Gottesman (1990) and is discussed in detail in Chapter 15.

Death from natural causes

The early mortality studies by Alström (1942) and Ødegård (1951) found that excess mortality in patients with mental illness resulted from respiratory and infectious diseases. In particular, mortality from tuberculosis led to the creation of special institutions for patients with both tuberculosis and mental disorders. Studies also generally found excess mortality from all other major causes of death with the exception of cancer. In more recent studies of schizophrenia, the major source of excess mortality is suicide (e.g. Tsuang, 1978; Evenson et al., 1982; Pokorny, 1983; Black et al., 1985; Allebeck and Wistedt, 1986; Roy, 1986; Mortensen and Juel, 1993), but an elevated mortality from natural causes has also been found in many of these studies. Some studies report increased mortality from cardiovascular disorders (Lindelius and Kay, 1973; Saugstad and Ødegård, 1979, 1985; Herrman et al., 1983; Brook, 1985; Wood et al., 1985; Allebeck and Wistedt, 1986; Mortensen and Juel, 1990, 1993; Saku et al., 1995). Ciompi and Müller (1976) found an increased cardiovascular mortality in male patients but a relative deficit in female patients. Zilber et al. (1989) found a significant deficit of death from cardiovascular and cerebrovascular causes. Giel et al. (1978) found a deficit of death from cerebrovascular diseases although this finding is difficult to interpret because this study had a large proportion of patients with undetermined cause of death. Mortensen and Juel (1990) found a significant reduction in cerebrovascular mortality in both males and females among a cohort of mainly chronic hospitalized schizophrenic patients. However, in their study of a different cohort of first-admitted patients (Mortensen and Juel, 1993), there was a nonsignificant trend towards an elevated risk among male patients. It is unclear whether this apparent change is caused by possible survival bias in the study of the cohort of long-stay patients or whether it is a consequence of changing exposure patterns to risk factors for cerebrovascular disorder, such as smoking. Mortality from respiratory diseases has consistently been found to be increased in schizophrenic patients (Alström 1942; Ødegård 1951; Weiner and Marvit, 1977; Wood et al., 1985; Allebeck and Wistedt, 1986; Mortensen and Juel, 1990, 1993). Allebeck and Wistedt (1986) reported a significant increase in gastrointestinal and urogenital death. With the exception of cancer and, as mentioned above, cerebrovascular diseases, Mortensen and Juel both in the study of chronic patients (1990) and that of first-admitted patients (1993) found an elevated mortality from all specific natural causes. This pattern is overall in line with the estimates presented by Harris and Barraclough (1998), but it should be noted that these estimates are heavily influenced by the two studies by Mortensen and Juel because of their relatively large sample size. Harris and Barraclough (1998) also concluded that there was a slight deficit of cancer mortality in schizophrenic males, whereas there was a slight excess in schizophrenic females. Individual studies generally have not found any significant excess or deficits in cancer mortality among schizophrenic patients. This will be discussed further below.

In summary, studies generally find that schizophrenic patients have elevated mortality rates from natural causes. However, there have been almost no studies of risk factors explaining this excess, and there have been no intervention studies of possible ways of reducing the excess mortality.

Suicide

The occurrence of and risk factors for suicide in schizophrenia have been reviewed several times (Drake et al., 1985; Simpson, 1988; Caldwell and Gottesman, 1990) and the topic is dealt with in detail in Chapter 15. Therefore, only a few key points will be mentioned here. Estimates of suicide risk in schizophrenic patients vary, but about 10% of all schizophrenic patients (range 2–13%) are reported to end their lives by suicide. In general, the risk of suicide among individuals with schizophrenia is estimated to be 10- to 20-fold higher than in the general population. Furthermore, studies have generally not been based upon first-episode cases and, since suicide risk in schizophrenia tends to be higher in young patients and higher early in the course of the illness, the lifetime risk for suicide may be closer to 20–25% (Mortensen, 1995a).

Many risk factors for suicide in schizophrenia have been identified and these are reviewed in Chapter 15. These include male gender, young age, social isolation, being single, unemployment, limited external support, and psychological factors such as recent loss or rejection. Clinically relevant variables include a history of previous suicide attempts, hopelessness or comorbid symptoms of depression, deteriorating course with high premorbid functioning, chronic course with many exacerbations, and high levels of psychopathology and functional impairment after discharge. In Denmark, suicide risk among schizophrenic patients has been found to be increasing in parallel with a decreasing number of available inpatient beds (Mortensen and Juel, 1993). It has been suggested that the increasing tendency to short admissions with frequent readmissions that has accompanied the decreased availability of inpatient beds may have contributed significantly to this increase (Rossau and Mortensen, 1997).

Although there is a large literature on suicide risk in schizophrenia, there have been no clinical trials of preventive interventions. Such trials would probably be very difficult to conduct with sufficient statistical power. Even in the subgroups of schizophrenic patients at highest risk, it would generally be less than 1 or 2% of patients who would commit suicide within a year. Controlled trials would have to include an unrealistically large number of patients followed-up for a long time. Therefore, preventive interventions in the future will probably have to be based on information from other epidemiological studies rather than clinical trials (Mortensen, 1995a).

Physical illness

The relatively consistent finding of elevated mortality rates from most natural causes would lead to the expectation that schizophrenic patients have higher risk of a broad area of physical disorders. However, the literature on the epidemiology of physical disorders in schizophrenic patients is not as clear and unequivocal as might be expected. Adler and Griffith (1991) reviewed some of the literature and outlined some of the difficulties of diagnosing and managing physical illness in schizophrenic patients. They generally found high levels of concurrent physical illness and low detection rates of those illnesses. They also reviewed some of the difficulties that arise from the effects of neuroleptic treatment on concurrent physical disorders. The problems associated with diagnosing physical illness in schizophrenic patients should be borne in mind when evaluating the literature on physical disease in schizophrenia. Any study of the occurrence of any particular physical disorder will be subject to methodological difficulties, in particular studies finding reduced occurrence of some physical disorders. This literature has been reviewed by Baldwin (1979), later by Tsuang et al. (1983), Harris (1988) and Jeste and coworkers (1996). Apart from the above-mentioned mortality studies, much of the literature consists of clinical observations or hypotheses about positive or, more frequently, negative associations between schizophrenia and specific physical disorders. Only one published study attempted to cover the full range of physical illnesses in an epidemiological sample, and the results of that study have only been published in part because of the death of the principal investigator (Baldwin and Wing, 1978).

Cardiovascular disease

Baldwin (1980) has reported an increased incidence of arteriosclerotic heart disease among schizophrenic patients. Increased cardiovascular morbidity and mortality would be expected in schizophrenic patients because of the frequency of heavy smoking, the possible effects of neuroleptic treatment on the cardiovascular system (Risch et al., 1981) and, presumably, poor diet (although there is little information about the dietary practices among schizophrenics that would be of relevance for cardiovascular illness). Unfortunately, no epidemiological studies of cardiovascular illness in schizophrenic patients exist where tobacco smoking or other important factors have been taken into acount. It would be very worthwhile to pursue such studies since cardiovascular illness is one of the major contributors to the excess mortality of schizophrenic patients.

Cancer

Studies of cancer incidence and mortality in schizophrenic patients fall into three main categories. First, there are studies of proportionate mortality, that is, the proportion of all deaths among schizophrenics that are caused by cancer compared with the proportionate cancer mortality in the general population. Second, there are studies that calculate cancer-specific SMRs among schizophrenic patients and, third, there are studies focusing on the incidence of cancer among schizophrenic patients. Many of the problems in studying physical illness in schizophrenia can be illustrated by the literature on cancer and schizophrenia, and a great deal of confusion in the literature regarding cancer and schizophrenia originates from the attempt to compare results between these three categories of study design.

The earliest reports on cancer risk in schizophrenia and the only studies finding reduced occurrence of cancer in schizophrenic patients prior to the introduction of neuroleptics were studies of proportionate cancer mortality (Büel, 1925; Hahnemann, 1931; Alström, 1942; Scheflen, 1951; Hussar, 1966). None of these found significant differences between schizophrenic patients and the general population. Of the mortality studies conducted in schizophrenia after the introduction of neuroleptics, Ciompi and Müller (1976) and Zilber et al. (1989) found a significantly reduced cancer mortality. The finding by Zilber et al. is complex, however, since they found a significantly reduced cancer risk in patients aged 40 years or more, whereas it was significantly increased in patients under 39 years of age. Furthermore, Giel et al. (1978) and Brook (1985) found significantly reduced cancer mortality rates, but their results were difficult to interpret because of a large proportion of patients in the studies who had undetermined causes of death. Studies not finding significant differences include Saugstad and Ødegård (1979), Tsuang et al. (1980), Herrman et al. (1983) and Allebeck and Wistedt (1986).

Mortality studies measure the joint effect of cancer incidence and survival time of cancer patients; this means that any difference in the prognosis of cancer between schizophrenics and the general population will complicate the interpretation of cancer mortality as cancer risk. There are relatively few studies of cancer incidence and the results are somewhat inconsistent. Ehrentheil (1957) and Baldwin (1980) found no difference in cancer incidence in schizophrenics compared with the general population. Nakane and Ohta (1986) reported an increased rate of breast cancer in younger females, but methodological problems make this finding difficult to interpret. Gulbinat et al. (1992) reported results from three World Health Organization (WHO) study centres. In the Hawaii centre, there was a nonsignificant trend towards increased incidence of cancer of the uterine cervix and breast cancer in schizophrenic patients of Japanese origin, but no differences for patients of Caucasian origin. In another centre from this WHO collaborative study, Dupont et al. (1986) reported an overall reduced incidence of cancer in males and a marginally significant reduced risk in females. No specific cancer occurred with an increased frequency, and cancer risk was significantly reduced, particularly for respiratory cancers, cancer of the uterine cervix and, in males, gastrointestinal cancers and cancer of the prostate. In a separate study of a younger cohort of first-admitted psychiatric patients, there was still a significantly reduced cancer incidence in male schizophrenic patients and a nonsignificant reduction in female patients. The only types of cancer occurring with a reduced incidence were melanoma, other skin cancers and testicular cancer. Because of the relatively low age of this cohort, it was difficult to document reduced incidence of any specific type of cancer, but respiratory cancers also occurred at a notably low rate, especially in the light of the high occurrence of tobacco smoking. The causes of this reduced cancer risk are not known and could not be ascribed to undiagnosed cancers. A number of animal studies, together with some casuistic reports of regression of cancers in patients treated with neuroleptics, have suggested that some neuroleptics may impair growth of tumours or reduce cancer risk (for reviews see Mortensen 1992, 1995b). In a case-control study, risk of prostate cancer was found to be reduced by treatment with phenothiazines. Although it has been suggested that neuroleptic treatment increases the risk of breast cancer through elevated prolactin levels (Schyve et al. 1978), the evidence is inconclusive (Mortensen, 1987; Halbreich et al., 1996).

The literature on cancer and schizophrenia illustrates a number of methodological issues. First, detection bias with problems in diagnosing specific illnesses in schizophrenic patients must be addressed specifically for every disease. Second, even comparatively common conditions like breast cancer or respiratory cancer require the follow-up of thousands of patients for decades in order to yield reasonably solid results. This means that such studies will be very difficult or impossible to conduct without access to epidemiological databases such as those used by Baldwin (Baldwin, 1980; Dupont et al., 1986) and Mortensen (1994). One such epidemiological study has recently been published and the findings do not agree with previous work. Lichtermann et al. (2001) identified a cohort of 26 996 individuals born between 1940 and 1969 in Helsinki, Finland who were treated for schizophrenia between 1969 and 1991. They were followed up for cancer from 1971 to 1996 by record linkage with the Finnish Cancer Registry, and standardized incidence ratios (SIRs) were calculated. In patients with schizophrenia, an increased overall cancer risk was found. Half of the excess cases were attributable to lung cancer, and the strongest relative increase in risk was in pharyngeal cancer, indicating that specific lifestyle factors, particularly tobacco smoking and alcohol consumption, were responsible. However, this study also studied the incidence of cancer in the relatives of schizophrenic patients and, interestingly, the cancer incidence in siblings and parents was consistently lower than that in the general population. The authors concluded that this finding would be compatible with a postulated genetic risk factor for schizophrenia offering selective advantage to unaffected relatives.

Rheumatoid arthritis

The literature on rheumatoid arthritis has been reviewed by Eaton et al. (1992). Generally, studies found that schizophrenic patients have less rheumatoid arthritis than expected on the basis of general population rates. This has also been confirmed in more recent studies by Mors et al. (1999) and Oken and Schulzer (1999).

In their study of autoimmune disorders in first-degree relatives of schizophrenic patients, Gilvarry and colleagues (1996) found a reduced occurrence of rheumatoid arthritis, but this did not reach statistical significance. The apparent negative relationship between rheumatoid arthritis and schizophrenia has led to hypotheses about an autoimmune component in the aetiology of schizophrenia or associations with specific HLA types. However, some studies (Mors et al., 1999) have also found a reduced occurrence of osteoarthritis, suggesting that the apparent low occurrence of rheumatoid arthritis in patients could be the result of a tendency not to detect the illness, perhaps because of elevated pain threshold or maybe less mechanical trauma in more sedentary patients.

Diabetes mellitus

It has been reported that there are elevated rates of diabetes in schizophrenic patients (McKee et al., 1986; Mukherjee et al., 1996) and diabetes appears to occur more frequently in the relatives of psychotic patients (Gilvarry et al., 1996). Diabetes may be a consequence of phenothiazine neuroleptic treatment in schizophrenic patients (Dynes, 1969; Marinow, 1971). Recently, some studies have suggested that treatment with clozapine may increase the risk of diabetes or impaired glucose tolerance (Hagg et al., 1998). Abnormalities in glucose metabolism have also been implied as a possible risk factor for tardive dyskinesia (Schultz et al., 1999). Generally, the epidemiological knowledge of the occurrence of diabetes in parents or relatives is still limited, and the exact relationship between diabetes and schizophrenia is not known.

Multiple sclerosis

Multiple sclerosis (MS) is of interest in relation to schizophrenia because of the autoimmune hypothesis mentioned above and because of the number of similarities in the epidemiological distribution of schizophrenia and MS. This literature has been reviewed by Stevens (1988a). Generally, however, there are no good studies of the cooccurrence of the two disorders, and the study by Gilvarry et al. (1996) did not have sufficient power to study the occurrence of MS in relatives of psychotic patients. So, in general, the relationship between schizophrenia and MS awaits empirical studies.

Epilepsy

Stevens (1988b) reviewed much of the literature regarding epilepsy and schizophrenia and concluded that studies had not found a greater incidence of schizophrenia among individuals with epilepsy, nor of epilepsy in those with schizophrenia. However, a more recent study by Bredkjaer et al. (1998) found a general increase in schizophrenia risk among patients ever hospitalized with epilepsy, and particularly in patients with temporal lobe epilepsy. At present, it is unclear if patients developing psychosis during the course of epilepsy constitute a subgroup distinct from other schizophrenic patients, or if the association indicates that aetiological factors for epilepsy also increase schizophrenia risk.

Human immunodeficiency virus

Recently, studies have suggested that psychotic patients constitute a high-risk group for infection with human immunodeficiency virus (HIV) (Susser et al., 1997; Walkup et al., 1999). Although it is possible that exposure to retrovirus contributes to the risk for developing schizophrenia and other psychoses (Yolken and Torrey, 1995; Hart et al., 1999), the opposite direction of causality is more likely, since schizophrenic patients may be exposed to risk factors for HIV infection, notably drug abuse and high-risk sexual activity (Cournos et al., 1994; Miller and Finnerty, 1996; Thompson et al., 1997; Grassi et al., 1999). These risk factors would be a reasonable target for preventive efforts (Weinhardt et al., 1997).

Other diseases

A suspected positive association between coeliac disease and schizophrenia has not been confirmed empirically (Stevens et al., 1977; Baldwin, 1980; Lambert et al., 1989). A single study has suggested a possible increased risk for amyotrophic lateral sclerosis among the relatives of patients with schizophrenia, but the finding has not so far been replicated (Goodman, 1994). Appendicitis was reported to occur with an unexpectedly low frequency among schizophrenic patients by Baldwin (1980) and Lauerma et al. (1998). Although there are methodological problems in those studies, the negative association seems to be confirmed in an ongoing study by Ewald et al. (2001). Lauerma et al. (1998) hypothesized that genes that predispose to schizophrenia may provide protection from appendicitis, thus providing a selective advantage during evolution.

Conclusions and suggestions for future studies

In general, the literature on physical illness and schizophrenia has contained more hypotheses than empirical data. Good epidemiological samples are hard to find, since the study of one relatively uncommon disorder in a patient group with another relatively uncommon disorder requires very large study populations to be followed up for a long time. In particular, negative associations may be very difficult to study. The best method of studying such associations is through linkage between records in historical cohorts as, for example, in the studies by Baldwin (1980), Mortensen (1994), Bredkjaer et al. (1998) and Lichterman et al. (2001). It is often difficult to exclude diagnostic bias where physical illness is detected less readily among schizophrenic patients. It is also difficult to separate the effect of schizophrenia from the effects of treatments, and generally little is known about long-term health effects of neuroleptic medication. Finally, studies have generally not controlled for confounders other than age and gender. Notably, studies have neither taken general social variables into account nor adjusted for such well-documented risk factors as smoking, diet or alcohol consumption.

It would seem obvious that the physical morbidity and mortality of schizophrenic patients cannot be understood as a phenomenon isolated from the changing treatment and general social conditions available to these individuals. Historically, it has become obvious that the high mortality rate from tuberculosis observed earlier (Alström, 1942) was not something specific for schizophrenia as a disease, but rather a feature of the general morbidity pattern linked to the living conditions available to patients inside as well as outside psychiatric hospitals. Today we see similar phenomena in Western countries where schizophrenic patients are more exposed to tobacco smoking, alcohol and drug abuse, and possibly high-risk sexual activity, which would be expected to lead to high incidence of cardiovascular diseases, respiratory diseases and HIV infections. At present, the research most likely to influence the life expectancy of patients are studies of the distribution of common risk factors for common diseases among patients with schizophrenia, as well as evaluations of preventive programmes aimed at reducing smoking, alcohol and drug abuse.

Studies of mortality are relatively unequivocal, confirming both an increased mortality from natural causes and a continued and possibly increasing elevation of suicide risk. In these areas, the greatest research need now seems to be identification of specific risk factors and intervention studies to provide practical guidelines for the prevention of excess mortality among schizophrenic patients.

REFERENCES

Adler LE, Griffith JM (1991) Concurrent medical illness in the schizophrenic patients: epidemiology, diagnosis, and management. Schizophrenia Research 4, 91–107.

Allebeck P (1989) Schizophrenia: a life-shortening disease. Schizophrenia Bulletin 15, 81–89.

Allebeck P, Wistedt B (1986) Mortality in schizophrenia. A ten-year follow-up based on the Stockholm County inpatient register. Archives of General Psychiatry 43, 650–653.

Alström CH (1942) Mortality in mental hospitals with especial regard to tuberculosis. Acta Psychiatrica et Neurologica Suppl. XXIV.

Büel ES (1925) Maligne Tumoren bei Geisterskrankheiten. Algemeine Zeitschrift für Psychiatrie 80, 312–321.

Baldwin JA (1979) Schizophrenia and physical disease. Psychological Medicine 9, 611–618.

Baldwin JA (1980) Schizophrenia and physical disease: a preliminary analysis of the data from the Oxford Record Linkage Study. In: Biochemistry of Schizophrenia and Addiction in Search of a Common Factor, Hemmings G, ed. Lancaster: MTP Press, pp. 297–317.

Baldwin JA, Wing J (1978) Disease associations in linked records: schizophrenia and accidental injury. British Journal of Psychiatry 133, 445–447.

Black DW, Winokur G, Warrack G (1985) Suicide in schizophrenia: the Iowa Record Linkage Study. Journal of Clinical Psychiatry 46, 14–17.

Bredkjaer SR, Mortensen PB, Parnas J (1998) Epilepsy and non-organic nonaffective psychosis. National epidemiologic study. British Journal of Psychiatry 172, 235–238.

Brook OH (1985) Mortality in the long-stay population of Dutch mental hospitals. Acta Psychiatrica Scandinavica 71, 626–635.

Caldwell CB, Gottesman II (1990) Schizophrenics kill themselves too: a review of risk factors for suicide. Schizophrenia Bulletin 16, 571–589.

Ciompi L, Müller C (1976) Lebensweg und Alter der Schizophrenen Eine katamnestische Langzeitstudie bis in Senium. Berlin: Springer-Verlag.

Cournos F, Guido JR, Coomaraswamy S, Meyer-Bahlburg H, Sugden R, Horwath E (1994) Sexual activity and risk of HIV infection among patients with schizophrenia. American Journal of Psychiatry 151, 228–232.

Drake RE, Gates C, Whitaker A, Cotton PG (1985) Suicide among schizophrenics: a review. Comprehensive Psychiatry 26, 90–100.

Dupont A, Jensen OM, Strömgren E, Jablensky A (1986) Incidence of cancer in patients diagnosed as schizophrenic in Denmark. In: Psychiatric Case Registers in Public Health. A Worldwide Inventory 1060–1985, Ten Horn GHMM, Giel R, Gulbinat WH, Henderson JH, eds. Amsterdam: Elsevier, pp. 229–239.

Dynes JB (1969) Sudden death. Diseases of the Nervous System 30, 24–28.

Eaton W, Hayward C, Ram R (1992) Schizophrenia and rheumatoid arthritis: a review. Schizophrenia Research 6, 181–192.

Ehrentheil OF (1957) Malignant tumors in psychotic patients. Archives of Neurology and Psychiatry 77, 178–186.

Evenson RC, Wood JB, Nuttall EA, Cho DW (1982) Suicide rates among public mental health patients. Acta Psychiatrica Scandinavica 66, 254–264.

Ewald H, Mortensen PB, Mors O (2001) Decreased risk of acute appendicitis in patients with schizophrenia or manic-depressive psychosis. Schizophrenia Research 49, 287–293.

Farr W (1841) Report on the mortality of lunatics. Journal of the Royal Statistical Society 4, 17. [Cited in Simpson, 1988.]

Giel R, Dijk S, van Weerden DJR (1978) Mortality in the long-stay population of all Dutch mental hospitals. Acta Psychiatrica Scandinavica 57, 361–368.

Gilvarry CM, Sham PC, Jones PB et al. (1996) Family history of autoimmune diseases in psychosis. Schizophrenia Research 19, 33–40.

Goodman AB (1994) Elevated risks for amyotrophic lateral sclerosis and blood disorders in Ashkenazi schizophrenic pedigrees suggest new candidate genes in schizophrenia. American Journal of Medical Genetics 54, 271–278.

Grassi L, Pavanati M, Cardelli R, Ferri S, Peron L (1999) HIV-risk behaviour and knowledge about HIV/AIDS among patients with schizophrenia. Psychological Medicine 29, 171–179.

Gulbinat W, Dupont A, Jablensky A et al. (1992) Cancer incidence of schizophrenic patients. Results of record linkage studies in three countries. British Journal of Psychiatry Suppl. 75–83.

Hagg S, Joelsson L, Mjorndal T, Spigset O, Oja G, Dahlqvist R (1998) Prevalence of diabetes and impaired glucose tolerance in patients treated with clozapine compared with patients treated with conventional depot neuroleptic medications. Journal of Clinical Psychiatry 59, 294–299.

Hahnemann V (1931) Undersøgelser over kræftdødeligheden hos sindssyge. Ugeskrift for Laeger 93, 1132–1139.

Halbreich U, Shen J, Panaro V (1996) Are chronic psychiatric patients at increased risk for developing breast cancer? American Journal of Psychiatry 153, 559–560.

Harris AE (1988) Physical disease and schizophrenia. Schizophrenia Bulletin 14, 85–96.

Harris EC, Barraclough B (1998) Excess mortality of mental disorder. British Journal of Psychiatry 173, 11–53.

Hart DJ, Heath RG, Sautter FJ Jr et al. (1999) Antiretroviral antibodies: implications for schizophrenia, schizophrenia spectrum disorders, and bipolar disorder. Biological Psychiatry 45, 704–714.

Herrman HE, Baldwin JA, Christie D (1983) A record-linkage study of mortality and general hospital discharge in patients diagnosed as schizophrenic. Psychological Medicine 13, 581–593.

Hussar A (1966) Leading causes of death in institutionalized chronic schizophrenic patients. Journal of Nervous and Mental Disease 142, 45–57.

Jeste DV, Gladsjo JA, Lindamer LA, Lacro JP (1996) Medical comorbidity in schizophrenia. Schizophrenia Bulletin 22, 413–430.

Lambert MT, Bjarnason I, Connelly J et al. (1989) Small intestine permeability in schizophrenia. British Journal of Psychiatry 155, 619–622.

Lauerma H, Lehtinen V, Joukamaa M, Jarvelin MR, Helenius H, Isohanni M (1998) Schizophrenia among patients treated for rheumatoid arthritis and appendicitis. Schizophrenia Research 29, 255–261.

Lichtermann D, Ekelund J, Pukkala E, Tanskanen A, Lönnqvist J (2001) Incidence of cancer among persons with schizophrenia and their relatives. Archives of General Psychiatry 58, 573–578.

Lindelius R, Kay DW (1973) Some changes in the pattern of mortality in schizophrenia in Sweden. Acta Psychiatrica Scandinavica 49, 315–323.

Marinow A (1971) Diabetes in chronic schizophrenia. Diseases of the Nervous System 32, 777–778.

McKee HA, D'Arcy PF, Wilson PJ (1986) Diabetes and schizophrenia – a preliminary study. Journal of Clinical Hospital Pharmacology 11, 297–299.

Miller LJ, Finnerty M (1996) Sexuality, pregnancy, and childrearing among women with schizophrenia-spectrum disorders. Psychiatric Services 47, 502–506.

Mors O, Mortensen PB, Ewald H (1999) A population-based register study of the association between schizophrenia and rheumatoid arthritis. Schizophrenia Research 40, 67–74.

Mortensen PB (1987) Neuroleptic treatment and other factors modifying cancer risk in schizophrenic patients. Acta Psychiatrica Scandinavica 75, 585–590.

Mortensen PB (1992) Neuroleptic medication and reduced risk of prostate cancer in schizophrenic patients. Acta Psychiatrica Scandinavica 85, 390–393.

Mortensen PB (1994) The occurrence of cancer in first admitted schizophrenic patients. Schizophrenia Research 12, 185–194.

Mortensen PB (1995a) Suicide among schizophrenic patients: occurrence and risk factors. Clinical Neuropharmacology 18, 1–8.

Mortensen PB (1995b) The Epidemiology of Cancer in Schizophrenic Patients. Aarhus: Aarhus University.

Mortensen PB, Juel K (1990) Mortality and causes of death in schizophrenic patients in Denmark. Acta Psychiatrica Scandinavica 81, 372–377.

Mortensen PB, Juel K (1993) Mortality and causes of death in first admitted schizophrenic patients. British Journal of Psychiatry 163, 183–189.

Mukherjee S, Decina P, Bocola V, Saraceni F, Scapicchio PL (1996) Diabetes mellitus in schizophrenic patients. Comprehensive Psychiatry 37, 68–73.

Nakane Y, Ohta Y (1986) The example of linkage with a cancer register. In: Psychiatric Case Registers in Public Health. A Worldwide Inventory 1960–1985, Ten Horn GHMM, Giel R, Gulbinat W, Henderson JH, eds. Amsterdam: Elsevier, pp. 240–245.

Ødegård Ø (1951) Mortality in Norwegian mental hospitals 1926–1941. Acta Genetica et Statistica Medica 2, 141–173.

Oken RJ, Schulzer M (1999) At issue: schizophrenia and rheumatoid arthritis. The negative association revisited. Schizophrenia Bulletin 25, 625–638.

Pokorny AD (1983) Prediction of suicide in psychiatric patients. Report of a prospective study. Archives of General Psychiatry 40, 249–257.

Risch SC, Groom GP, Janowsky DS (1981) Interfaces of psychopharmacology and cardiology – Part two [review article]. Journal of Clinical Psychiatry 42, 47–59.

Rossau CD, Mortensen PB (1997) Risk factors for suicide in schizophrenic patients. A nested case-control study. British Journal of Psychiatry 171, 355–359.

Roy A (1986) Depression, attempted suicide, and suicide in patients with chronic schizophrenia. Psychiatric Clinics of North America 9, 193–206.

Saku M, Tokudome S, Ikeda M et al. (1995) Mortality in psychiatric patients, with a specific focus on cancer mortality associated with schizophrenia. International Journal of Epidemiology 24, 366–372.

Saugstad LF, Ødegård, Ø (1979) Mortality in psychiatric hospitals in Norway 1950–74. Acta Psychiatrica Scandinavica 59, 431–447.

Saugstad L, Ødegård Ø (1985) Recent rise in supposedly stress dependent causes of death in psychiatric hospitals in Norway indicating increased 'stress' in hospitals? Acta Psychiatrica Scandinavica 71, 402–409.

Scheflen AE (1951) Maglinant tumors in the institutionalized psychotic population. Archives of Neurology and Psychiatry 66, 145–155.

Schultz SK, Arndt S, Ho BC, Oliver SE, Andreasen NC (1999) Impaired glucose tolerance and abnormal movements in patients with schizophrenia. American Journal of Psychiatry 156, 640–642.

Schyve PM, Smithline F, Meltzer HY (1978) Neuroleptic-induced prolactin level elevation and breast cancer: an emerging clinical issue. Archives of General Psychiatry 35, 1291–1301.

Simpson JC (1988) Mortality studies in schizophrenia. In: Handbook of Schizophrenia.

Nosology, Epidemiology and Genetics of Schizophrenia, Tsuang MT, Simpson JC, eds. Amsterdam: Elsevier, pp. 245–274.

Stevens FM, Lloyd RS, Geraghty SM et al. (1977) Schizophrenia and coeliac disease – the nature of the relationship. Psychological Medicine 7, 259–263.

Stevens JR (1988a) Schizophrenia and multiple sclerosis. Schizophrenia Bulletin 14, 231–241.

Stevens JR (1988b) Epilepsy, psychosis and schizophrenia. Schizophrenia Research 1, 79–89.

Susser E, Colson P, Jandorf L et al. (1997) HIV infection among young adults with psychotic disorders. American Journal of Psychiatry 154, 864–866.

Thompson SC, Checkley GE, Hocking JS, Crofts N, Mijch AM, Judd FK (1997) HIV risk behaviour and HIV testing of psychiatric patients in Melbourne. Australian and New Zealand Journal of Psychiatry 31, 566–576.

Tsuang MT (1978) Suicide in schizophrenics, manics, depressives, and surgical controls. A comparison with general population suicide mortality. Archives of General Psychiatry 35, 153–155.

Tsuang MT, Woolson RF, Fleming JA (1980) Causes of death in schizophrenia and manic-depression. British Journal of Psychiatry 136, 239–242.

Tsuang MT, Perkins K, Simpson JC (1983) Physical diseases in schizophrenia and affective disorder. Journal of Clinical Psychiatry 44, 42–46.

Walkup J, Crystal S, Sambamoorthi U (1999) Schizophrenia and major affective disorder among Medicaid recipients with HIV/AIDS in New Jersey. American Journal of Public Health 89, 1101–1103.

Weiner BP, Marvit RC (1977) Schizophrenia in Hawaii: analysis of cohort mortality risk in a multi-ethnic population. British Journal of Psychiatry 131, 497–503.

Weinhardt LS, Carey MP, Carey KB (1997) HIV risk reduction for the seriously mentally ill: pilot investigation and call for research. Journal of Behavior Therapy and Experimental Psychiatry 28, 87–95.

Wood JB, Evenson RC, Cho DW, Hagan BJ (1985) Mortality variations among public mental health patients. Acta Psychiatrica Scandinavica 72, 218–229.

Yolken RH, Torrey EF (1995) Viruses, schizophrenia, and bipolar disorder. Clinical Microbiology Reviews 8, 131–145.

Zilber N, Schufman N, Lerner Y (1989) Mortality among psychiatric patients – the groups at risk. Acta Psychiatrica Scandinavica 79, 248–256.

15

The clinical epidemiology of suicide in schizophrenia

Hannele Heilä and Jouko Lönnqvist

National Public Health Institute, Helsinki, Finland

Numerous studies have found that persons with mental disorders are at signifi-cantly higher risk for suicide than the general population. In 'psychological autopsy' studies (Table 15.1) the prevalence for current mental disorders among suicide victims has been as high as 81 to 100%. The heightened suicide risk has been associated with many types of mental disorder, most often with affective disorders, substance abuse and schizophrenic disorders (Miles, 1977; Black et al., 1985; Harris and Barraclough, 1997). Suicide is the most common cause of premature death in schizophrenia: 28% of the excess mortality in schizophrenia, and 11–38% of all deaths in schizophrenia are attributable to suicide (Leff et al., 1992; Brown, 1997; Baxter and Appleby, 1999).

Methodological aspects of suicide research

Definition of suicide

As with all human behaviour, suicide is complex and multifaceted in nature. From the research point of view, studying suicide is fraught with many methodological problems. There is no single, unanimously accepted definition of suicide. Definitions often include three components: the death occurs as a result of an injury, which is both self-inflicted and intentionally inflicted. The least ambiguous factor is that the outcome of the injury is death. It has been suggested that suicidal intent may represent the varying degree of consciousness and determination to die in suicide (Stengel, 1960; O'Carroll et al., 1996). However, the retrospective evalu-ation of the victim's mental intention to die at the time of suicide is usually very difficult, unless obvious from the circumstances (Hirschfield and Davidson, 1988; Rosenberg et al., 1988; O'Carroll et al., 1996).

Classification of suicide

Most member nations of the World Health Organization (WHO) currently use the standardized International Classification of Diseases (ICD) to code mortality data.

However, official ascertainment of suicide varies a lot between different countries. Different levels of evidence may be needed between medical or legal systems for classification of suicide as cause of death, and also within countries there may have been changes in the legal classifications for suicide during time course (Hirschfield and Davidson, 1988; Garrison, 1992; Neeleman and Wessely, 1997). Suicidal deaths may be officially classified as accidental or undetermined deaths if the evidence for suicidal intention has not been considered adequate (Lönnqvist, 1977) or to allow insurance compensation (Cheng and Lee, 2000), thus leading to underestimation of suicide. In a large case register-based study by Ruschena and colleagues (1998), schizophrenic patients were eight times over-represented among those deaths classified as 'open' verdicts by coroners. Furthermore, the classification of suicide is likely to be affected by the mode of death, overall rate of postmortems performed in the country, regional cultural and religious concepts, age and sex of the deceased (Sainsbury and Jenkins, 1982; Litman, 1989, Neeleman and Wessely, 1997; Canetto and Sakinofsky, 1998). Conversely, deaths preceded by mental illness or suicidal threats may lead to overcounting in suicide (Kleck, 1988). All in all, however, the varying official suicide rates are suggested to be affected in less than 10% by biases of estimation, allowing comparisons of the rates between countries and over time (Lönnqvist, 1977; Sainsbury and Jenkins, 1982; Kleck, 1988; Litman, 1989; Mościcki, 1997).

Research designs in suicidology

The most obvious problem in suicide research is the lack of self-reported data from suicide victims. Follow-up studies, either prospective or retrospective, are not usually able to collect information close to the time of death of the deceased, and knowledge of recent antecedents of suicide may be missed. The frequent use of patient record-based data is compromised by information biases owing to varying levels of information obtained, or information with varying levels of accuracy. In these studies, the quality of missing information concerning suicide process is especially problematic: is the information truly absent or just not noted (Brent, 1989)?

Psychological autopsy

The psychological autopsy study method answers some of the problems caused by the use of retrospective record data, making feasible the study of circumstances of suicide in an attempt to gain knowledge of motivation for suicide (Shneidman, 1981). The use of the psychological autopsy method originates from the late 1950s in Los Angeles, USA, where it was first used as a method for determining the mode of death in equivocal cases of death. The suicidal process was reconstructed through interviews with informants important to the deceased (Litman et al., 1963; Shneidman, 1981). Since then, psychological autopsy has been used for studying suicide as a method of obtaining detailed information on the victim's psychological state, psychiatric status, behaviour, health, interpersonal relations, religious commitments and life events (Shneidman, 1981; Hawton et al., 1998). Other available data, such as hospital and other health-care records, and information from police and social services are also used for synthesizing and validating the information received (Shneidman, 1981; Beskow et al., 1990; Clark and Horton-Deutsch, 1992). The major methodological problem of psychological autopsy studies relates to information bias, with the interview-based information coming from persons other than the deceased. These biases may lead to under- or over-reporting of information (Brent, 1989; Clark and Horton-Deutsch, 1992; Hawton et al., 1998). However, the use of different sources of information and integrating all available data are likely to enhance the general level of information and improve its validity (Brent, 1989; Clark and Horton-Deutsch, 1992).

Most studies have been retrospective in nature, because the ideal prospective study designs would be extremely costly, time consuming, and inefficient owing to the low base rate of suicide in the population. Studying risk factors for suicide would require large and representative populations in order to avoid selection biases, as the cases and/or controls should be representative of the population at risk (Pokorny, 1983; Brent, 1989). For these reasons, suicide research has been compromised by the frequent use of individual-level studies that have been based on small clinical samples at high risk, or ecological studies that have been on the population level and thus correlational in nature in regard to risk factors (Pokorny, 1983).

A problematic area in suicide research is the study of the effectiveness of preventive interventions, which would require the use of randomization, blinding and/or placebo techniques. These would often be unethical and thus unfeasible, for example randomization of suicidal patients to different forms of treatment conditions (Linehan, 1997; Mościcki, 1997).

Prevalence of schizophrenia among general population suicides

The prevalence of schizophrenia among general population suicides has varied from 2% to 12% in psychological autopsy studies (Table 15.1). In older studies, the proportion of schizophrenic suicides is smaller, but most recent studies from Europe and Asia with clearly defined diagnoses estimate that about 7% of all suicide victims have had schizophrenia (Table 15.1). This rate is supported by a primary care record-based study of suicides in Scotland, which found that 9% of suicides were committed by people with schizophrenia (Milne et al., 1994). The standardized mortality ratio (SMR) represents the risk of death compared with a general population of similar age and sex. In recent meta-analyses, SMR values for suicide in schizophrenia have been shown to be about nine times higher than in the general population (Brown, 1997; Harris and Barraclough, 1997, 1998). Some studies have reported

Table 15.1. Prevalence of suicide in schizophrenia in community-based psychological postmortem studies of nonselected completed suicides

Reference	Country, area (time period)	Sample size (suicide rate in the area)	No. schizophrenics (%)	Diagnostic criteria for schizophrenia	Definition of suicide
Robins et al. (1959)	USA, St Louis (1956–57: 12 months)	134	3/134 (2)	Clinical diagnosis	Confirmed by coroner
Dorpat and Ripley (1960)	USA, Seattle: 1 county (1957–58: 12 months)	114	14/114 (12)	Not specified	Confirmed by coroner
Barraclough et al. (1974)	UK, 2 counties (1966–68)	100	3/100 (3)	Not specified	Confirmed by coroner
Hagnell and Rorsman (1979)	Sweden, Lundby (1947–72)	28	1/28 (4)	Woodruff et al. (1974)	Official statistics
Chynoweth et al. (1980)	Australia, Brisbane (1973–74: 12 months)	135 (16/100000)	5/135 (4)	Not specified	Confirmed by coroner
Mitterauer (1981)	Austria, Salzburg (1978)	121	5/99 (5)	Not specified	Police
Rich et al. (1986)	USA, San Diego (1981–83: 20 months)	283	9/283 (3)	DSM-III sch	Definite and possible suicides judged by the coroner were reviewed by researchers
Arato et al. (1988)	Hungary, Budapest (1985)	217 (47/100000)	16/200 (8)	RDC sch	Not specified
Cheng (1995)	Taiwan, eastern part 2 counties (1989–91: 30 months)	116 (15.6/100000 (Ami); 68.2/100000 (Atayl))	7/116 (6)	DSM-III-R sch, sch-aff	Coroner and prosecutor were interviewed; joint discussion among research team
Heilä et al. (1997)	Finland (1987–88: 12 months)	1397 (28.3/100000)	92/1397 (7)	DSM-III-R sch	Police and medicolegal examination
Foster et al. (1997)	Northern Ireland (1992–93: 12 months)	154 (12.4/100000)	7/118(6)	DSM-III-R sch	All deaths reported to the coroners screened by researcher; judged on clinical grounds referred as suicides
Vijayakumar and Rajkumar (1999)	India, Madras (1994–95: 13 months)	120 (17.2/100000)	4/100(4)	DSM-III-R sch	Official death certificate by the police or the magistrate

sch, schizophrenia; sch-aff, schizoaffective.

higher SMR for women with schizophrenia than for men with schizophrenia
(Allebeck and Wistedt, 1986a; Black and Fisher, 1992; Mortensen and Juel, 1993).

Suicide rate in follow-up studies of people with schizophrenia

The lifetime suicide rate among people with schizophrenia is high: 10–13% have
been estimated to end their lives by committing suicide (Miles, 1977; Caldwell and
Gottesman, 1990). It has been claimed that this estimate is too high because of
selection of patients from inpatient samples and incomplete lifetime follow-ups of
cohorts (Inskip et al., 1998). Geddes and Kendell (1995) found a low suicide rate
among a cohort of never-hospitalized schizophrenic patients over 2–13 years of
follow-up. Reviews of the topic (Harris and Barraclough, 1997; Inskip et al., 1998)
are compromised by the use of mixed cohorts of first-episode and chronic patient
populations, which probably underestimates the suicide rate. Also, the great variance in diagnostic classifications of schizophrenia (Harris and Barraclough, 1997;
Inskip et al., 1998) makes it difficult to compare suicide rates between different
studies. Studies using clinical registers for case identification may cause underestimation by missing the early cases of schizophrenia. Application of diagnostic criteria for first admissions may also differ between clinical samples, producing both
false-negative and false-positive diagnoses of schizophrenia (Kelly et al., 1998; Reid
et al., 1998; Baxter and Appleby, 1999).

Selection of patients from different treatment settings may also affect the estimate of suicide rate. Monitoring care may be better when patients are currently in
treatment contact. This may have a suicide preventive effect, especially when clinical short-term follow-up studies are concerned. It is possible that suicidal patients
drop out or are not served by their health-care system before suicide (Reid et al.,
1998), although it seems that the majority of suicides have occurred while patient
are in psychiatric treatment (Heilä et al., 1999a). Overestimation of suicide rate
among hospital-based samples could be caused by more frequent admissions of
suicidal high-risk patients with schizophrenia.

Consequently, it is difficult to draw conclusions of reliable estimates for lifetime
suicide rate in schizophrenia. It would be ideal to have large, representative first-
contact follow-up cohorts of people with schizophrenia for estimating suicide rate.
For this chapter, we carried out a literature review from 1966 to 1999 of mortality
studies, follow-up studies and suicide studies, in cohorts of first-contact patients
and mixed cohorts (both first-episode and multiple-episode patients). This produced 33 studies in which the suicide rate in a schizophrenia cohort was reported
and which used modern diagnostic classifications for schizophrenia (ICD-8 (World
Health Organization, 1967) and newer, RDC (Research Diagnostic Criteria; Spitzer
et al., 1990), DSM-III (American Psychiatric Association, 1980) and newer). These
studies are presented in Tables 15.2 and 15.3.

Table 15.2. Suicide rate in follow-up and cohort studies of people with first-contact or early-phase schizophrenia

Reference	Sample area	Sample (no.)	Data source (time period)	Diagnostic criteria (mean age (years) at onset	Mean follow-up time; lost in follow-up (%) (other than deaths)	Suicide rate (%) (suicide risk)
Lee et al. (1998)[b]	Hong Kong, 3 clinics	Random sample (100)	Interview (1977–78)	ICD-9 (26.5)	Retrospective: 15 yr; 19 (19%)	10/100 (10%)
Murray and van Os (1998)[c]	3 hospitals in London	Consecutive aged 16–50 yr (191)	Interview (1987–88, 1988–89)	RDC (23.7)	Prospective: 4 yr; 16 (8.4%)	7/191 (3.6%)
Räsänen et al. (1998)	Northern Finland	Unselected birth cohort 1966	Case records and registers (1980–94)	DSM-III-R sch	Prospective: up to 24 yr	4/25 (16%)
Wiersma et al. (1998)	Two northern provinces, the Netherlands (502)	Consecutive (82)	Interview and case records (1978–79)	ICD-9: 295, 297, 298.3–9 (most <25)	Prospective: 15 yr and 5 yr; (7.3%)	9/82 (11%) and 7/82 (8.5%)
Peuskens et al. (1997)	1 hospital in Kortenberg, Belgium	Consecutive (502)	Case records (1979–88)	DSM-III-R sch, sch-aff (24.1)	Retrospective: 6 yr	27/502 (5.3%) and sch: 23/437 (5.3%)
Mason et al. (1996)[b]	Nottingham area of UK	Consecutive aged 15–54 yr (67)	Interview, case records and registers (1978–80: 24 months)	ICD-9 sch (29; range 15–54	Prospective: 13 yr; 4 (6%)	3/67 (4.5%)
Geddes and Kendell (1995)	Edinburgh, Scotland	No hospital admission (66)	Charts and interview (1978–89)	Clinical diagnosis (38.9)	Retrospective: 2–14 yr	1/66 (2%)
Krausz et al. (1995)	Child and adolescent hospital in Hamburg, Germany	Random sample (61)	Interview (1972–78)	ICD-9/ PSE (median 17; range 14–18)	Prospective: 5 yr and 18 yr	2/61 (3.2%) and 9/61 (13.1%)

Table 15.2 (cont.)

Reference	Sample area	Sample (no.)	Data source (time period)	Diagnostic criteria (mean age (years) at onset)	Mean follow-up time; lost in follow-up (%) (other than deaths)	Suicide rate (%) (suicide risk)
Thara et al. (1994)	1 clinic in Madras, India	Consecutive (90)	Interview (1981–82: 12 months)	ICD-9 sch/PSE (most <24 yr)	Prospective: 10 yr; 4 (4%)	4/90 (4.4%)
Mortensen and Juel (1993)	All Danish psychiatric hospitals	Consecutive (9156)	Registers (1970–87)	ICD-8 clinical diagnosis	Retrospective: 1–18 yr	508/9156 (5.5%) (SMR = 20.7)
Carone et al. (1991)[d]	2 hospitals in Chicago, USA	Consecutive aged 17–30 yr (79)	Interview	DSM-III sch (23.1)	Prospective: 4.9 yr and 2.5 yr	8/79 (10%) and 6/79 (8%)
Lim and Tsoi (1991)	1 hospital in Singapore	Consecutive (482)	Index hospitalization records and registers (1975)	DSM-III-R sch (26.7)	Prospective: 15 yr	41/482 (8.5%) (567/100 000; RR = 50)
Cohen et al. (1990)	2 community clinics in 1 county, Wisconsin, USA	Young, nonalcoholic aged 18–30 yr (122)	Interview (1978–86)	RDC: sch,sch-aff or DSM-III: sch-typal (20.3)	Prospective: 8.3 yr	8/122 (6.6%)
Helgason (1990)	All patients in Iceland	Consecutive (107)	Interview, registers and case records (1966–67)	ICD-9 sch (33.5)	Prospective: 21–22 yr	10/107 (9.3%) (RR = 20); admitted: 6/80 (7.5%); never admitted: 4/27 (14.8%)

Study	Setting	Sample	Source	Diagnostic criteria	Follow-up	Suicides
Achté et al. (1986)	All hospitals in Helsinki, Finland	5 random sample cohorts (494)	Case records and interview (1–4): 1950, 1960, 1965, 1970; 5: 1975	1–4: clinical diagnosis of sch and paranoid psychosis 5: DSM-III sch, sch-form (27.4) (34.3, 36.2, 35.5, 38.0)	Retrospective: each cohort 5 yr; 8 (1.6%)	1–4: 3/100; (3%); 2/100; (2%); 2/100; (2%); 2/100 (2%) 5: 4/94 (4.3%)
Wilkinson (1982)	Camberwell, London, UK	Consecutive hospital and GP patients (43)	Case records and registers (1965–69)	RDC (32)	Retrospective: 10–15 yr; 4 (9.3%)	3/43 (7%) (500–750/100; 000; RR = 56–83)
Bland and Orn (1978)	Major psychiatric hospital in northern Alberta, Canada	Consecutive, nonalcoholic (45)	Interview and charts (1963)	ICD-8: 295 (32.6)	Retrospective: 14 yr; 2 (4.4%)	1/45 (2.2%)
Bland et al. (1976)	Major hospital in southern Alberta, Canada	Consecutive, non-abuse (92)	Interview and charts (1963)	ICD-8 and DSM-II sch (34)	Retrospective: 10 yr; 4 (4%)	2/88 (2.3%) (RR = 28)

sch, schizophrenia; sch-aff, schizoaffective disorder; PSE, Present State Examination; yr, year; RR, relative risk; SMR, standardized mortality ratio.

[a] Criteria used were ICD-8, ICD-9, DSM-III, DSM-III-R, RDC: see text for details.

[b] International Study on Schizophrenia (IsoS).

[c] Camberwell Collaborative Psychosis Study.

[d] Chigaco (III) Follow-up Study.

Table 15.3. Suicide rate in follow-up and cohort studies of people with mixed-episode schizophrenia

Reference	Sample area	Sample (No.)	Time period (mean age, years)	Diagnostic criteria[a] and data source	Mean follow-up time; non-traceable (%)	Suicide rate (%) suicide risk
Baxter and Appleby (1999)	Salford, UK	All patients (1410)	1969–75	ICD-8/ICD9: registers	Retrospective: up to 18 yr	44/1410 (3.1%) RR = 14.2
Kelly et al. (1998)	Nithsdale, southwest Scotland	All patients in 1 clinic (133)	48 yrs 1981: 1 day (48)	ICD-9: clinical diagnosis, survey and interview	Prospective: 16 yr; 4 (3%)	1/133 (0.75%)
Reid et al. (1998)	Texas, USA	All public patients (30/130)	1993–95	Clinical diagnosis of sch, sch-aff: registers	Retrospective: 2 yr	38/30130 (0.013%) (63/100000; RR = 5.3)
Ruschena et al. (1998)	Victoria, Australia	All public patients (25/202)	1995 (43.2)	ICD-9: 295, 297: registers	Retrospective: 1 yr	50/25202 (0.2%) (RR = 13.5; 95% confidence interval 10.1–18.1)
Parker and Hadzi-Pavlovic (1995)	Sydney, Australia	Consecutive patients in 2 hospitals (157)	1990: 6 months (34.8)	Clinical diagnosis: interview	Prospective: 1 yr; 24 (15%)	2/157 (1.3%)
Black and Fisher (1992)	Iowa, USA	Consecutive admissions in 1 hospital (356)	At index hospital 1970–81 (30.1)	DSM-III-R: case records and registers	Retrospective: 1–18 yr	16/359 (4.5%) (SMR = 23.2)
Leff et al. (1992)[b]	8 countries	Consecutive admissions to psychiatric facilities in study centres (1065)	1968–69	ICD-8/ CATEGO: interview	Prospective: 5 yr; 258 (24%)	20/1065 (1.9%) (suspected and ascertained suicide)
Breier et al. (1991)	USA	Selected young research patients (74)	1976–84 (26)	RDC: sch, sch-aff: interview	Prospective: 6 yr; 7 (9.5%)	3/74 (4%)

Study	Location	Sample	Period (mean age)	Criteria: source	Follow-up	Suicides/total (%) (SMR)
Anderson et al. (1991)	UK	Discharged or day patients in 2 hospitals (532)	(28.6 yr at index hospital)	ICD-9: 295, 297: case records and registers	Retrospective: 4–14 yr; 81 (15%)	7/532 (1.3%) (females SMR = 12.8; males SMR = 19.5)
Fenton and McGlashan (1991)[c]	Maryland, USA	Consecutive discharges in 1 hospital (187)	1950–75 (27.9 at admission)	DSM-III: case records and interview	Retrospective: 19 yr	10/174 (5.7%)
Newman and Bland (1991)	Alberta, USA	All public patients (3623)	1976–85 (37.3)	ICD-8/ICD9 295: registers	Retrospective 6 yr (1–10yr)	97/3623 (2.6%) SMR = 19.6; SMR = 22.8 (1–5 yr follow-up); SMR = 11.2 (6–10 yr follow-up)
Shepherd et al. (1989)	Buckinghamshire, UK	Consecutive admissions (121)	18 months (36.3)	PSE: interview	Prospective: 5 yr; 1/121 (0.8%)	3/121 (2.5%)
Prudo and Plum (1987)[b]	London, UK	Nonchronic, admissions in 3 hospitals (100)	1968–69: 12 months (71%: 15–34)	ICD-8: interview and case records	Prospective: 5 yr; 12 (12%)	5/100 (5%)
Allebeck and Wistedt (1986a)	Sweden	All discharges in Stockholm county (1190)	1971	ICD-8: 295: registers	Retrospective: 10 yr	33/1190 (2.8%) (SMR = 12.5)
Black et al. (1985)[d]	Iowa, USA	Consecutive admissions in 1 hospital (688)	1972–81	ICD-9: 295: registers	Prospective: 10yr; N>41 (6%), not known	14/688 (2.0%) (males SMR = 31; females SMR = 625)

sch, schizophrenia; sch-aff, schizoaffective disorder; PSE, Present State Examination; yr, year; SMR, standardized mortality ratio.

[a] Criteria used were ICD-8, ICD-9, DSM-III, DSM-III-R, RDC: see text for details.

[b] International Pilot Study of Schizophrenia.

[c] Chestnudge Lodge Follow-up Study.

[d] Iowa record linkage Study.

Suicide rate and follow-up time

Suicide risk has been found to be particularly elevated during the first year after the index admission in cohorts of first-admission schizophrenic patients (Mortensen and Juel, 1993). A survey of mortality carried out in Laos, a rural society with no psychiatric services, found a high rate of suicide particularly in the first years of illness (Westermayer, 1978). The high risk of suicide during the early years of illness in the follow-up studies of first contact or early phase patients with schizophrenia is shown in Table 15.2. The suicide rate averages 5.5% (range 3.2–10%) during the first 5 years and 7.9% (range 2.2–13%) when follow-up is extended for 10 years or more. Mixed cohorts of first- and multiple-episode patients also give support for higher suicide risk in early follow-up compared with late (Table 15.3), but average suicide rates derived from these studies are considerably lower (2–3%), both in short-term (5 years) and in long-term (10 years or more) follow-up studies, compared with first-contact samples.

However, increased mortality from suicide has been found throughout the whole span of the illness in long-term follow-up studies (Tsuang and Woolson, 1978). Many suicide victims with schizophrenia have had a prior duration of illness of 5–10 years before suicide (Caldwell and Gottesman, 1990). Suicide occurrence over large age and illness duration ranges was found in a representative nationwide sample of all schizophrenic suicides over a 12-month period (Heilä et al., 1997).

Risk factors for suicide in schizophrenia

Many studies of risk factors for suicide and clinical characteristics of suicide victims with schizophrenia have been compromised by the relatively small numbers of subjects, the heterogeneous diagnostic criteria, and the use of casenote data only. Studies using ICD-8, ICD-9 (World Health Organization, 1987), RDC, DSM-III or DSM-III-R (American Psychiatric Association, 1987) diagnostic criteria, with a sample size over 15 and with a comparison group are shown in Table 15.4

Cultural factors

Suicide is an endpoint of a complex multifactorial process, including sociocultural and society-related factors, as reflected in great differences between suicide rates in various countries and regions (Robins and Kulbock, 1988; World Health Organization, 1999). The interaction between the impact of cultural factors and the illness itself in contributing to suicide in schizophrenia is unknown.

Very little research knowledge exists on this issue. In psychological autopsy studies using DSM-III-R criteria, the proportion of schizophrenic suicides among all suicides was lower in India compared with European countries and Taiwan (Table 15.1). In line with this, the overall outcome of schizophrenia has been suggested to be better in developing countries than in developed countries (Kulhara, 1994). Better outcome may be reflected by low suicide mortality in schizophrenia, as reported in one 10-year follow-up study from India (Thara et al., 1994). Factors such as social network, cohesiveness of families and expressed emotions probably vary from culture to culture and influence functional and symptomatic outcome in schizophrenia (Kulhara, 1994). These may also play some role in affecting suicide rates among people with schizophrenia.

Sociodemographic risk factors

Female sex and older age at onset have been associated with characteristics of good outcome in general among schizophrenic patients (Bardenstein and McGlashan, 1990). Male sex and younger age are usually associated with increased suicide risk in schizophrenia (Caldwell and Gottesman, 1990). The mean age at time of suicide ranges from 23.3 to 43 years (Table 15.4). However, the overall effect of young age as a risk factor for suicide appears to be of less importance when compared with other risk factors such as male sex and clinical illness history (previous suicide attempts, depression, severe physical disorders, and psychiatric hospitalization patterns) (Rossau and Mortensen, 1997).

Persons with schizophrenia frequently are unmarried and living alone, and this applies more often to men than women (Bardenstein and McGlashan, 1990). In schizophrenia, the relative risk for suicide among single males has not been found to be elevated (Breier and Astrachan, 1984; Drake et al., 1984) but unmarried, divorced or widowed status raises the risk for suicide by tenfold among women with schizophrenia (Allebeck et al., 1987).

Duration of schizophrenia, illness course and illness phase

ICD-8 and ICD-9 are broader diagnostic classifications for schizophrenia than DSM-III or DSM-III-R definitions, which require a longer duration of disorder and deterioration in the level of premorbid functioning. First-contact studies based on DSM reported suicide rates that were higher (5.7%) during 5–6 years of illness (Table 15.2: Achté et al., 1986; Carone et al., 1991; Peuskens et al., 1997) than those reported in studies using ICD (3.7%) (Table 15.2: Krausz et al., 1995; Wiersma et al., 1998). In long-term follow-up studies of mixed-episode patient samples, a similar trend is also found between the diagnostic classifications used (Table 15.3) DSM giving 4.9% (26/533) (Fenton and McGlashan, 1991; Black and Fisher, 1992) and ICD giving 2.9% (78/2653) (Allebeck and Wistedt, 1986a; Kelly et al., 1998; Baxter and Appleby, 1999).

These disparities in suicide rates between the diagnostic systems may be explained by the fact that some factors that affect suicide risk are already included in the diagnostic classification. Some established suicide risk factors, such as illness

Table 15.4. Controlled studies on suicide in schizophrenia[a] with sample size of 15 or more

Author	Country, group	Follow-up (No. suicides)	Sample	Controls of study (No.)	Data source	History of depressive episode/depressive symptoms at last contact (%)	Suicide attempts (%)	Inpatients (%)
Roy (1982)	Toronto, Canada: Clarke Institute of Psychiatry	1968–79 (30)	Retrospective follow-up of inpatients and outpatients with subchronic and chronic sch	DSM-III sch; matched for age, sex, sch type (30)	All available patient records	57/53	40	23
Breier and Astrachan (1984)	New Haven, USA: Mental Health Center	1970–81 (20)	Retrospective follow-up of patients with DSM-III sch psychoses	1. Non-sch suicidal group (18) 2. Randomly selected sch group (81) 3. Sch patients matched for sex (20)	All available patient records	?	60	?
Drake et al. (1984)	Massachusetts, USA: Cambridge-Somerville Health System	1976–80 (15)	Retrospective follow-up of DSM-III sch inpatients	Inpatients; excluding long-stay, elderly and patients with brief admission (160)	Hospital records from admission before suicide or first admission	80/?	73	33
Wilkinson and Bacon (1984)	Edinburgh, UK: all patients	1968–81 (17)	Retrospective follow-up of admitted ICD-8/ICD-9 patients	Matched for patient records and age, sex, admission year (17)	Case records and registers, including death causes	?	59	35
Allebeck et al. (1987)	Sweden: Stockholm County: all inpatients	1971–81 (32)	Cohort of discharged DSM-III sch patients	Representing a 10% random sample of the cohort (64)	Inpatient registers, medical records, death certificates and national cause-of-register	13/?	72	44
Wolfersdorf et al. (1989)	Germany, Weissenau county: all inpatients	1986–87 (115)	Inpatients with ICD-9 (295) sch	Living sch patients matched for age, sex and diagnosis (115)	Hospital records	?/25	>55	All
Cheng et al. (1990)	Hong Kong: two outpatient clinics	1981–85 (74)	Retrospective follow-up of Chinese chronic and subchronic DSM-III sch	Matched for age and sex (74)	All available patient records	27/9	38	0

Study	Setting	Period (n)	Design	Comparison group (n)	Source of data			
Hu et al. (1991)	Taiwan, Taipei: Taipei Psychiatric Center	1972–87 (42)	Retrospective follow-up of inpatients and outpatients with DSM-III sch	1. Matched for age, sex, and outpatient care length (84) 2. First outpatient clinic visit in 1982, non-suicidal sch patients; follow-up of at least 5 years (60)	Patient records and family interviews	48/24	55	31
Lim and Tsoi (1991)	Singapore: Woodbridge Hospital	1975–90 (41)	Prospective follow-up of a DSM-III-R sch first-admission cohort	(411)	Inpatient register, inpatient records at first admission and death cause register	>12/?	>28	?
Modestin et al. (1992)	Switzerland: two hospitals	1973–87 (53)	Retrospective sample of RDC sch inpatients	Matched for diagnosis, sex index admission year, inpatient status (53)	Clinical records and police records	?	53	All
Fenton et al. (1997)	USA, Maryland: Chestnudge Lodge Hospital	1950–75 + 19 years follow-up (19)	Retrospective follow-up of a cohort of discharged patients with DSM-III sch psychoses and sch typal personality	(276)	Medical records and interviews with subjects and/or significant others	?	?	?
Peuskens et al. (1997)	Belgium: Kortenberg; one hospital	1979–89 (27)	Retrospective follow-up of young inpatients with DSM-III-R sch and sch affective	Patients matched for age, sex, diagnosis subtype and time of first admission (27)	Hospital records and controls contacted	?/67	63	41
Rossau and Mortensen (1997)	Denmark: all inpatients	1970–88 (508)	Retrospective follow-up of ICD-8 sch from the Danish Psychiatric Case Register	Individually matched living controls with sch (5080)	Inpatient psychiatric case register and register of death certificates	?	?	33

sch, schizophrenia.

[a] Criteria used were ICD-8, ICD-9, DSM-III, DSM-III-R, RDC: see text for details.

severity, chronic illness course with acute exacerbations (Roy, 1982) and high number of psychiatric admissions during the last year (Rossau and Mortensen, 1997) may be more characteristic for DSM than ICD schizophrenia. There is also a suggestion that suicide risk would be higher in chronic courses of RDC schizophrenia than in acute schizophrenic disorders early in the course of the illness (Westermeyer et al., 1991). At the time of suicide, the majority of suicide victims with DSM-III-R-defined schizophrenia were suffering from active psychotic symptoms (78%) and two-fifths were experiencing an acute exacerbation of illness, regardless of illness duration (Heilä et al., 1997).

Schizophrenia subtypes and symptoms

Earlier descriptive studies suggested an association of suicide risk with paranoid features of schizophrenia (Drake et al., 1985); this is supported by a controlled study by Fenton et al. (1997). There is some evidence for lowered suicide risk among patients with prominent negative symptoms, and particularly for the deficit type of schizophrenia (Black and Fisher, 1992; Fenton et al., 1997).

Comorbidity and suicide risk

Depression among patients with schizophrenia is found in approximately 25% during the longitudinal course of schizophrenia, but its presence varies according to the diagnostic methods and patient samples used; it is associated with functional impairment, morbidity and mortality (Siris, 1995). Comorbid depressive symptoms are one of the most frequently cited features of schizophrenic patients who commit suicide (Caldwell and Gottesman, 1990). Between 9 and 80% of suicide victims with schizophrenia were noted as having depressive symptoms in the patient records of last contact before suicide (Table 15.4). This large range in the reported level of depressive symptoms may be a consequence of variation in patient samples, classification of depressive states and the accuracy and volume of information in patient records. A history of depressive episodes has been reported in 27–58% of suicide victims with schizophrenia, significantly more often than among living comparison patients with schizophrenia (Roy, 1982; Cheng et al., 1990; Hu et al., 1991). The majority of suicide victims with schizophrenia (64%) had been suffering from depressive symptoms shortly before suicide (Heilä et al., 1997).

Findings linking substance abuse and suicide risk in schizophrenia are less consistent. Rossau and Mortensen (1997) did not find comorbid substance abuse associated with high suicide risk, when some other suicide risk factors were taken into account. Some studies have found a history of substance abuse less often among suicide victims with schizophrenia than among living subjects with schizophrenia (Drake et al., 1984; Wolfersdorf et al., 1989), whereas one study found a history of substance abuse increasing the risk for suicide, but only among men (Allebeck et al., 1987).

The extent and consequences of comorbidity with physical illness in patients with schizophrenia are generally under-recognized (Jeste et al., 1996) and this topic is discussed in detail in Chapter 14. A case-control study based on register data found that schizophrenic patients with a previous general hospital admission for physical disorders were at increased risk of suicide, suggesting that poor physical health may be an important risk factor for suicide (Rossau and Mortensen, 1997). Comorbidity patterns and suicide risk may vary with age, sex and their interaction among suicide victims with schizophrenia, but these are largely unknown as yet (Heilä et al., 1997).

Previous suicidality and suicide risk in schizophrenia

Schizophrenia is associated with a very high rate of suicidal behaviour. Lifetime estimates for a history of suicide attempts have ranged from 21% to 40% in clinical samples of schizophrenics (Planansky and Johnston, 1971; Niskanen et al., 1973; Roy et al., 1984; Nyman and Jonsson, 1986; Landmark et al., 1987; Keith et al., 1991; Jones et al., 1994; Fenton et al., 1997; Harkavy-Friedman et al., 1999; Radomsky et al., 1999). Previous suicidal behaviour is a strong risk factor for subsequent suicide: it has been estimated that 20–50% of people with schizophrenia who have attempted suicide ultimately kill themselves (Haas, 1997). Contrary to the common view that schizophrenic suicide occurs without warning (Breier and Astrachan, 1984; Johns et al., 1986), we found, in a nationwide suicide population, that communication of suicidal intent shortly before death occurred as often among suicide victims with schizophrenia as among nonschizophrenic victims (Heilä et al., 1998).

Adverse life events and suicide

The onset of schizophrenic illness and changes in its symptoms have both been associated with stressful life events (Lukoff et al., 1984; Bebbington et al., 1993; Norman and Malla, 1993). Adverse life events are an established risk factor for suicide in the general population. The proportions of subjects with schizophrenia who had experienced life events prior to suicide varies from 12 to 64% (Shaffer et al., 1974; Yarden, 1974; Breier and Astrachan, 1984; Rich et al., 1988; Salama, 1988; Cheng et al., 1989; Modestin et al., 1992; Heilä et al., 1999b; De Hert and Peuskens, 2000). This large variation is partly the result of methodological differences between the studies. Studies involving comparison groups have reported fewer life events for schizophrenic suicides compared with nonschizophrenic suicides (Breier and Astrachan, 1984; Rich et al., 1988; Heilä et al., 1999b). The rate of life events among schizophrenic suicides shortly before suicide was found to be similar to that in other psychotic suicide victims (Heilä et al., 1999b). When compared with the general population, the impact of life events among schizophrenic subjects seems of less importance in their suicide process.

Familial factors and suicide in schizophrenia

Family history of suicide has been shown to be associated with suicide among psychiatric patients, particularly among those with depression, but the evidence for higher familial suicide risk in schizophrenia has not been very impressive (Winokur et al., 1972; Roy, 1983; Tsuang, 1983). Most studies on clinical patient samples (Roy, 1982; Breier and Astrachan, 1984; Drake et al., 1984; Cheng et al., 1990; Hu et al., 1991), but not all (de Hert and Peuskens, 2000), found no significant differences in presence of family history of schizophrenia between living patients and suicide victims with schizophrenia, although under-reporting may cause bias in these studies.

Treatment-related factors

In contrast with nonpsychotic mental disorders, the majority of people with schizophrenia have been in contact with health-care services and also received treatment during their illness (Regier et al., 1993). Suicide in people with schizophrenia has usually occurred in the context of psychiatric treatment. In clinical samples of suicide victims with schizophrenia, a high proportion (10–44%) of suicides occurred during inpatient treatment (Yarden, 1974; Roy, 1982; Drake et al., 1984; Wilkinson and Bacon, 1984; Allebeck et al., 1986b; Hu et al., 1991; Heilä et al., 1997). Patients with schizophrenia have usually constituted the largest proportion (31–76%) of psychiatric hospital suicides (Lönnqvist et al., 1974; Copas and Robin, 1982; Goh et al., 1989; Wolfersdorf et al., 1989; Taiminen and Lehtinen, 1990; Modestin et al., 1992; Roy and Draper, 1995; Proulx et al., 1997). Further, a substantial proportion (33–55%) of suicides among clinical samples of schizophrenics have occurred within 3 months of discharge (Yarden, 1974; Roy, 1982; Drake et al., 1984), the risk being highest immediately after discharge (Rossau and Mortensen, 1997).

Suicide in patients with schizophrenia during psychiatric inpatient treatment is often preceded by more severe illness and a history of suicidal behaviour (Wolfersdorf et al., 1989; Modestin et al., 1992). Treatment changes, particularly among long-stay patients, and problems in the treatment relationship have been common shortly before suicide among inpatients with schizophrenia (Niskanen et al., 1974; Virkkunen, 1976; Goh et al., 1989; Roy and Draper, 1995; Heilä et al., 1998).

The risk for suicide is particularly high after discharge from psychiatric inpatient care (Goldacre et al., 1993, Rossau and Mortensen, 1997). The reasons for this are not known. High levels of psychopathology and functional impairment, suicide attempts during the preceding year and brief hospitalizations are all associated with suicide after discharge (Lindelius and Kay, 1973; Caldwell and Gottesman, 1992; Heilä et al., 1998). Frequent psychiatric admissions during the previous year has been found to increase suicide risk in schizophrenia, suggesting that 'revolving door' admission patterns are associated with high suicide risk (Rossau and Mortensen, 1997). Register-based studies from Denmark have also reported an increase in suicide rate in patient cohorts of first-contact schizophrenia corresponding with reductions in facilities for inpatient treatment. It has been suggested that increased suicide rate among patients with schizophrenia may be an indicator of adverse effects of deinstitutionalization (Munk-Jørgensen and Mortensen, 1992; Mortensen and Juel, 1993; Österberg et al., 2000).

Drug treatment

Most suicide victims with schizophrenia have been receiving antipsychotic medication at the time of suicide (Yarden, 1974; Roy, 1982; Drake et al., 1984; Wilkinson and Bacon, 1984; Heilä et al., 1999a); however the role of such treatment in suicides still remains unclear. A follow-up outcome study of first-episode hospitalized schizophrenic patients across 1950–80 did not show differences in suicide rate despite the different treatment practices over this period (Achté et al., 1986). Interestingly, a long-term follow-up study in the USA between 1913 and 1940 and of schizophrenic inpatients who were not treated with drugs reported the same risk factors for suicide as current studies of treated patients, such as previous suicidal behaviour, depressive symptoms during hospitalization and poor premorbid functioning (Stephens et al., 1999).

It has been suggested that high doses of neuroleptics may be associated with suicidal behaviour because of side effects, especially akathisia (Hogan and Awad, 1983; Drake and Ehrlich, 1985; Schulte, 1985), and some studies in living patients have shown an association between neuroleptics and depressive states (Siris, 1996). Comparisons of dosages of prescribed neuroleptics between suicide victims and living patients with schizophrenia have yielded inconsistent findings. Some studies found that higher dosages were prescribed before suicide; others found that lower doses were prescribed. The higher doses prescribed to some suicide victims may be because they had more severe illness, while lower doses in others may imply concurrent treatment for depressive symptoms (Cohen et al., 1964; Warnes, 1968; Roy, 1982; Hogan and Awad, 1983; Cheng et al., 1990; Taiminen and Kujari, 1994). However, pharmacological undertreatment of psychotic symptoms may be a serious problem in the management of suicidal schizophrenics. In a Finnish nationwide study, most suicides (78%) occurred during the active illness phase of schizophrenia (Heilä et al., 1997) and a significant proportion of suicide victims in the active illness phase had received inadequate antipsychotic treatment before suicide, whether in terms of dosage of neuroleptic treatment and noncompliance (57%) or poor treatment response (23%) (Heilä et al., 1999a).

Register-based linkage studies have provided some evidence for a protective effect of clozapine against suicidality and suicide, at least in certain patient subpopulations (Walker et al., 1997; Reid et al., 1998; Munro et al., 1999). Meltzer and Okayli (1995) found the risk of suicidal ideation and suicide attempts decreased during maintenance treatment with clozapine among treatment-resistant patients with schizophrenia. The specific nature of this 'suicide-reducing' effect is still unknown; it may relate to drug efficacy, treatment setting, and/or selection of patients.

The issue of noncompliance has rarely been addressed in the context of suicide. A study by Peuskens et al. (1997) reported higher risk of suicide for noncompliant than compliant patients in a young adult patient cohort. Helgason (1990) reported that the suicide rate was higher among never-admitted patients compared with patients admitted at least once to psychiatric hospital (Table 15.2). Many of these never-admitted patients had been advised to accept admission, but they had refused. It has been suggested that treatment resistance may be associated with increased suicide risk in schizophrenia (Haas, 1997; Meltzer, 1998), but a study comparing neuroleptic-responsive and neuroleptic-resistant patients showed no difference between the groups for history of suicidal behaviour (Meltzer and Okayli, 1995).

Although depressive symptoms are an important risk factor for suicide in schizophrenia, there is a lack of knowledge about the role of antidepressant treatment in suicide prevention among depressive patients with schizophrenia. There is some evidence that tricyclic antidepressants can be effective when used in conjunction with neuroleptic medication after the the acute phase has resolved (Siris, 1996), and atypical neuroleptics may reduce depressive symptoms during the active illness phase in patients with schizophrenia (Levinson et al., 1999).

Limitations of current studies and future implications for research

The current knowledge of suicide risk factors during the longitudinal course and different illness phases of schizophrenia is still quite limited. The heterogeneity in symptoms, outcomes and illness course within and between persons with schizophrenia is likely to encompass several high-risk subgroups for suicide with different risk factors and characteristics. Little is known about suicide risk factors among specific subgroups of patients.

Follow-up studies of first-episode schizophrenia (Ch. 8), would provide valuable information on suicide rates in schizophrenia in varying settings and cultural environments and on protective and risk factors for suicide. Very little research on suicidal behaviour has been performed in developing countries. Furthermore, suicide as an outcome in schizophrenia has often been neglected in follow-up studies, as suicide rates or detailed information on suicide subjects is seldom reported.

The study of short- and long-term risk and protective factors for suicide would be of great value for clinicians treating schizophrenic patients. So far, clinical retrospective studies with sufficient numbers of suicide victims for individual-level analyses have been mainly cross-sectional evaluations of factors or markers at index hospitalization, or at other clinical reference points using record-based data. Psychological autopsy studies using controlled study designs would provide information close to the time of suicide to estimate short-term risk factors for suicide in schizophrenia.

Treatment-related risk factors for suicide are feasible targets for further study and improved suicide prevention in schizophrenia. Suicide risk appears to vary during different treatment phases among patients with schizophrenia. There is some preliminary evidence for the efficacy of atypical antipsychotic medication in reducing suicide and suicidal behaviour in schizophrenia. These issues would be crucial for further studies with high-risk patients and controls. Finally, as depression is an important risk factor for suicide in schizophrenia, the role of treating depression for suicide prevention in schizophrenia should be addressed.

Conclusions

Schizophrenia is a lifelong disorder known to have severe disabling effects on people who suffer from it. It could also be viewed as a life-threatening disorder because of the high rates of suicidal behaviour and suicide, especially early in the illness course. Suicide is the worst outcome for chronic and severe illness course among younger adults with schizophrenia. However, suicide can occur throughout the entire course of schizophrenia, particularly in the high-risk periods of relapse, active illness phase or depressive episode. People with schizophrenia communicate warning signs of suicidal intent shortly before suicide just as often as suicide victims without schizophrenia. Psychiatric care should be supportive and tailored to the needs of the individual patient especially during these times. It is important to offer hope for patients by optimizing both psychosocial and pharmacological treatment. The high rate of inadequate treatment (inadequate dosing, noncompliance and nonresponse) among suicide victims with schizophrenia is worrying and indicates a need for further controlled follow-up studies addressing the potential protective effect of adequate antipsychotic treatment and the role of antidepressants in treating the

depressive syndrome in schizophrenia. Specific pharmacological interventions
such as clozapine treatment may have some suicide preventive effect. Finally, the
possible effects of changes in treatment provision, such as de-institutionalization,
on suicide rates should be urgently addressed, since there are indications that
suicide among people with schizophrenia is increasing.

REFERENCES

Achté K, Lönnqvist J, Kuusi K, Piirtola O, Niskanen P (1986) Outcome studies on schizophrenic psychoses in Helsinki. Psychopathology 19, 60–67.

Allebeck P, Wistedt B (1986a) Mortality in schizophrenia. A ten-year follow-up based on the Stockholm county inpatient register. Archives of General Psychiatry 43, 650–653.

Allebeck P, Varla A, Wistedt B (1986b) Suicide and violent death among patients with schizophrenia. Acta Psychiatrica Scandinavica 74, 43–49.

Allebeck P, Varla A, Kristjansson E, Wistedt B (1987) Risk factors for suicide among patients with schizophrenia. Acta Psychiatrica Scandinavica 76, 414–419.

American Psychiatric Association (1980) Diagnostic and Statistical Manual of Mental Disorders, 3rd edn. Washington, DC: American Psychiatric Press.

American Psychiatric Association (1987) Diagnostic and Statistical Manual III–Revised. Washington, DC: American Psychiatric Press.

Anderson C, Connelly J, Johnstone EC, Owens DGC (1991) V. Cause of death. British Journal of Psychiatry 159(Suppl. 13), 30–33.

Arato M, Demeter E, Rihmer Z, Somogyi E (1988) Retrospective psychiatric assessment of 200 suicides in Budapest. Acta Psychiatrica Scandinavica 77, 454–456.

Bardenstein KK, McGlashan TH (1990) Gender differences in affective, schizoaffective, and schizophrenic disorders: a review. Schizophrenia Research 3, 159–172.

Barraclough BM, Bunch B, Nelson B, Sainsbury P (1974) A hundred cases of suicide: clinical aspects. British Journal of Psychiatry 125, 355–373.

Baxter D, Appleby L (1999) Case register study of suicide risk in mental disorders. British Journal of Psychiatry 175, 322–326.

Bebbington P, Wilkins S, Jones P et al. (1993) Life events and psychosis. Initial results from the Camberwell Collaborative Psychosis Study. British Journal of Psychiatry 162, 72–79.

Beskow J, Runeson B, Åsgård U (1990) Psychological autopsies: methods and ethics. Suicide and Life Threatening Behavior 20, 307–323.

Black DW, Fisher R (1992) Mortality in DSM-III-R schizophrenia. Schizophrenia Research 7, 109–116.

Black DW, Warrack G, Winokur G (1985) The Iowa record-linkage study. I. Suicides and accidental deaths among psychiatric patients. Archives of General Psychiatry 42, 71–75.

Bland RC, Orn H (1978) 14-year outcome in early schizophrenia. Acta Psychiatrica Scandinavica 58, 327–338.

Bland RC, Parker JH, Orn H (1976) Prognosis in schizophrenia. A ten year follow-up of first admissions. Archives of General Psychiatry 33, 949–954.

Breier A, Astrachan BM (1984) Characterization of schizophrenic patients who commit suicide. American Journal of Psychiatry 141, 206–209.

Breier A, Schreiber JL, Dyer J, Pickar D (1991) National Institute of Mental Health longitudinal study of chronic schizophrenia. Archives of General Psychiatry 48, 239–246.

Brent DA (1989) The psychological autopsy: methodological considerations for the study of adolescent suicide. Suicide and Life Threatening Behavior 19, 43–57.

Brown S (1997) Excess mortality of schizophrenia. A meta-analysis. British Journal of Psychiatry 171, 502–508.

Caldwell CB, Gottesman II (1990) Schizophrenics kill themselves too: a review of risk factors for suicide. Schizophrenia Bulletin 16, 571–588.

Caldwell CB, Gottesman II (1992) Schizophrenia – a high risk factor for suicide: clues to risk reduction. Suicide and Life Threatening Behavior 22, 479–493.

Canetto SS, Sakinofsky I (1998) The gender paradox in suicide. Suicide and Life Threatening Behavior 28, 1–23.

Carone BJ, Harrow M, Westermayer JF (1991) Posthospital course and outcome in schizophrenia. Archives of General Psychiatry 48, 247–253.

Cheng ATA (1995) Mental illness and suicide. A case-control study in East Taiwan. Archives of General Psychiatry 52, 594–603.

Cheng ATA, Lee C-S (2000) Suicide in Asia and the Far East. In: The International Handbook of Suicide and Attempted Suicide, Understanding Suicidal Behaviour, Hawton K, van Heeringen K, eds. Chichester: Wiley, pp. 29–48.

Cheng KK, Leung CM, Lo WH, Lam TH (1989) Suicide among Chinese schizophrenics in Hong Kong. British Journal of Psychiatry 154, 243–246.

Cheng KK, Leung CM, Lam TH (1990) Risk factors of suicide among schizophrenics. Acta Psychiatrica Scandinavica 81, 220–224.

Chynoweth R, Tonge JI, Armstrong J (1980) Suicide in Brisbane – a retrospective psychological study. Australian and New Zealand Journal of Psychiatry 14, 37–45.

Clark DC, Horton-Deutsch SL (1992) Assessment in absentia: The value of psychological autopsy method for studying antecedents of suicide and predicting future suicides. In: Assessment and Prediction of Suicide, Maris RW, Berman AL, Maltsberger JT, Yufit RI, eds. New York: Guilford Press, pp. 144–182.

Cohen LJ, Test MA, Brown RL (1990) Suicide and schizophrenia: data from a prospective community treatment study. American Journal of Psychiatry 147, 602–607.

Cohen S, Leonard CV, Farberow NL, Shneidman ES (1964) Tranquilizers and suicide in the schizophrenic patient. Archives of General Psychiatry 11, 312–321.

Copas JB, Robin A (1982) Suicide in psychiatric in-patients. British Journal of Psychiatry 141, 503–511.

de Hert M, Peuskens J (2000) Psychiatric aspects of suicidal behaviour: schizophrenia. In: The International Handbook of Suicide and Attempted Suicide, Hawton K, van Heeringen K, eds. Chichester: Wiley, pp. 121–134.

Dorpat TL, Ripley HS (1960) A study of suicide in the Seattle area. Comprehensive Psychiatry 1, 349–359.

Drake RE, Ehrlich J (1985) Suicide attempts associated with akathisia. American Journal of Psychiatry 142, 499–501.

Drake RE, Gates C, Cotton PG, Whitaker A (1984) Suicide among schizophrenics. Who is at risk? Journal of Nervous and Mental Disease 172, 613–617.

Drake RE, Gates C, Whitaker A, Cotton PG (1985) Suicide among schizophrenics: a review. Comprehensive Psychiatry 26, 90–100.

Fenton WS, McGlashan TH (1991) Natural history of schizophrenia subtypes. I. Longitudinal study of paranoid, hebefrenic, and undifferentiated schizophrenia. Archives of General Psychiatry 48, 969–977.

Fenton WS, McGlashan TH, Victor BJ, Blyler CR (1997) Symptoms, subtype, and suicidality in patients with schizophrenia spectrum disorders. American Journal of Psychiatry 154, 199–204.

Foster T, Gillespie K, McClelland R (1997) Mental disorders and suicide in Northern Ireland. British Journal of Psychiatry 170, 447–452.

Garrison CZ (1992) Demographic predictors of suicide. In: Assessment and Prediction of Suicide, Maris RW, Berman AL, Maltsberger JT, Yufit RI, eds. New York: Guilford Press, pp. 484–498.

Geddes JR, Kendell RE (1995) Schizophrenic subjects with no history of admission to hospital. Psychological Medicine 25, 859–868.

Goh SE, Salmons PH, Whittington RM (1989) Hospital suicides: are there preventable factors? Profile of the psychiatric hospital suicide. British Journal of Psychiatry 154, 247–249.

Goldacre M, Seagroatt V, Hawton K (1993) Suicide after discharge from psychiatric inpatient care. Lancet 31, 283–286.

Haas GL (1997) Suicidal behavior in schizophrenia. In: Review of Suicidology, Maris RW, Silverman MM, Canetto SS, eds. New York: Guilford Press, pp. 206–236.

Hagnell O, Rorsman B (1979) Suicide in the Lundby Study: a comparative investigation of clinical aspects. Neuropsychobiology 5, 61–73.

Harkavy-Friedman JM, Restifo K, Malaspina D et al. (1999) Suicidal behavior in schizophrenia: characteristics of individuals who had and had not attempted suicide. American Journal of Psychiatry 156, 1276–1278.

Harris EC, Barraclough B (1997) Suicide as an outcome for mental disorders. A meta-analysis. British Journal of Psychiatry 170, 205–228.

Harris EC, Barraclough B (1998) Excess mortality of mental disorder. British Journal of Psychiatry 173, 11–53.

Hawton K, Appleby L, Platt S et al. (1998) The psychological autopsy approach to studying suicide: a review of methodological issues. Journal of Affective Disorders 50, 269–276.

Heilä H, Isometsä ET, Henriksson MM, Heikkinen MH, Marttunen MJ, Lönnqvist JK (1997) Suicide and schizophrenia: a nationwide psychological autopsy study on age- and sex-specific clinical characteristics of 92 suicide victims with schizophrenia. American Journal of Psychiatry 154, 1235–1242.

Heilä H, Isometsä ET, Henriksson MM, Heikkinen MH, Marttunen MJ, Lönnqvist JK (1998) Antecedents of suicide among people with schizophrenia. British Journal of Psychiatry 173, 330–333.

Heilä H, Isometsä ET, Henriksson MM, Heikkinen MH, Marttunen MJ, Lönnqvist JK (1999a) Suicide victims with schizophrenia in different treatment phases and adequacy of antipsychotic medication. Journal of Clinical Psychiatry 60, 200–208.

Heilä H, Heikkinen MH, Isometsä ET, Henriksson MM, Marttunen MJ, Lönnqvist JK (1999b) Life events and completed suicide in schizophrenia. A comparison of suicide victims with and without schizophrenia. Schizophrenia Bulletin 25, 519–531.

Helgason L (1990) Twenty years' follow-up of first psychiatric presentation for schizophrenia: what could have been prevented? Acta Psychiatrica Scandinavica 81, 231–235.

Hirschfield RMA, Davidson L (1988) Risk factors for suicide. In: Review of Psychiatry, Vol. 7, Frances AJ, Hales R, eds. Washington, DC: American Psychiatric Press, pp. 307–333.

Hogan TP, Awad AG (1983) Pharmacotherapy and suicide risk in schizophrenia. Canadian Journal of Psychiatry 28, 277–281.

Hu W-H, Sun C-M, Lee C-T, Peng S-L, Lin S-K, Shen WW (1991) A clinical study of schizophrenic suicides. 42 cases in Taiwan. Schizophrenia Research 5, 43–50.

Inskip HM, Harris C, Barraclough B (1998) Lifetime risk of suicide for affective disorder, alcoholism and schizophrenia. British Journal of Psychiatry 172, 35–37.

Jeste DV, Gladsjo JA, Lindamer LA, Lacro JP (1996) Medical comorbidity in schizophrenia. Schizophrenia Bulletin 22, 413–430.

Johns CA, Stanley M, Stanley B (1986) Suicide in schizophrenia. Annals of New York Academy Sciences 487, 294–300.

Jones JS, Stein DJ, Stanley B, Guido JR, Winchel R, Stanley M (1994) Negative and depressive symptoms in suicidal schizophrenics. Acta Psychiatrica Scandinavica 89, 81–87.

Keith SJ, Regier DA, Rae DS (1991) Schizophrenic disorders. In: Psychiatric Disorders in America: The Epidemiologic Catchment Area Study, Robins LN, Regier DA, eds. New York: The Free Press, pp. 33–53.

Kelly C, McCreadie RG, MacEwan T, Carey S (1998) Nithsdale schizophrenia surveys 17. Fifteen year review. British Journal of Psychiatry 172, 513–517.

Kleck G (1988) Miscounting suicides. Suicide and Life Threatening Behavior 18, 219–236.

Krausz M, Müller-Thomsen T, Haasen C (1995) Suicide among schizophrenic adolescents in the long-term course of illness. Psychopathology 28, 95–103.

Kulhara P (1994) Outcome of schizophrenia: some transcultural observations with particular reference to developing countries. European Archives of Psychiatry and Clinical Neurosciences 244, 227–235.

Landmark J, Cernovsky ZZ, Merskey H (1987) Correlates of suicide attempts and ideation in schizophrenia. British Journal of Psychiatry 151, 18–20.

Lee PWH, Lieh-Mak F, Wong MC, Fung ASM, Mak KY, Lam J (1998) The 15-year outcome of Chinese patients with schizophrenia in Hong Kong. Canadian Journal of Psychiatry 43, 706–713.

Leff J, Sartorius N, Jablensky A, Korten A, Ernberg G (1992) The International Pilot Study of Schizophrenia: five year follow-up findings. Psychological Medicine 22, 131–145.

Levinson DF, Umapathy C, Musthaq M (1999) Treatment of schizo-affective disorder and schizophrenia with mood symptoms. American Journal of Psychiatry 156, 1138–1148.

Lim LCC, Tsoi WF (1991) Suicide and schizophrenia in Singapore – a fifteen year follow-up study. Annals Academy of Medicine 20, 201–203.

Lindelius R, Kay WK (1973) Some changes in the pattern of mortality in schizophrenia in Sweden. Acta Psychiatrica Scandinavica 49, 315–323.

Linehan MM (1997) Behavioral treatments of suicidal behaviors. Definitional obfuscation and treatment outcomes. Annals of the New York Academy of Sciences 836, 302–328.

Litman RE (1989) 500 psychological autopsies. Journal of Forensic Sciences 34, 638–646.

Litman RE, Curphey T, Shneidman ES, Farberow NL, Tabachnik N (1963) Investigations of equivocal suicides. Journal of American Medical Association 184, 924–929.

Lukoff D, Snyder K, Ventura J, Nuechterlein KH (1984) Life events, familial stress, and coping in the developmental course of schizophrenia. Schizophrenia Bulletin 10, 258–292.

Lönnqvist J (1977) Suicide in Helsinki: an epidemiological and social psychiatric study of suicides in Helsinki in 1960–61 and 1970–71. Helsinki: Monographs of Psychiatrica Fennica No. 8.

Lönnqvist J, Niskanen P, Rinta-Mänty R, Achté K, Kärhä E (1974) Suicides in psychiatric hospitals in different therapeutic eras. A review of literature and own study. Psychiatrica Fennica 265–273.

Mason P, Harrison G, Glazebrook C, Medley I, Croudace T (1996) The course of schizophrenia over 13 years. A report from the International Study on Schizophrenia (ISoS) coordinated by the world Health Organization. British Journal of Psychiatry 169, 580–586.

Meltzer HY (1998) Suicide in schizophrenia: risk factors and clozapine treatment. Journal of Clinical Psychiatry 59, 15–20.

Meltzer HY, Okayli G (1995) Reduction of suicidality during clozapine treatment of neuroleptic-resistant schizophrenia: impact on risk-benefit assessment. American Journal of Psychiatry 152, 183–190.

Miles CP (1977) Conditions predisposing to suicide: a review. Journal of Nervous and Mental Disease 164, 231–246.

Milne S, Matthews K, Ashcroft GW (1994) Suicide in Scotland 1988–1989. Psychiatric and physical morbidity according to primary care case notes. British Journal of Psychiatry 165, 541–544.

Mitterauer B (1981) Mehrdimensionale diagnostik von 121 suiziden im bundesland Salzburg im jahre 1978. Wiener Medizinische Wochenschrift 131, 229–234.

Modestin J, Zarro I, Waldvogel D (1992) A study of suicide in schizophrenic in-patients. British Journal of Psychiatry 160, 398–401.

Mortensen PB, Juel K (1993) Mortality and causes of death in first admitted schizophrenic patients. British Journal of Psychiatry 163, 183–189.

Mościcki EK (1997) Identification of suicide risk factors using epidemiologic studies. Psychiatric Clinics of North America 20, 499–517.

Munk-Jørgensen P, Mortensen PB (1992) Incidence and other aspects of the epidemiology of schizophrenia in Denmark, 1971–87. British Journal of Psychiatry 161, 489–495.

Munro J, O'Sullivan D, Andrews C, Arana A, Mortimer A, Kerwin R (1999) Active monitoring of 12760 clozapine recipients in the UK and Ireland. British Journal of Psychiatry 175, 576–580.

Murray RM, van Os J (1998) Predictors of outcome in schizophrenia. Journal of Clinical Psychopharmacology 18, 2S–4S.

Neeleman J, Wessely S (1997) Changes in classification of suicide in England and Wales: time trends and associations with coroners´ professional backgrounds. Psychological Medicine 27, 467–472.

Newman SC, Bland RC (1991) Mortality in a cohort of patients with schizophrenia: a record linkage study. Canadian Journal of Psychiatry 36, 239–245.

Niskanen P, Lönnqvist J, Achté K (1973) Schizophrenia and suicides. Psychiatrica Fennica 223–229.

Niskanen P, Lönnqvist J, Achté K, Rinta-Mänty R (1974) Suicides in Helsinki psychiatric hospitals in 1964–1972. Psychiatrica Fennica 275–280.

Norman RMG, Malla AK (1993) Stressful life events and schizophrenia. I: A review of the research. British Journal of Psychiatry 162, 161–166.

Nyman AK, Jonsson H (1986) Patterns of self-destructive behavior in schizophrenia. Acta Psychiatrica Scandinavica 73, 252–262.

O'Carroll PW, Berman AL, Maris RW, Moscicki EK, Tanney BL, Silverman MM (1996) Beyond the tower of Babel: a nomenclature for suicidology. Suicide and Life Threatening Behavior 26, 237–252.

Ösby U, Correia N, Brandt L, Ekborn A, Sparén P (2000) Time trends in schizophrenia mortality in Stockholm County, Sweden: cohort study. British Medical Journal 321, 483–484.

Parker G, Hadzi-Pavlovic D (1995) The capacity of a measure of disability (the LSP) to predict hospital readmission in those with schizophrenia. Psychological Medicine 25, 157–163.

Peuskens J, De Hert M, Cosyns P, Pieters G, Theys P, Vermonte R (1997) Suicide in young schizophrenic patients during and after inpatient treatment. International Journal of Mental Health 25, 39–44.

Planansky K, Johnston R (1971) The occurrence and characteristics of suicidal preoccupation and acts in schizophrenia. Acta Psychiatrica Scandinavica 47, 473–483.

Pokorny AD (1983) Prediction of suicide in psychiatric patients. Report from a prospective study. Archives of General Psychiatry 40, 249–257.

Proulx F, Lesage AD, Grunberg F (1997) One hundred in-patient suicides. British Journal of Psychiatry 171, 247–250.

Prudo R, Blum HM (1987) Five-year outcome and prognosis in schizophrenia: a report from the London field research centre of the International Pilot Study of schizophrenia. British Journal of Psychiatry 150, 345–354.

Radomsky ED, Haas GL, Mann JJ, Sweeney JA (1999) Suicidal behavior in patients with schizophrenia and other psychotic disorders. American Journal of Psychiatry 156, 1590–1595.

Räsänen P, Tiihonen J, Isohanni M, Moring J, Koiranen M (1998) Juvenile mortality, mental disturbances and criminality: a prospective study of the Northern Finland 1966 birth cohort. Acta Psychiatrica Scandinavica 97, 5–9.

Regier DA, Narrow WE, Rae DS, Manderscheid RW, Locke BZ, Goodwin FK (1993) The de Facto US Mental and Addictive Disorders Service System. Epidemiologic catchment area prospective 1-year prevalence rates of disorders and services. Archives of General Psychiatry 50, 85–94,

Reid WH, Mason M, Hogan T (1998) Suicide prevention effects associated with clozapine therapy in schizophrenia and schizoaffective disorder. Psychiatric Services 49, 1029–1033.

Rich CL, Young D, Fowler RC (1986) San Diego suicide study: I. Young vs old subjects. Archives of General Psychiatry 43, 577–582.

Rich CL, Motooka MS, Fowler RC, Young D (1988) Suicide by psychotics. Biological Psychiatry 23, 595–601.

Robins E, Murphy GE, Wilkinson RH, Gassner S, Kayes J (1959) Some clinical considerations in the prevention of suicide based on a study of 134 successful suicides. American Journal of Public Health 49, 888–899.

Robins LN, Kulbok PA (1988) Epidemiologic studies in suicide. In: Review of Psychiatry, Vol. 7, Frances AJ, Hales R, eds. Washington, DC: American Psychiatric Press, pp. 289–306.

Rosenberg ML, Davidson LE, Smith JC et al. (1988) Operational criteria for the determination of suicide. Journal of Forensic Sciences 32, 1445–1455.

Rossau CD, Mortensen PB (1997) Risk factors for suicide in patients with schizophrenia: nested case-control study. British Journal of Psychiatry 171, 355–359.

Roy A (1982) Suicide in chronic schizophrenia. British Journal of Psychiatry 141, 171–177.

Roy A (1983) Family history of suicide. Archives of General Psychiatry 40, 971–974.

Roy A, Draper R (1995) Suicide among psychiatric hospital in-patients. Psychological Medicine 25, 199–202.

Roy A, Mazonson A, Pickar D (1984) Attempted suicide in chronic schizophrenia. British Journal of Psychiatry 144, 303–306.

Ruschena D, Mullen PE, Burgess P et al. (1998) Sudden death in psychiatric patients. British Journal of Psychiatry 172, 331–336.

Sainsbury P, Jenkins J (1982) The accuracy of official reported suicide statistics for purposes of epidemiological research. Journal of Epidemiological Community Health 36, 43–48.

Salama A (1988) Research note. Depression and suicide in schizophrenic patients. Suicide and Life Threatening Behavior 18, 379–384.

Schulte JL (1985) Homicide and suicide associated with akathisia and haloperidol. American Journal of Forensic Psychiatry 6, 3–7.

Shaffer JW, Perlin S, Schmidt CW, Stephens JH (1974) The prediction of suicide in schizophrenia. Journal of Nervous and Mental Disease 159, 349–355.

Shepherd M, Watt D, Falloon I, Smeeton N (1989) The natural history of schizophrenia: a five-year follow-up study of outcome and prediction in a representative sample of schizophrenics. Psychological Medicine, Monograph Supplement 15. Cambridge: Cambridge University Press.

Shneidman ES (1981) The psychological autopsy study. Suicide and Life Threatening Behavior 11, 325–340.

Siris SG (1995) Depression and schizophrenia. In: Schizophrenia, Hirsch SR, Weinberger DR, eds. Oxford: Blackwell Science, pp. 128–145.

Siris SG (1996) Treatment of depression in patients with schizophrenia. In: The New Pharmacotherapy of Schizophrenia, Breier A, ed. Washington, DC: American Psychiatric Press, pp. 205–221.

Spitzer RL, Williams JBW, Gibbon M (1990) User's Guide for the Structured Clinical Interview for DSM-III-R (SCID). Washington, DC: American Psychiatric Press.

Stengel E (1960) Some unexplored aspects of suicide and attempted suicide. Comprehensive Psychiatry 1, 71–79.

Stephens JH, Richard P, McHugh PR (1999) Suicide in patients hospitalized for schizophrenia: 1913–1940. Journal of Nervous and Mental Disease 187, 10–14.

Taiminen TJ, Kujari H (1994) Antipsychotic medication and suicide risk among schizophrenic and paranoid inpatients. A controlled retrospective study. Acta Psychiatrica Scandinavica 90, 247–251.

Taiminen TJ, Lehtinen K (1990) Suicides in Turku psychiatric hospitals in 1971–1987. Psychiatrica Fennica 21, 235–247.

Thara R, Henrietta M, Joseph A, Rajkumar S, Eaton WW (1994) Ten-year course of schizophrenia – the Madras longitudinal study. Acta Psychiatrica Scandinavica 90, 329–336.

Tsuang MT (1983) Risk of suicide in the relatives of schizophrenics, manics, depressives and controls. Journal of Clinical Psychiatry 44, 396–400.

Tsuang MT, Woolson RF (1978) Excess mortality in schizophrenia and affective disorders. Do suicides and accidental deaths solely account for this excess? Archives of General Psychiatry 35, 1181–1185.

Vijayakumar L, Rajkumar S (1999) Are risk factors for suicide universal? A case-control study in India. Acta Psychiatrica Scandinavica 99, 407–411.

Virkkunen M (1976) Attitude to psychiatric treatment before suicide in schizophrenia and paranoid psychoses. British Journal of Psychiatry 128, 47–49.

Walker AM, Lanza LL, Arellano F, Rothman KJ (1997) Mortality in current and former users of clozapine. Epidemiology 8, 671–677.

Warnes H (1968) Suicide in schizophrenics. Diseases of Nervous System 29(Suppl. 5), 35–40.

Westermayer J (1978) Mortality and psychosis in a peasant society. Journal of Nervous and Mental Disease 166, 769–773.

Westermeyer JF, Harrow M, Marengo J (1991) Risk for suicide in schizophrenia and other psychotic and nonpsychotic disorders. Journal of Nervous and Mental Disease 179, 259–266.

Wiersma D, Nienhuis FJ, Slooff CJ, Giel R (1998) Natural course of schizophrenic disorders: a 15-year follow-up of a Dutch incidence cohort. Schizophrenia Bulletin 24, 75–85.

Wilkinson DG (1982) The suicide rate in schizophrenia. British Journal of Psychiatry 40, 138–141.

Wilkinson G, Bacon NA (1984) A clinical and epidemiological survey of parasuicide and suicide in Edinburgh schizophrenics. Psychological Medicine 14, 899–912.

Winokur G, Morrison J, Clancy J, Crowe R, Iowa City (1972). The Iowa 500. II. A blind family history comparison of mania, depression, and schizophrenia. Archives of General Psychiatry 27, 462–464.

Wolfersdorf M, Barth P, Steiner B et al. (1989) Schizophrenia and suicide in psychiatric inpatients. In: Current Research on Suicide and Parasuicide, Platt S, Kreitman N, eds. Edinburgh: Edinburgh University Press, pp. 67–77.

Woodruff RA, Goodwin DW, Guze SB (1974) Psychiatric Diagnosis. London: Oxford University Press.

World Health Organization (1967) Manual of International Statistical Classification of Diseases, Injuries and Causes of Death, 8th edn. Geneva: World Health Organization.

World Health Organization (1987) Manual of International Statistical Classification of Diseases, Injuries and Causes of Death, 9th edn. Geneva: World Health Organization.

World Health Organization (1999) Figures and facts about suicide. Geneva: WHO, Department of Mental Health.

Yarden PE (1974) Observations on suicide in chronic schizophrenics. Comprehensive Psychiatry 15, 325–333.

16

What is the relationship between substance abuse and schizophrenia?

Robin M. Murray[1], Anton Grech[2], Peter Phillips[3] and Sonia Johnson[3]

[1]Institute of Psychiatry, King's College London, UK
[2]Victoria, Gozo, Malta
[3]Royal Free and University College London Medical Schools, London, UK

Abuse of alcohol and illicit drugs is on the increase in many parts of the world and, not surprisingly, people with psychosis participate in this general trend. But do people with schizophrenia abuse substances over and above the frequency of abuse in the general population, and, if so, do they abuse all or only some drugs? Unfortunately, much of the research in this area is subject to a range of methodological biases. First, these studies have commonly been carried out in unrepresentative samples such as inpatients in hospitals for veterans of the armed forces. Second, inadequate attention has often been paid to either the measurement of the substance abuse or the diagnosis of schizophrenia. Third, many samples mix together first-onset, relapsing and chronic patients. Fourth, very few studies are prospective.

Finally, even when the facts are established, they are often obscured by the clamorous debate between those who believe that substance abuse can cause schizophrenia and those who believe that schizophrenia predisposes to increase in abuse of substances. These opposing views are frequently held with a certainty that goes way beyond the evidence. As we shall see, different mechanisms may underlie the association between schizophrenia and substance misuse in different situations, and the way in which comorbidity develops may vary from substance to substance.

From an epidemiological point of view, there are a number of possible explanations for a reported association between a substance of abuse and schizophrenia (Thornicroft, 1990; Blanchard et al., 2000). First, the reported relationship may be spurious. Second, the substance abuse may cause schizophrenia; either de novo or by revealing a previously latent psychosis. Third, schizophrenia may lead to an increased consumption of the drug; this could occur either through self-medication for unpleasant symptoms or because of the psychological and social difficulties associated with schizophrenia. Fourth, schizophrenia and substance abuse may share common aetiological factors. We shall discuss each of these in turn before examining the particular characteristics of those schizophrenic patients who abuse substances. Finally, we will consider the effect of substance abuse on outcome of the psychosis.

Is there an association between substance abuse and schizophrenia?

International evidence

USA

Many studies carried out in the USA have reported that people with schizophrenia frequently abuse substances. Blanchard et al. (2000) reviewed nine recent, mostly American, studies that met basic standards of methodological competence and concluded that approximately 40–50% of schizophrenic patients in the USA have a lifetime history of substance abuse disorder. Unfortunately, relatively few of these studies included comparisons with an appropriate general population control group or took adequate account of potential confounding factors such as unemployment and current socioeconomic status.

There have also been two large epidemiological studies in the USA. In the first, the Epidemiologic Catchment Area (ECA) study (Regier et al., 1990; Robins and Regier, 1991), 47% of persons meeting criteria for schizophrenia also met criteria for substance use disorder compared with a rate of 17% for the latter in the general population. Age, sex and ethnic group were controlled for in this study, but current socioeconomic status was not. A similar association between substance abuse and schizophrenia was found in the National Comorbidity Study. Unfortunately, comparisons with assessments made by clinicians cast some doubt on the validity of diagnoses of schizophrenia made by lay interviewers in both the above studies (Kendler et al., 1996).

UK

The British National Psychiatric Morbidity Study compared drug and alcohol use among residents of institutions who were suffering from schizophrenia and delusional disorders with that among people living in private households (Farrell et al., 1998). In the 'institutional' sample, people with schizophrenia showed slightly higher rates of alcohol dependence than the general population (6% versus 5%) and were also more likely than the general population to be abstinent from alcohol. The rate for any drug use in past years was 7% in the residents with schizophrenia compared with 5% in the people in private households.

Of course, one must ask whether those schizophrenic patients who are living in institutions are likely to be representative of the whole population of people with schizophrenia. More generalizable findings come from a study in south London, where Menezes et al. (1996) attempted to interview all patients with psychotic illness from a defined area who were in contact with psychiatric services. The 1-year prevalence rate for any substance abuse in the 171 patients they interviewed was 36%. Unfortunately, this study did not have a general population comparison group.

Europe

Elsewhere in Europe, studies on this topic have tended to be small with unrepresentative samples. However, their evidence indicates that patterns do not always mirror those found in US samples, and that there is substantial variation between the different European countries. As in the UK, reported rates are rarely as high as those in US studies. For example, Soyka et al. (1993) found a lifetime prevalence of substance misuse disorders of 22% among inpatients with schizophrenia at a university clinic in Munich and 43% among their equivalents at a Bavarian State hospital. Verdoux et al. (1996) studied 92 people with psychotic disorders recruited via inpatient and day patient services in Nantes, France; the lifetime prevalence was 25% for substance misuse (according to DSM-III-R criteria; American Psychiatric Association, 1987). Modestin et al. (1997) noted that 12% of a series of consecutively admitted inpatients in Switzerland with schizophrenia were frequent cannabis users and 8% frequent users of opiates or cocaine. Cassano et al. (1998) examined 96 people admitted to hospital with psychotic disorders in Pisa, Italy; 12% were identified as having substance misuse or dependence.

Australia

Fowler et al. (1998) reported the 6-month and lifetime prevalences of substance abuse/dependence among patients suffering from schizophrenia were 26.8% and 59.8%, respectively. Jablensky et al. (2000) sampled 980 Australians with psychosis and reported that 39% of the men and 17% of the women met lifetime criteria for alcohol abuse or dependence; the figures for drug abuse or dependence were 36% of men and 16% of women. In decreasing order of frequency, the most commonly abused drugs were cannabis, amphetamines, lysergic acid diethylamide (LSD), heroin and tranquillizers.

Temporal and geographic variations

National differences in the relative availability of drugs clearly affect the choice of drugs abused by psychotic patients. This was the explanation given by Fowler et al. (1998) for their finding that patients suffering from schizophrenia in USA were more likely to abuse cocaine than those living in Australia. The prevalence of drug abuse in the general population in the USA is, no doubt, the reason why drug abuse by schizophrenic patients attracts more clinical attention and research interest there than in any other country.

To a considerable extent, the substance preferences of people with schizophrenia also reflect the changing habits of the general population (Regier et al., 1990). Nowhere is this more obvious than in relation to stimulants. For example, Patkar et al. (1999) assessed 1700 hospital admissions for schizophrenia and schizoaffective disorder in Philadelphia, USA over 12 years and reported that over this period cocaine replaced amphetamine as the preferred drug of abuse among this patient population. This change was a consequence of a crack-cocaine epidemic in Philadelphia.

Cultural factors also strongly influence the choice of drugs abused by psychotic patients. For example, the chewing of the stimulant leaf khat is widespread in northeast Africa and the Arabian peninsula. As a consequence, in the UK, khat consumption and so-called 'khat-induced psychosis' is encountered mainly in immigrants from these areas (Yousef et al., 1995).

The different substances

The term substance abuse covers a range of diverse psychoactive substances with widely different actions on the nervous system. One cannot expect that all these drugs will show similar associations with schizophrenia. We will, therefore, consider each of the major groups of substances in turn. In reading this, the reader might like to bear in mind the epidemiological criteria outlined by Hill (1965), and quoted by Thornicroft (1990), for determining the nature of the association between an environmental risk factor and a disease: the strength of the association, its consistency, specificity, temporality, biological gradient, plausibility and coherence.

Alcohol abuse

Apart from nicotine, alcohol is the drug most commonly abused throughout the world by both the sane and the not so sane. Many authors, particularly from the USA, have found that patients with psychotic illness are especially likely to abuse alcohol (Mueser et al., 1990; Dixon et al., 1991; Rolfe et al., 1993). The ECA study in the USA found that 34% of those meeting criteria for schizophrenia also met criteria for alcohol abuse. Although there are methodological defects in the ECA study, its conclusions are very similar to those that Blanchard et al. (2000) came to in their review of nine studies of schizophrenic patients: the median lifetime prevalence of alcohol abuse was 35%.

As noted earlier, studies of patients with schizophrenia often mix together all patients from the first contact to the chronic. In an exception to this, Häfner et al. (1999) investigated a series of first-episode schizophrenic patients drawn from a defined population in Germany and compared them with a control sample matched for age, sex and population of origin. The lifetime prevalence for alcohol abuse was about 24% in first-episode schizophrenic patients compared with 12%

in the control population. In the UK, Cantwell et al. (1999) measured the prevalence of substance misuse among 168 individuals with first-episode psychosis presenting to services in Nottingham. They found a 1-year prevalence of alcohol misuse among these subjects of 11.7% and a 1-year prevalence of drug misuse of 19.5%; these figures included 8.4% who eventually received a primary diagnosis of substance-related psychotic disorder.

Some studies have not found that schizophrenic patients drink significantly more than the general population (Schneier and Siris, 1987, el-Guebaly and Hodgins, 1992). These include the UK study of institutionalized schizophrenic patients (Farrell et al., 1998) discussed above and two studies of patients admitted to psychiatric hospitals in south London (Bernadt and Murray, 1986; A. Grech and R. M. Murray, unpublished data). The more recent of these found an odds ratio (OR) of 0.76 for alcohol abuse among psychotic patients: that is, if anything psychotic patients were less likely to abuse alcohol than the general population.

It is possible that some of the disparities in the results of inpatient studies reflect aspects of the local referral and admission patterns of patients with dual diagnosis. The strength of any association between schizophrenia and alcohol misuse may also vary from place to place, depending on social conditions experienced by people with schizophrenia and the settings in which they live. For example, living with family or in supported accommodation may decrease the likelihood of alcohol abuse.

We conclude that the balance of probability is that in the USA there is a weak association between alcoholism and schizophrenia. However, this association is neither strong nor universal, and findings from elsewhere, the UK in particular, tend to be more negative.

Cannabis

Cannabis is the illicit drug most commonly abused by people with psychosis; this is not surprising since its use is widespread in the general population in many countries. In the study of Häfner et al. (1999) just considered, cannabis was the illicit drug most commonly used: by 88% of those schizophrenic patients who were taking drugs. Cannabis was also the illicit drug most commonly taken in the south London study of Menezes et al. (1996), and in the Australian study of Fowler et al. (1998).

Most studies report a positive association between cannabis consumption and psychosis. (Andreasen et al., 1987; Schneier and Siris, 1987; Dixon et al., 1991; Mathers et al., 1991; Rolfe et al., 1993; Linszen et al., 1994; Longhurst et al., 1997). Such reports stretch back many years and come from many countries. For example, the Indian Hemp Drugs Commission (1894) noted that 'excessive use indicates and intensifies instability of the mind: it may even lead to insanity'. Similar reports have come from South Africa (Rottanburg et al., 1982) and the West Indies (Knight, 1976).

Grech et al. (1998) compared psychotic patients from two different cultural settings, London and Malta; cannabis (and indeed all illicit drugs) consumption was much more widespread in the former. In both centres, psychotic patients abused substances more than controls. A particularly strong association between cannabis abuse and psychosis was shown by the fact that the OR for cannabis abuse in patients over controls was greater in both centres than the OR for substance abuse in general or for any other type of substance. Therefore, in terms of Hill's criteria, quoted above, the association between psychosis and cannabis is fairly consistently reported (with a few exceptions, e.g. Mueser et al., 1990).

Stimulants

After cannabis, stimulants are the illicit drugs most commonly abused by schizophrenic patients in the USA and in Pacific countries. Mueser et al. (1990) reviewed the literature and compared their own data on a sample of people with schizophrenia with results of a US national household survey of patterns of substance use; they concluded that people with schizophrenia used stimulants and hallucinogens more than the general population. Many reports have come from Japan and Taiwan. These have been reviewed by Chen (2001), who was also able to identify 174 individuals presenting with methamphetamine-induced psychosis within a 2-year period in Tapei.

Opiates

There is no evident association between opiate abuse and psychosis in the USA (Schneier and Siris, 1987; Rolfe et al., 1993; Soyka et al. 1993) with opiate use being reported only at low levels. In Europe, however, there is rather more variability, with opiate use sometimes exceeding that of cocaine and amphetamine. For example, in a survey of individuals known to community teams in the environs of Paris, Launay et al. (1998) reported that alcohol was the most frequently used substance, followed by cannabis and then opiates, with little evidence of cocaine or stimulant use.

In Hamburg, Lambert et al. (1997) described the drug choices of 222 substance users who were in contact with a variety of general psychiatric facilities. Alcohol (by 52%) and cannabis (by 25%) were the predominant substances used. There was very little evidence of stimulant consumption, with just one individual (0.5%) using cocaine, compared with 4.1% using opiates.

Nicotine

Cigarette smoking has not been mentioned so far; indeed most studies of substance abuse ignore it since, by some curious convention, nicotine is not usually considered as a substance of abuse. More importantly, many mental health professionals acquiesce in the nicotine addiction shown by their psychotic patients and, shamefully, in institutional settings such as wards and hostels, cigarettes are still sometimes used as a means of rewarding desired behaviours. Nevertheless, dependence on nicotine is the most common form of dependence among patients with schizophrenia. Studies of smoking habits in schizophrenic patients have reported prevalence rates as high as 90%, with the greatest rates and heaviest addiction tending to be found among those with chronic illness (Leon et al., 1995; Diwan et al., 1998).

Ziedonis and George (1997) summarized the American literature as indicating that, while 25–30% of the general population smoke, approximately 40–50% of patients with depression and anxiety disorders do so, rising to 70–90% for schizophrenic patients. In an Australian survey of 980 people with psychosis, cigarette smoking was reported by 73% of men and 56% of women with psychosis as opposed to 27% and 20%, respectively, in the general population (Jablensky et al., 2000). Kelly and McCreadie (1999) examined the smoking habits of all known schizophrenic patients within a discrete geographical area in southern Scotland; the prevalence of smoking (and the level of nicotine addiction) was greater in schizophrenic patients (58%) than in the general population (28%).

Summary

In short, there is evidence that, on the whole, patients with schizophrenia are more likely to abuse substances than is the general population. Their drug preferences tend to reflect that of the population from which they come. Cigarette consumption is both extremely common and strongly associated with schizophrenia; alcohol abuse is next most common, but the association with schizophrenia is weak at best. Cannabis and stimulant abuse are generally reported to be associated with schizophrenia in countries where their use is common. These facts are not generally disputed. What different authors tend to disagree on is the reason for the associations. We now turn to these reasons.

Can substance abuse cause schizophrenia?

The question of whether substance abuse can cause or precipitate psychotic illness remains hotly disputed, some authors maintaining that sufferers consume substances to ameliorate negative or dysphoric symptoms (Peralta and Cuesta, 1992) or to counteract the unpleasant effects of antipsychotic drugs. What is the evidence that substance abuse can cause psychosis? A number of studies have attempted to examine the temporal relationship between onset of substance misuse and schizophrenia in an effort to clarify the direction of any aetiological relationship between the two. Unfortunately, both disorders tend to begin in a relatively gradual way so that a time of onset is difficult to pinpoint.

Temporal relationship between substance use and schizophrenia

The ABC study of Häfner and colleagues (1999) does, however, try to avoid some of these problems by a very detailed history-taking, including collateral reports from relatives. Thus, in an attempt to assess 'whether substance abuse via possible dopaminergic effects might trigger a psychotic episode', these investigators reported that 80% of drug abusers began their abuse before the onset of positive symptoms of psychosis, 3% in the same month and 14% following the onset of positive symptoms, findings compatible with their hypothesis. However, a different picture emerges when time of onset of drug use is compared with the emergence of the first sign of schizophrenia of any sort, including more nonspecific indications of deterioration; Hambrecht and Häfner (1996) report that drug misuse preceded the first symptom of any sort in 27.5%, followed it in 37.9%, and emerged in the same month in 34.6%. They conclude that the concurrence of onsets of schizophrenia and drug use in a substantial number of patients suggests a causal relationship, though one where the direction is unclear.

Other reports have included an Israeli study by Silver and Abboud (1994) of 42 subjects who had schizophrenia and used drugs; 24 had begun before their first admission. Rabinowitz et al. (1998) describe a cohort of individuals with psychosis and moderate or severe substance misuse studied at the time of their first hospital admission. According to their retrospective evaluation, 49 of the 52 males in their sample had begun substance misuse before the appearance of their first positive symptom, although only 3 out of 15 women appeared already to be substance misusers at this point. By their nature, these samples obviously did not include people with psychotic illness who developed substance misuse subsequent to their first admission.

Can stimulant use cause psychosis?

Amphetamines, cocaine and hallucinogens have all been associated with psychosis (Schneier and Siris, 1987; Boutros and Bowers, 1996). Turner and Tsuang (1990) and Poole and Brabbins (1996) have reviewed the substantial evidence that stimulants both trigger brief psychotic episodes and intensify pre-existing psychotic symptoms. Of particular interest are reports that progressive sensitization occurs with cocaine use, with short-term psychotic symptoms triggered more rapidly and after smaller amounts of cocaine as subjects continue to use cocaine (Satel et al., 1991; Bartlett et al., 1997).

Whether there is a link between stimulant misuse and psychotic states that are indistinguishable in their psychopathology from schizophrenia and persist long term after abstinence from substances is more difficult to establish. The evidence put forward for this mainly consists of case series of stimulant users who have developed psychotic illnesses. Often comparable control groups are lacking and a

major problem for causal inference is the possibility that the stimulant use has
developed because of prodromal manifestations of schizophrenia.

In a classic report, Connell (1958) described a series of 36 patients with symptoms suggestive of paranoid schizophrenia who were abusing amphetamines; nine
developed protracted psychotic syndromes persisting at least 2 months after withdrawal from amphetamines and three had psychotic syndromes that persisted
'indefinitely'. Both amphetamine abuse and the resultant psychosis are still
common in Japan and Taiwan (Chen, 2001), but amphetamine-induced psychosis
appears to have become less common in Western Europe and North America. In
contrast, cocaine has emerged as a problem among schizophrenic patients, particularly in the USA.

A number of case series have been used as the basis for an argument that chronic
amphetamine and cocaine use can result in a minority of users in a chronic psychotic syndrome indistinguishable from chronic psychosis (Boutros and Bowers,
1996; Flaum and Schultz, 1996). McLellan et al. (1979) describe a study that is particularly interesting in that it is longitudinal and makes comparisons between stimulant users and control groups of depressant or narcotic users. They studied 51
subjects, none of whom showed evidence of psychotic symptoms at baseline assessment. Of the 11 stimulant users, six had developed chronic psychotic states resembling schizophrenia at follow-up, and five had been hospitalized for this, whereas
no such states were reported among the control subjects.

These descriptions of chronic psychosis developing among stimulant users have
persuaded some to argue for the existence of long-term psychotic states in which
substance misuse is a significant aetiological factor (e.g. Boutros and Bowers, 1996).
It could well be that a spectrum exists from individuals who require very large quantities of drugs to induce psychosis, to others those who become chronically psychotic on minimal use. However, the accumulated evidence for this probably does
not as yet pass rigorous methodological scrutiny (Turner and Tsuang, 1990); the
problems include the paucity of longitudinal data, the possibility of reverse causality, the paucity of good data about the proportion of regular substance users who
develop psychotic illnesses, and the lack of appropriate control groups.

There is a rather smaller body of evidence linking LSD with transient psychotic
states. Similarly, less evidence is available on hallucinogens and chronic psychotic
states, but Boutros and Bowers (1996) reviewed a few case reports and case series
describing development of chronic psychotic states following LSD or solvent use.

Can cannabis use cause psychosis?

Thornicroft (1990) reviewed studies of cannabis consumption in the general population and concluded that it can produce paranoid ideas and occasional hallucinations; an organic toxic state can also occur with mild impairment of

concentration, poor concentration and orientation. Indeed, there is little dispute that cannabis intoxication can trigger brief episodes of psychotic symptoms and that it can produce short-term exacerbations or recurrences of pre-existing psychotic symptoms (Negrete et al., 1986; Thornicroft, 1990; Mathers and Ghodse, 1992). However, there remains controversy over the existence of chronic psychotic states persisting beyond cessation of cannabis use and resembling schizophrenia (Johns, 2001).

For many years it was unclear how cannabis induced its psychotropic effects. However, recent evidence has demonstrated that Δ^9-tetrahydrocannabidiol (THC), the principal active metabolite of cannabis, increases the release of dopamine from the nucleus accumbens and prefrontal cortex and raises the level of cerebral dopamine (Patel et al., 1985; Gardner and Lowinson, 1991; Tanda et al., 1997). This is likely to be the basis for its reinforcing properties and recreational use (Ashton, 2000) and could, of course, be a mechanism for inducing psychosis.

Thornicroft (1990) pointed out that if cannabis is causally associated with psychosis, then we should expect to find a dose–response relationship of greater morbidity with higher dose. Such a dose–response relationship was found in a prospective study in which Andreasson and his colleagues (1987) followed 45 570 Swedish 18-year-olds who were interviewed about their drug consumption at the time they were conscripted into the army. The relative risk of developing schizophrenia over the next 15 years was 2.4 for cannabis users compared with nonusers (at time of conscription) and rose to 6.0 for heavy users. Of course, it is possible to argue that these individuals were already unwell at age 18 and were taking cannabis as an attempt at self-medication. Andreasson et al. (1987) noted that 430 of the 730 'high consumers' did indeed have a psychiatric diagnosis other than psychosis (mainly neurosis and personality disorder) when they were conscripted at age 18 years. When this confound was controlled for, the relative risk was roughly halved to 2.9 but remained significant. This is a well-designed and executed study but as Johns (2001) points out 'There is a large temporal gap between self-reported cannabis use on conscription and the development of schizophrenia over 15 years, and no data as to whether the cannabis use continued during this time.'

One possibility is that cannabis on its own is insufficient to cause psychosis but it can trigger psychosis in predisposed individuals. This is compatible with the findings of Andreasson et al. (1987) in that only a small proportion of heavy cannabis-using conscripts went on to present with schizophrenia. Support for this view can also be drawn from a study by McGuire et al. (1995), who found that patients with cannabis-associated psychosis had a significantly increased familial morbid risk for schizophrenia. This might be taken to imply that cannabis abuse acts on genetic predisposition to schizophrenia to trigger psychosis; of course, one might also speculate that several members of the same family could have been abusing cannabis and thus increased their risk of psychosis.

Our interpretation of the studies reviewed above is that people vulnerable to psychiatric disorder are more likely to abuse cannabis than the rest of the population but that heavy abuse of cannabis also acts as an independent risk factor for psychosis. Heavy abuse of cannabis can not only cause a brief organic reaction but probably also acts as a further risk factor to which those with biological predisposition to psychosis are especially vulnerable. However, this case would not yet withstand really rigorous methodological scrutiny.

Can alcohol use cause psychosis?

Kraepelin, the originator of the concept of dementia praecox/schizophrenia, was passionately interested in the adverse consequences of alcohol on mental health and was so convinced by these that he became a total abstainer. In his memoirs (Hippius et al., 1987), he states that this unusual habit involved him in endless discussions on alcohol and '... caused a sensation. I am quite sure that my entire scientific work did not make my name as famous as the plain fact that I did not drink alcohol'. However, the consensus so far has been that alcohol misuse is unlikely to be a cause of schizophrenia (Mueser et al., 1998).

An exception to this consensus is the ABC study of Häfner et al. (1999), which investigated a series of first-episode schizophrenic patients and a well-matched control population; the schizophrenics showed a doubling in the lifetime prevalence of alcohol abuse. In at least some cases, the alcohol abuse preceded the positive symptoms of schizophrenia, leading the authors to suspect that it can play an aetiological role.

Can nicotine use cause psychosis?

The reason why more people with schizophrenia smoke so much more than the general population is unclear. Nicotine may reduce negative symptoms of schizophrenia or ameliorate some of the side effects of typical antipsychotic drugs (Ziedonis and George, 1997). However, cigarette smoking is one of the major causes of disability and death among schizophrenic patients. In addition, as McCreadie and Kelly (2000) point out, people with chronic schizophrenia are among those who can least afford the habit; these authors found that more of their smoking than nonsmoking patients had financial difficulties.

In the study of Kelly and McCreadie (1999), 90% of the patients who smoked had started smoking before the onset of schizophrenia. Patients who smoked were younger than nonsmokers, more of them were male, they had more hospitalizations and poorer childhood social adjustment. Among the female patients, there was a positive correlation between age at starting smoking and age of onset of schizophrenia. The authors speculated that smoking may be a risk-increasing factor for schizophrenia in vulnerable individuals. Although nicotine has dopaminergic effects, this view that has not received much endorsement.

An explanatory model

One can best understand how substance abuse might contribute to the onset of psychosis by reflecting on the current view of schizophrenia as a multifactorial disorder in which genes and early environmental brain insults interact to cause neurodevelopmental impairment and to set preschizophrenic children on a trajectory of ever increasing deviance (Jones et al., 1994; Murray and Fearon, 1999). Risk factors more proximal to the onset of the illness may compound this vulnerability and project the susceptible individual over the threshold for the expression of frank psychosis.

There is good evidence that certain types of social adversity (Sharpley et al., 2001) and abuse of drugs such as amphetamines, cocaine and possibly cannabis can act as such proximal risk factors; presumably the mechanism is by their dopamine-releasing or agonist effects. It is not difficult to understand that the compromised brain of a person with neurodevelopmental impairment may show greater vulnerability to the actions of dopaminergic drugs. However, unlike such drugs, alcohol does not appear to induce psychosis in the short term. Nevertheless, aspects of alcoholism could compound the neurodevelopmental damage – epilepsy, malnutrition, delirium tremens – and also result in the social stresses likely to contribute to breakdown.

Certain terms are sometimes used for the psychoses associated with substance abuse (e.g. alcoholic hallucinosis and cannabis psychosis). These can most usefully be considered in the light of the evidence that there are developmental and nondevelopmental components to the schizophrenia syndrome (Murray et al., 1992; van Os et al., 1998). Much evidence suggests that negative symptoms and disorganization (thought disorder) have their origins in neurodevelopmental impairment. However, positive symptoms such as hallucinations and delusions have not been so clearly associated with developmental impairment.

The phenomenology said to be characteristic of alcoholic hallucinosis (i.e. hallucinations in the absence of prominent negative symptoms or thought disorder) is compatible with a schizophrenic syndrome in which nondevelopmental factors play a major role. We take a similar view of the so-called 'cannabis psychosis', since there is no evidence for its existence as a distinct phenomenon (Thornicroft, 1990).

One can best consider such so-called special conditions in the light of the evidence presented elsewhere in this book that liability to psychosis is a continuously distributed trait in the general population (i.e. like hypertension). This helps us to understand why it has been so difficult to define alcoholic hallucinosis or cannabis psychosis as discrete categories. We can postulate that in those with only a small genetic loading for schizophrenia (perhaps one or two susceptibility genes), then the psychotic symptoms may only be temporary; but in those with a heavier genetic loading then the illness may proceed to become indistinguishable from classical schizophrenia.

Does established psychosis lead to an increase in substance abuse?

The self-medication hypothesis

Given the extent of their suffering, it would not be surprising if schizophrenic patients discovered that substances of abuse can offer temporary relief from their distress, and then proceeded to become over-reliant on them. This self-medication hypothesis suggests that patients suffering from schizophrenia use substances to alleviate aspects of psychosis, and the resultant short-term beneficial effects reinforce the drive towards taking these substances (Buckley, 1998).

This hypothesis has two main variants, the first postulating that patients select specific substances to alleviate specific symptoms of schizophrenia, and the second referring to a much broader idea that patients take substances because they alleviate general dysphoria.

Since alcohol and the various illicit drugs act on different receptors, one cannot expect them to act in a uniform manner. For example, substances with sedative effects can be used by anxious or overaroused psychotic patients as anxiolytics. By comparison, those suffering from negative symptoms may value substances for their stimulant actions, a view particularly emphasized by Khantzian (1997). It is also possible that stimulant drugs make patients feel better by counteracting the dopamine D_2 blockade of antipsychotic drugs.

However, as discussed above, the substances abused by patients seem to reflect local availability and patterns of use in the general population more than a specific tendency for individuals with particular symptom profiles to select particular substances. Consequently, Mueser et al. (1998) conclude that there is little support for the narrow form of the self-medication hypothesis.

Dixon et al. (1990) found few self-reports in the literature of use of substances to alleviate positive symptoms of psychosis, perhaps not surprising as many drugs of abuse are known to exacerbate them. Whether subjects are seeking to alleviate negative symptoms through substance use is rather harder to ascertain, as it is difficult to elicit clear self-reports of such symptoms and difficult to judge whether self-medication is occurring for a symptom of which the subject may not be fully aware. Alleviation of general dysphoria of a variety of forms, including low mood, boredom and loneliness, is an effect reported for a range of substances used by people with schizophrenia in a number of studies (e.g. Noordsy et al., 1991; Carey and Carey, 1995; Mueser et al., 1998).

Surprisingly, few studies have enquired of patients why they take nonprescribed drugs. Fowler et al. (1998) asked their patients open-ended questions about their reasons for substance use and grouped their responses into four categories: drug intoxication effects (e.g. 'to get a lift'), dysphoria relief ('feel less anxious'), social effects ('be part of a group'), illness and medication-related effects ('get away from voices'). Among amphetamine abusers, 79% nominated drug intoxication effects; cannabis was used both to relieve dysphoria (62%) and for its intoxication effects (41%); alcohol was equally likely to be used for dysphoria relief and for social reasons (58%). Surprisingly, illness-related reasons, including the relief of antipsychotic drug side effects, were nominated by only a minority of substance users. However, those who abused rather than used alcohol were more likely to nominate illness and medication-related reasons for their consumption (14% versus 3%); this was also the case for abusers versus users of cannabis (16% versus 0%).

Of course, some drugs can both alleviate symptoms in the short term or at low dose and exacerbate them in the longer term or at higher dosages. This was shown by two studies of the effects of cannabis. In a prospective study, Linszen et al. (1994) showed that schizophrenics abusing low amounts of cannabis had fewer symptoms of anxiety and depression but that cannabis abuse resulted in significantly more and earlier psychotic relapses, the latter effect occurring particularly in those who abused high amounts of cannabis. Peralta and Cuesta (1992) also showed that low levels of consumption of cannabis by schizophrenic patients could attenuate negative symptoms but did not have an effect on positive symptoms. Therefore, it can be postulated that at low dosages the main action of cannabis on psychosis is attenuating anxiety and negative symptoms, while at high dosages it can precipitate positive symptoms.

Effects of the social milieu

Another possibility, less often considered, is that the social conditions in which many people with schizophrenia live, their unrewarding social lives and the problems they encounter in coping with daily life predispose them to substance use. This view proposes that patterns of substance use may be influenced by factors such as social isolation, difficulty in establishing a satisfactory social identity, boredom and lack of activity, and difficulty coping with social situations (Phillips and Johnson, 2001).

Bachrach (1989) considers substance misuse as one of a cluster of problems experienced by a generation of 'young chronic' patients who, although not institutionalized long term, have nonetheless not adjusted well to community living. The problems include erratic engagement with services, impulsive substance misuse and offending, poor social support, alienation from conventional authority and difficulty in establishing a clear role and identity. She views substance misuse as one of the dysfunctional coping strategies or antisocial behaviours engaged in by this generally alienated and chaotic group. Many of the characteristics described are those of the difficult-to-engage patients now identified as appropriate for assertive outreach teams. This conceptualization of the relationship between psychosis and substance misuse has implications for treatment strategies, suggesting that a broad focus is required on social difficulties and identity rather than a narrow one on treatment of substance misuse.

Dixon et al. (1990) examined the possibility that substance abuse provides isolated, socially handicapped individuals with an identity and a social group. Around half of their subjects endorsed an item suggesting that their drug use was a way of 'going along with the group'; they also point out, however, that drug use was solitary in many cases, so a purely social explanation is inadequate. Cuffel et al. (1993) mention boredom, lack of activity and difficulty initiating social contacts as factors in substance misuse among people with psychotic illnesses. Test et al. (1989) carried out semi-structured interviews with 29 young adults with schizophrenic illnesses who abused substances; the most frequently cited reason for using substances was to relieve boredom, followed by having something to do with friends, and then feeling more relaxed. Subjects were also asked to identify negative consequences of substance use and most frequently cited money problems, trouble keeping appointments, legal problems and hospitalization.

Finally, individuals with mental illness often meet and socialize with one another, both in and outside treatment settings. It is possible that drug and alcohol misuse may be disseminated, in part, in treatment settings and through the social networks of the mentally ill. For example, Sandford (1995) reported that 68% of the UK psychiatric nurses in their sample were aware of illicit drug use on the premises where they worked, which were mainly inpatient units, and that drug dealing was also taking place in these settings.

Is there a common factor underlying both schizophrenia and substance misuse?

Given the evidence of a major genetic component to schizophrenia (e.g. Cardno et al., 1999; see also Chs. 10 and 11) and a lesser but nevertheless important influence on substance abuse (Merikangas et al., 1998), there has been speculation that the conditions might have genes in common (e.g. Blanchard et al., 2000). Kendler (1985), in particular, has addressed this question, but so far the findings have not been very positive. It is unlikely that the question will be resolved until the genes responsible for the two conditions have been identified.

One way in which a shared genetic mechanism might operate is via inherited personality characteristics. Mueser et al. (1998) point out that there is a well-documented link between antisocial personality disorder and substance misuse and speculate that antisocial personality disorder may underlie both schizophrenia and substance misuse. They argue this on the basis of raised prevalence of antisocial personality disorder and the conduct disorder, which is frequently its precursor in childhood, among people with schizophrenia. We are not convinced by this argument, which is not supported by cohort studies (e.g. Jones et al., 1994).

One factor undoubtedly associated with both schizophrenia and substance misuse is low socioeconomic status. Most of the studies cited above that have made comparisons with general population samples have not taken socioeconomic status into account; consequently the extent to which substance abuse among people with schizophrenia may be at comparable levels to that among others with similar experiences of social deprivation and unemployment has not been clearly established.

Characteristics of schizophrenic patients who abuse substances

Sex

Substance abuse is more common in male than female patients (Drake et al., 1989, 1996; Pulver et al., 1989; Hambrecht et al., 1992; Cuffel et al., 1993; De-Quadro et al., 1994). For example, Menezes et al. (1996) found that male psychotic patients in south London were twice as likely as their female counterparts to abuse any substance, presumably a reflection of sex differences in the alcohol and drug consumption of the general population.

Age at onset

Psychotic patients who abuse drugs have an earlier age of onset of psychosis than those who do not (Breakey et al., 1974; Drake et al., 1989; Pulver et al., 1989; Cuffel et al., 1993; De-Quadro et al., 1994; Menezes et al., 1996). In the study of Häfner et al. (1999) discussed above, the mean age of onset of psychosis in patients abusing drugs before their first admission was 24.6 years, while that of those who did not abuse drugs was 31.1 years. Although this difference is a consistent finding, it has been difficult to disentangle the possible role of drug abuse in precipitating the psychosis from the fact that younger people tend to abuse drugs more than their elders, and males more than females. Indeed, Rabinowitz et al. (1998) draw attention to the fact that many of the comparisons of age of onset have been made without controlling for sex (males with schizophrenia both have an earlier mean age of onset than females and are more likely to have comorbid substance abuse).

Premorbid personality

Amminger et al. (1999) suggested that the premorbid characteristics of patients with schizophrenia who abuse substances are different from those of patients who do not. These authors followed up the offspring of parents with psychosis and divided those offspring who developed schizophrenia-related psychoses into those with and without comorbid substance abuse. Childhood behavioural problems were found to have been more common among the psychotic patients who did not abuse drugs. Possibly related to these findings are reports of better premorbid personality and social adjustment in people with schizophrenia and substance misuse than those with schizophrenia only (Turner and Tsuang, 1990; Arndt et al., 1992).

The probable explanation is that those preschizophrenic individuals who have shown noticeably abnormal childhood function require little or no additional stress to become frankly psychotic in adult life; by comparison, those with little or no neurodevelopmental impairment are likely to need more in the way of proximal risk factors such as drug abuse before they become psychotic. An additional argument is that those schizophrenic patients with childhood impairment are less likely to have acquired the social skills and initiative necessary first to be exposed to substance abuse and then to obtain and fund the consumption of large quantities of alcohol and/or drugs.

Chen (2001) compared 174 methamphetamine abusers who developed psychosis with 261 who did not. Those who became psychotic had more disordered personality, tended also to abuse other drugs, and their mothers rated their childhood personality more highly on a schizoid–schizotypal inventory. Furthermore, those whose psychosis persisted for more than 6 months were especially likely to have had a deviant childhood personality, and their relatives were more likely to have had a psychotic illness.

Effect of substance abuse on outcome of psychosis

There is little doubt that a person with schizophrenia in remission who then returns to abusing substances can be precipitated into a relapse of his/her psychosis This may be through a direct effect on psychotic symptoms as with the dopaminergic effects or indirectly by an increase in depression or anxiety, which are known to predispose to relapse of psychosis. In addition, when individuals return to substance abuse, their compliance with antipsychotic medication often declines, their self-care deteriorates and increasing poverty often ensues, with the resultant social crisis acting as a trigger.

Use of services

In south London, Menezes et al. (1996) reported that patients who abused substances had attended the psychiatric emergency services 1.3 times more frequently over the previous 2 years and had spent 1.8 times as many days in hospital as their nonabusing counterparts. Gerding et al. (1999a,b) found that psychotic patients with alcohol dependence were at a higher risk for hospital admission and had longer hospital stays than those who were not dependent on alcohol. Greater use of inpatient and emergency facilities tends to be accompanied by higher overall treatment costs. For example, examining costs associated with treatment of severe mental illness in public sector facilities, Dickey and Azeni (1996) concluded that people with schizophrenia and substance misuse incurred costs 60% higher than those with psychotic illness alone.

In the ABC study, Häfner et al. (1999) compared the outcome of 133 first-admitted schizophrenic patients who had been drug/alcohol abusers at first episode with those who had not. At first admission, patients who abused alcohol or drugs had significantly more delusions and hallucinations. Over the subsequent 5 years, there were no differences in the global SANS (scale for the assessment of negative symptoms) score or in total days hospitalized or in social disability. However, the comorbid patients were much less compliant with prescribed medication or with rehabilitation programmes. This study can be criticized on the basis that the analysis of effects of substance abuse on outcome was based solely on data concerning substance abuse habits at first admission.

Fortunately, other studies have collected data on drug abuse throughout the period of follow-up. In Holland, Linszen et al. (1994) compared cannabis-abusing schizophrenic outpatients with their nonabusing counterparts over a 12-month follow-up period. The abusers, particularly the heavier abusers, were more likely to have a relapse and, indeed, many reported an increase in their psychotic symptoms soon after taking cannabis. Caspari et al. (1999) followed 27 schizophrenic patients with a history of cannabis use for a mean of 69 months and compared their outcome with that of schizophrenic patients without such a history. About half of the cannabis users ceased their consumption or switched to alcohol. Nevertheless, those with a history of cannabis use had significantly more hospitalizations, tended to worse psychosocial functioning and showed more thought disorder and hostility. Grech et al. (1999) replicated these findings in a prospective 4-year follow-up of 98 patients with recent onset of psychosis in south London. Those who were noted to abuse cannabis at both index and follow-up interviews had the most chronic outcome. There was a dose-dependent adverse influence of cannabis intake on subsequent positive, but not negative, psychotic symptoms.

Kovasznay et al. (1997) reported similar findings from a study of patients suffering their first episode of schizophrenia. Those patients who had a lifetime history of substance use disorder showed worse clinical functioning, as reflected in worse GAF (global assessment of functioning) scores. After 6 months of follow-up, the authors concluded that further cannabis use 'may exacerbate overall symptoms, as represented by the BPRS score, while showing little effect on the negative symptoms as represented by the SANS'.

Owen et al. (1996) reported a significant association between substance abuse and medication noncompliance among people with schizophrenia, a relationship that may to some extent mediate the relationship between schizophrenia and some of its other adverse associations. They suggest that reasons for this increased rate of noncompliance may include neglecting to take medication when intoxicated and increased side effects because of an interaction between antipsychotic drugs and the substances taken. They also suggest that some substance misusers with schizophrenia stop taking medication because they have been told not to combine medication with substances of abuse.

Risk of violence

Many studies have reported that psychotic patients who also abuse drugs or alcohol are more likely to be violent and are more likely to be imprisoned (Ch. 17). Cross-sectional data from the ECA study also indicated a higher prevalence of self-reported violence among individuals with schizophrenia and substance misuse (24.5% with alcohol use, 37.4% with drug use) than among people with schizophrenia only (12.7%; Regier et al., 1990).

There have also been two careful prospective studies. Rasanen et al. (1998) prospectively followed a birth cohort of 11 017 individuals born in northern Finland in 1996 to age 26 years and collected data on psychiatric disorders and crime from the comprehensive Finnish national registers. Men who were diagnosed as having both schizophrenia and alcoholism were 25 times more likely to commit violent crimes than mentally healthy men; the risk for schizophrenic men who did not abuse alcohol was 3.6. Therefore, schizophrenic men with concomitant alcoholism were seven times more likely to commit such a crime than sober schizophrenic men.

In another birth cohort study, Arsenault et al. (2000) studied all 1037 individuals born in Dunedin, New Zealand in the year 1972–73 and successfully followed up 94% of them to age 21 years. Within the sample, 11.3% of the risk of becoming a violent offender was attributable to alcohol dependence, 28.2% to marijuana dependence and 9.6% to schizophrenia spectrum disorder. Having two of these together doubled the risk compared with having one of them. The OR for being a violent offender was 8.3 (95% confidence interval (CI) 3.3–21.5) for alcohol dependence plus schizophrenia spectrum disorder; for marijuana dependence plus schizophrenia spectrum disorder it was 18.4 (95% CI 7.5–45.3).

Other outcomes

Compared with their nonabusing counterparts, those with coexisting substance abuse have higher rates of homelessness (Drake et al., 1991) and more unemployment (Seibyl et al., 1993). Relationships with some other indicators of adverse outcome are less strong and consistently found. For example, study results have varied considerably in findings about whether comorbidity is associated with worse positive symptoms (Arndt et al., 1992; Cuffel et al., 1993; Rabinowitz et al., 1998). It should also be borne in mind that sometimes the associations found might be explained by a number of different causal mechanisms. For example, the finding that comorbid substance misuse in schizophrenia is associated with an increased prevalence of low mood and suicidal behaviour (e.g. Pulver et al., 1989; Kovaznay et al., 1993) might be explained by substance use causing low mood. However, the reverse of this causal link is also a possibility: it may be that those people with schizophrenia who are more depressed are more likely to resort to substance use as a way of coping with this depression. In the USA, several studies have found high rates of infection with human immunodeficiency virus among people with dual diagnosis (RachBeisel et al., 1999).

Future studies

As this review has shown, progress has been bedevilled by the large number of poorly designed studies available so far. In future, it will be preferable to have a small number of large well-designed prospective studies. These should examine how substance misuse and its correlates develop among people with schizophrenia and also the rates and patterns of development of psychotic symptoms among cohorts of substance users. Epidemiologically based follow-up studies need to be conducted both on patients suffering from schizophrenia in whom substance abuse predates the onset of psychosis and on patients with schizophrenia who started to abuse substances after the onset of psychotic illness. Such studies could clarify how the one condition can influence the development of the other.

It is also desirable that future studies should differentiate more clearly between the abuse of different substances (though obviously polysubstance use can make this difficult) and also the quantities of individual substances abused by the probands. This is to allow for the possible different effects caused by the same substance at different levels of intake. Detailed information needs to be collected on the symptoms of schizophrenia that probands are suffering from, in order to ascertain if a particular substance of abuse is associated or not with a particular symptom. The social contexts in which substance misuse develops and continues, and the reasons for use that patients themselves report, also warrant more attention.

Finally, a major problem that we have not yet considered is the likely unreliability of much of the information collected about substance use. In future studies, this problem could be partly resolved by using analysis of blood, urine or hair. Hair analysis has the advantages of being easier to obtain than blood or urine, and of giving information on substance intake over a longer period of time (Marsh, 1997). While such toxicological analyses provide some evidence as to whether an individual is using a drug and over what time, the information provided on pattern of use and associated problems is obviously very limited. Therefore, full assessment of whether dependence or misuse are present will always require further information. Use of multiple methods of assessment, including the perspectives of patients, clinicians and carers, as well as physical examination and laboratory tests is the best way of accurately detecting and assessing substance use disorders (Drake et al., 1991).

REFERENCES

American Psychiatric Association (1987) Diagnostic and Statistical Manual III–Revised. Washington, DC: American Psychiatric Press.

Amminger GP, Pape S, Rock D et al. (1999) Relationship between childhood behavioral disturbance and later schizophrenia in the New York High-Risk Project. American Journal of Psychiatry 156, 525–530.

Andreasson S, Alleback P, Engstrom A, Rydberg U (1987) Cannabis and Schizophrenia: a longitudinal study of Swedish conscripts. Lancet ii, 1483–1486.

Arndt S, Tyrrell G, Flaum M et al. (1992) Comorbidity of substance abuse and schizophrenia: the role of premorbid adjustment. Psychological Medicine 22, 379–388.

Arsenault L, Moffitt TE, Caspi A, Taylor PJ, Silva PA (2000) Mental disorders and violence in a total birth cohort. Archives of General Psychiatry 57, 979–986.

Ashton CH (2000) Pharmacology and effects of cannabis. British Journal of Psychiatry 177, 469–472.

Bachrach L (1989) Sociological factors associated with substance abuse among new chronic patients. In: Adolescent Psychiatry: Developmental and Clinical Studies, Vol. 16, Feinstein S, Esman A, eds. Chicago, IL: University of Chicago, pp. 189–201.

Bartlett E, Hallin E, Chapman B, Angirst B (1997) Selective-sensitisation to the psychosis-inducing effects of cocaine. A possible marker for addiction relapse vulnerability? Neuropsychopharmacology 16, 77–82.

Bernadt MW, Murray RM (1986) Psychiatric disorder, drinking and alcoholism: What are the links? British Journal of Psychiatry 148, 393–400.

Blanchard JJ, Brown SA, Horan WP, Sherwood AR (2000) Substance use disorders in schizophrenia: review, integration, and a proposed model. Clinical Psychology Review 20, 207–234.

Boutros N, Bowers M (1996) Chronic substance-induced psychotic disorders: state of the literature. Journal of Neuropsychiatry and Clinical Neurosciences 8, 262–269.

Breakey WR, Goodell H, Lorenz PC, McHugh P (1974) Hallucinogenic drugs as precipitants of schizophrenia. Psychological Medicine 4, 255–261.

Buckley PF (1998) Substance abuse in schizophrenia: a review. Journal of Clinical Psychiatry 59(Suppl. 3), 26–30.

Cantwell R, Brewin J, Glazebrok C et al. (1999) Prevalence of substance abuse in first episode psychosis. British Journal of Psychiatry 174, 150–153.

Cardno A, Marshall J, Coid B et al. (1999) Heritability estimates for psychotic disorders: the Maudsley Twin Psychosis Series. Archives of General Psychiatry 56, 162–168.

Carey K, Carey M (1995) Reasons for drinking among psychiatric outpatients: relationship to drinking patterns. Psychology of Addictive Behaviors 9, 251–257.

Caspari D (1999) Cannabis and schizophrenia: results of a follow-up study. European Archives of Psychiatry and Clinical Neuroscience 249, 45–50.

Cassano CB, Pini S, Saettoni M et al. (1998) Occurrence and clinical correlates of psychiatric comorbidity in patients with psychotic disorders. Journal of Clinical Psychiatry 59, 60–68.

Chen C-K (2001) Predisposing factors to methamphetamine psychosis. PhD thesis, University of London, UK.

Connell PH (1958) Amphetamine Psychosis. Glasgow: Chapman Hall for the Institute of Psychiatry.

Cuffel BJ, Heithoff KA, Lawson W (1993) Correlates of patterns of abuse among patients with schizophrenia. Hospital and Community Psychiatry 44, 247–251.

DeQuadro JR, Carpenter CF, Tandon R (1994) Patterns of substance abuse in schizophrenia: nature and significance. Journal of Psychiatric Research 28, 267–275.

Dickey B, Azeni H (1996) Persons with dual diagnoses of substance abuse and major mental illness: their excess costs of psychiatric care. American Journal of Public Health 86, 973–977.

Diwan A, Castine M, Pomerleau CS, Meador-Woodruff JH, Dalack GW (1998) Differential prevalence of cigarette smoking in patients with schizophrenic vs mood disorders. Schizophrenia Research 33, 113–118.

Dixon L, Haas G, Weiden P, Sweeney J, Allen F (1990) Acute effects of drug abuse in schizophrenic patients: clinical observations and patients' self-reports. Schizophrenia Bulletin 16, 69–79.

Dixon L, Haas G, Weiden PJ, Sweeney J, Frances AJ (1991) Drug abuse in schizophrenic patients: clinical correlates and reasons for use. American Journal of Psychiatry 148, 224–230.

Drake RE, Osher FC, Wallach MA (1989) Alcohol use and abuse in schizophrenia. A prospective community study. Journal of Nervous and Mental Disease 177, 408–414.

Drake R, Antosca LM, Noordsy DL, Bartels SJ, Osher FC (1991) New Hampshire's specialised services for the dually diagnosed. New Directions for Mental Health Services 50, 57–67.

Drake R, Rosenberg S, Mueser K (1996) Assessing substance use disorder in persons with severe mental illness. New Directions for Mental Health Services 70, 3–17.

el-Guebaly N, Hodgins DC (1992) Schizophrenia and substance abuse: Prevalence issues. Canadian Journal of Psychiatry 37, 704–710.

Farrell M, Howes S, Taylor C et al. (1998) Substance misuse and psychiatric comorbidity: an overview of the OPCS National Psychiatric Morbidity Survey. Addictive Behaviours 23, 909–918.

Flaum M, Schultz SK (1996) When does amphetamine-induced psychosis become schizophrenia? American Journal of Psychiatry 153, 812–815.

Fowler IL, Carr VJ, Carter NT, Lewin TJ (1998) Patterns of current and lifetime substance use in schizophrenia. Schizophrenia Bulletin 24, 443–455.

Gardner EL, Lowinson JH (1991) Marijuana's interaction with brain reward systems: update 1991. Pharmacology, Biochemistry and Behavior 40, 571–580.

Gerding LB, Labbate LA, Measom MO, Santos AB, Arana GW (1999a) Alcohol dependence and hospitalization in schizophrenia. Schizophrenia Research 38, 71–75.

Gerding LB, Labbate LA, Measom MO, Santos AB, Arana GW (1999b) Alcohol dependence and hospitalization in schizophrenia. Schizophrenia Research 38, 71–75.

Grech A, Takei N, Murray R (1998) Comparison of cannabis use in psychotic patients and controls in London and Malta. Schizophrenia Research 29, 22.

Grech A, van Os J, Murray RM (1999) Influence of cannabis on the outcome of psychosis. Schizophrenia Research 36, 41.

Häfner H, Maurer K, Loffler W et al. (1999) Onset and prodromal phase as Determinants of Course. In: Search for the Causes of Schizophrenia, Vol. IV, Balance of the Century, Gattaz W, Häfner H, eds. Berlin: Springer-Verlag, pp. 35–58.

Hambrecht M, Häfner H (1996) Substance abuse and the onset of schizophrenia. Biological Psychiatry 40, 1155–1163.

Hambrecht M, Maurer K, Häfner H (1992) Gender differences in schizophrenia in three cultures. Results of the WHO collaborative study on psychiatric disability. Social Psychiatry and Psychiatric Epidemiology 27, 117–121.

Hill AB (1965) The environment and disease: association or causation? Proceedings of the Royal Society of Medicine 58, 295–300.

Hippius H, Peters G, Ploog D (eds) (1987) Kraepelin Memoirs. Berlin: Springer-Verlag, p. 71.

Indian Hemp Drugs Commission (1894) Report. Simla: IHDC.

Jablensky A, McGrath J, Herrman, Castle D, Gureje et al. (2000) Psychotic disorders in urban areas. Australian and New Zealand Journal of Psychiatry 34, 221–236.

Johns A (2001) Psychiatric effects of cannabis. British Journal of Psychiatry 178, 116–122.

Jones PB, Rodgers B, Murray RM, Marmot M (1994) Child developmental risk factors for adult schizophrenia in the British 1946 birth cohort. Lancet 344, 1398–1402.

Kelly C, McCreadie RG (1999) Smoking habits, current symptoms, and premorbid characteristics of schizophrenic patients in Nithsdale, Scotland. American Journal of Psychiatry 56, 1751–1757.

Kendler KS (1985) A twin study of individuals with both schizophrenia and alcoholism. British Journal of Psychiatry 147, 48–53.

Kendler KS, Gallagher TJ, Abelson JM, Kessler R (1996) Lifetime prevalence, demographic risk factors and diagnostic validity of nonaffective psychosis as assessed in a US community sample. Archives of General Psychiatry 53, 1022–1031.

Khantzian EJ (1997) The self-medication hypothesis of substance abuse disorders. Harvard Review of Psychiatry 4, 231–244.

Knight F (1976) Role of cannabis in psychiatric disturbance. Annals of New York Academy of Science 282, 64–71.

Kovasznay B, Bromet E, Schwartz JE, Ram R, Lavelle J, Brandon L (1993) Substance abuse and onset of psychotic illness. Hospital and Community Psychiatry 44, 567–571.

Kovasznay B, Fleischer J, Tanenberg-Karant M, Jandorf L, Miller AD, Bromet E (1997) Substance use disorder and the early course of illness in schizophrenia and affective psychosis. Schizophrenia Bulletin 23, 195–201.

Lambert M, Haasen C, Mass R et al. (1997) Konsummuster und Konsummotivation des Suchtmittelgebrauchs bei schizophrenen Patienten. Psychiatrische Praxis 27, 185–189.

Launay C, Petitjean F, Perdereau F, Antoine D (1998) Conduites toxicomaniaques chez les malades mentaux: une enquete en Ile-de-France. Annales Medico-Psychologiques 156, 482–486.

Leon D, Dadvand M, Canuso C, White AO, Stanilla JK, Simpson GM (1995) Schizophrenia and smoking; an epidemiological study in a state hospital. American Journal of Psychiatry 152, 453–455.

Linszen DH, Dingemans PM, Lenior MA (1994) Cannabis abuse and the course of recent-onset schizophrenic disorders. Archives of General Psychiatry 51, 273–279.

Longhurst JG, Boutros NN, Bowers MB (1997) Australian and New Zealand Journal of Psychiatry 31, 305–306.

McCreadie RM, Kelly C (2000) Patients with schizophrenia who smoke: private disaster, public resource. British Journal of Psychiatry 176, 109.

McGuire P, Jones P, Harvey I, Williams M, McGuffin P, Murray R (1995) Morbid risk of schizophrenia for relatives of patients with cannabis-associated psychosis. Schizophrenia Research 15, 277–281.

McLellan AT, Woody GE, O'Brien CP (1979) Development of psychotic illness in drug abusers: possible role of drug preference. New England Journal of Medicine 301, 1310–1314.

Marsh A (1997) Hair analysis for drugs of abuse. Syva Drug Monitor 2, 1–4.

Mathers DC, Ghodse AH (1992) Cannabis and psychotic illness. British Journal of Psychiatry 161, 648–653.

Mathers DC, Ghodse AH, Caan AW, Scott SA (1991) Cannabis use in a large sample of acute psychiatric admissions. British Journal of Addiction 86, 779–784.

Menezes P, Johnson S, Thornicroft G et al. (1996) Drug and alcohol problems among individuals with severe mental illness in South London. British Journal of Psychiatry 168, 612–619.

Merikangas KR, Stolar M, Stephens DE et al. (1998) Familial transmission of substance use disorders. Archives of General Psychiatry 55, 973–979.

Modestin J, Nussbaumer C, Angst D, Scheidegger P, Hell D (1997) Use of potentially abusive psychotropic substances in psychiatric inpatients. European Archives of Psychiatry and Clinical Neurosciences 247, 146–153.

Mueser K, Yarnold P, Levinson D et al. (1990) Prevalence of substance use in schizophrenia: demographic and clinical correlates. Schizophrenia Bulletin 16, 31–56.

Mueser K, Drake RE, Wallach MA (1998) Dual diagnosis: a review of etiological theories. Addictive Behaviors 23, 717–734.

Murray RM, Fearon P (1999) The developmental 'risk factor' model of schizophrenia. Journal of Psychiatric Research 33, 497–499.

Murray RM, O'Callaghan E, Castle DJ, Lewis SW (1992) A neurodevelopmental approach to the classification of schizophrenia. Schizophrenia Bulletin 18, 319–332.

Negrete J, Knapp W, Douglas D, Smith W (1986) Cannabis affects the severity of schizophrenic symptoms: results of a clinical survey. Psychological Medicine 16, 515–520.

Noordsy D, Drake RE, Teague G et al. (1991) Subjective experiences related to alcohol use among schizophrenics. Journal of Nervous and Mental Disease 179, 410–414.

Owen R, Fischer E, Booth B, Cuffel B (1996) Medication noncompliance and substance abuse among patients with schizophrenia. Psychiatric Services 47, 853–858.

Patel V, Borysenko M, Kumar MS (1985) Effects of delta THC on brain and plasma cathecolamine levels as measured by HPLC. Brain Research Bulletin 14, 85–90.

Patkar AA, Alexander RC, Lundy A, Certa KM (1999) Changing patterns of illicit substance use among schizophrenic patients: 1984–1996. American Journal of Addiction 8, 65–71.

Peralta V, Cuesta MJ (1992) Influence of cannabis abuse on schizophrenic psychopathology. Acta Psychiatrica Scandinavica 85, 127–130.

Phillips P, Johnson S (2001) How does drug and alcohol abuse develop among people with schizophrenia? Social Psychiatry and Psychiatric Epidemiology 36, 269–276.

Poole R, Brabbins C (1996) Drug induced psychosis. British Journal of Psychiatry 168, 1350–1358.

Pulver AE, Wolyniec PS, Wagner MG, Moorman CC, McGarath JA (1989) An epidemiologic investigation of alcohol dependent schizophrenics. Acta Psychiatrica Scandinavica 79, 603–612.

Rabinowitz J, Bromet EJ, Lavelle J, Carlson G, Kovasznay B, Schwartz JE (1998) Prevalence and severity of substance use disorders and onset of psychosis in first-admission psychotic patients. Psychological Medicine 28, 1411–1419.

RachBeisel J, Scott J, Dixon L (1999) Co-occurring severe mental illness and substance use disorders: a review of recent research. Psychiatric Services 50, 1427–1434.

Rasanen P, Tihonen J, Isohanni M, Rantakakallio P, Lehtonen J, Moring J (1998) Schizophrenia, alcohol abuse, and violent behaviour. Schizophrenia Bulletin 24, 437–441.

Regier DA, Farmer ME, Rae DS et al. (1990) Comorbidity of mental disorders with alcohol and other drug abuse. Results from the Epidemiological Catchment Area (ECA) Study. Journal of the American Medical Association 264, 2511–2518.

Robins LN, Reiger DA (eds.) (1991) Psychiatric Disorders in America: The Epidemiological Catchment Area Study. New York: Free Press.

Rolfe M, Tang CM, Sabally S, Todd JE, Sam EB, Hstib NJB (1993) Psychosis and cannabis abuse in the Gambia. A case-control study. British Journal of Psychiatry 163, 798–801.

Rottanburg D, Robins A, Ben-Arie O et al. (1982) Cannabis-associated psychosis with manic features. Lancet ii, 1364–1366.

Sandford T (1995) Drug use is increasing. Nursing Standard 9, 16.

Satel SL, Seibyl JP, Charney DS (1991) Prolonged cocaine abuse implies underlying major psychopathology. Journal of Clinical Psychiatry 52, 349–350.

Schneier FR, Siris SG (1987) A review of psychoactive substance use and abuse in schizophrenia. Patterns of drug choice. Journal of Nervous and Mental Disease 175, 641–652.

Seibyl JP, Satel SL, Anthony D, Southwick SM, Krystal JH, Charney DS (1993) Effects of cocaine on hospital course in schizophrenia. Journal of Nervous and Mental Disease 181, 31–37.

Sharpley MS, Hutchinson G, McKenzie K, Murray RM (2001) Understanding the excess of psychosis among the African-Caribbean population in England: review of current hypotheses. British Journal of Psychiatry 178 (Suppl. 40), S60–S68.

Silver H, Abboud E (1994) Drug abuse in schizophrenia: comparison of patients who began drug abuse before their first admission with those who began abusing drugs after their first admission. Schizophrenia Research 13, 57–63.

Soyka M, Albus M, Kathmann M et al. (1993) Prevalence of alcohol and drug abuse in schizophrenic in-patients. European Archives of Psychiatry and Clinical Neurosciences 242, 362–372.

Tanda G, Pontieri FE, Di Chiara G (1997) Cannabinoid and heroin activation of mesolimbic dopamine transmission by a common μ_1 opioid receptor mechanism. Science 276, 2048–2050.

Test M, Wallisch L, Allness D, Ripp K (1989) Substance use in young adults with schizophrenic disorders. Schizophrenia Bulletin 15, 465–476.

Thornicroft G (1990) Cannabis and psychosis. Is there epidemiological evidence for an association? British Journal of Psychiatry 157, 25–33.

Turner W, Tsuang M (1990) Impact of substance abuse on course and outcome of schizophrenia. Schizophrenia Bulletin 16, 87–95.

van Os J, Jones P, Sham P, Bebbington P, Murray R M (1998) Risk factors for onset and persistence of psychosis. Social Psychiatry and Psychiatric Epidemiology 33, 596–605.

Verdoux H, Mury M, Besancon G, Bourgeois M (1996) Etude comparative des conduites toxicomaniaques dans les trouble bipolaires, schizophreniques et schizoaffectifs. L'Encephale 22, 95–101.

Yousef G, Huq Z, Lambert T (1995) Khat chewing as a cause of psychosis. British Journal of Hospital Medicine 54, 322–326.

Ziedonis DM, George TP (1997) Smoking and nicotine use. Schizophrenia Bulletin 23, 247–254.

17

Criminal and violent behaviour in schizophrenia

Elizabeth Walsh and Alec Buchanan

Institute of Psychiatry, Kings College London, UK

The conclusions of those researching the putative link between schizophrenia and violence changed in the second half of the 20th century. Up until the early 1980s, the general consensus was that those with schizophrenia were no more likely than the general population to be violent. New epidemiological evidence has emerged, however, in recent years that has radically challenged this view. It is now generally accepted that people with schizophrenia, albeit by virtue of the activity of a small subgroup, are significantly more likely to be violent than members of the general population, but the proportion of societal violence attributable to this group is small. This chapter reviews the influential epidemiological studies in this area and provides an appraisal of the difficulties inherent in this type of research, with suggestions of how these might be overcome. We attempt to differentiate those most at risk of behaving violently and identify the likely victims of such acts. We conclude with some estimate of the absolute risk posed to the community by those with schizophrenia.

Review of studies investigating violent behaviour in schizophrenia

Three different approaches have been used to examine the association between schizophrenia and violence:
1 Studies estimating the prevalence of violent acts in those with schizophrenia
2 Studies estimating the prevalence of schizophrenia in individuals who have committed violent acts
3 Community-based epidemiological studies estimating the prevalence of violence in those with and without schizophrenia regardless of involvement with the mental health or criminal justice systems.

Studies estimating the prevalence of violent acts among those with schizophrenia

Two main study designs have been used to estimate the prevalence of violent acts among those with schizophrenia: first, cross-sectional studies before admission, during the course of hospitalization and following discharge from hospital; and second, cohort studies using case-linkage techniques.

Cross-sectional studies

With violence being a main selection criteria for admission to hospital, studies of violence committed before and during hospitalization are of limited usefulness as they will overestimate any association.

Before hospitalization

Humphreys et al. (1992) estimated that 20% of first-admission patients with Present State Examination (PSE)-diagnosed schizophrenia (Wing et al., 1974) had behaved in a life-threatening manner prior to admission. Volvavka et al. (1997), as part of the World Health Organization (WHO) study on determinants of outcome of severe mental disorders, estimated that 20% of first-contact patients with ICD-9 (World Health Organization, 1978) schizophrenia had assaulted another person at some time in the past. The assault (according to a combination of self-report, informant and case note information) coincided with the reported onset of illness in 58% of patients. An interesting finding in this study was the threefold elevated risk of violence among those from developing relative to developed countries.

During hospitalization

Violence among inpatients is a well-researched topic. These studies have suggested relatively high rates of assaultiveness, especially among patients with schizophrenia (Karson & Bigelow, 1987; Walker & Seifert, 1994). Results must be viewed with particular caution as violence may be more a response to the contextual setting of a confined ward than to an individual's mental state.

Following discharge

Discharged patients are a selected group as they are generally judged not to pose a threat or to pose less threat than those retained in hospital. As such, one would expect lower rates of violence to be recorded at this time than prior to admission.

The two most comprehensive studies published to date on violence risk postdischarge fail to provide separate data for schizophrenia (Steadman et al., 1998, Link et al., 1992; see below). Steadman et al. (1998) compared the prevalence of community violence in a sample of patients with a range of diagnoses, including schizophrenia, discharged from three acute psychiatric facilities with a group of residents living in one of the three areas. Violence was measured from multiple sources every 10 weeks for 1 year in patients and once for community controls. Although outcome violence measures used in this study have been the best to date, the study had a number of limitations, referred to below. Monahan & Applebaum (2000) have subsequently examined violence prevalence in the sample by diagnosis in the first 20 weeks following discharge. In their group, 17% of patients had a diagnosis of schizophrenia and of these 9% were violent. This compares with 19% for depression, 15% for bipolar disorder, 17.2% for other psychotic disorders, 29% for substance misuse disorders and 25% for personality disorder alone. The fact that this and other studies have found rates of violence to be lower in those with schizophrenia than in those with other diagnoses (Harris et al., 1993; Wallace et al., 1998) should not be misinterpreted to suggest schizophrenia may be irrelevant or even a protective factor against violence. It is probably true that schizophrenia is less of a violence risk than substance misuse, personality disorder and possibly other mental disorders, but when compared with the general population, as this review demonstrates, the evidence is overwhelmingly in favour of an increased rate of violent behaviour in schizophrenia.

Using a case-control design and at least one previous hospital admission as inclusion criteria, Modestin & Ammann (1996) compared lifetime prevalence of criminal behaviour in males with Research Diagnostic Criteria (RDC)-defined schizophrenia (Spitzer et al., 1990) with matched catchment area controls. After a search for criminal histories in the Swiss Central Criminal Records Department, the schizophrenic group were up to four times more likely to have been convicted of a violent offence.

Cohort studies

The cohort studies fall into two categories: retrospective studies of those diagnosed with schizophrenia traced on criminal registers and studies of prospective unselected birth cohorts where both psychiatric and criminal status are established from case registers and linked. The cohort studies are summarized in Table 17.1.

Retrospective cohorts using case linkage

Three studies using slightly different methodologies have drawn similar conclusions. In the first, a search was conducted up to 15 years later on the police register for 644 patients with ICD-8-defined schizophrenia (World Health Organization, 1967) discharged during 1 year and born between 1920 and 1959 in Sweden. The risk of violent offences in this group was estimated relative to the general population. Violent crimes were found to be four times more frequent among those with schizophrenia than in the general population (Lindqvist & Allebeck, 1990).

The second controlled for time at liberty to offend and compared the rate of criminal convictions among 538 incident cases of schizophrenia with that of nonpsychotic psychiatric controls matched for age and sex (Wessely et al., 1994). The risk of being convicted of violent offences for males with schizophrenia was at least twice that of men with other mental disorders. This was despite the control group

Table 17.1. Cohort studies on the prevalence of violence among psychiatric patients[a]

Authors	Location	No.	Diagnostic group[b]	Time period	Definition of violence
Retrospective					
Lindqvist and Allebeck (1990)	Sweden	790	Schizophrenia (ICD-8)	1971–86	Violent offences (criminal records)
Wessely et al. (1994)	England	538	Schizophrenia (ICD-9/DSM-III-R)	1964–84	Violent convictions (official records)
Mullen et al. (2000)	Australia	1084	Schizophrenia (ICD-9)	1975–95	Violent convictions (official records)
Prospective					
Hodgins (1992)	Sweden	15 117	All disorders	1953–83	Violent offences (official records)
Hodgins et al. (1996)	Denmark	324 401	All disorders (ICD-8)	1944–47	Violent convictions (official records)
Tiihonen et al. (1997)	Finland	12 058	All disorders	1966–92	Violent crimes (criminal records)
Brennan et al. (2000)	Denmark	335 990	Major mental disorders (ICD-8)	1944–47	Violent convictions (criminal records)
Arseneault et al. (2000)	New Zealand	961	All disorders (DSM-III-R)	1972–94	Court convictions and self-reported violence

Notes:

[a] Both male and female patients.

[b] See text for diagnostic criteria.

containing a substantial minority of individuals with psychiatric disorders with an established and noncontroversial association with crime. Women with schizophrenia were also significantly more likely to be convicted of violent crime than controls.

In the third study, Mullen et al. (2000) in Australia studied two groups of patients with schizophrenia first admitted in either 1975 (before major deinstitutionalization) or 1985 (when community care was becoming the norm). Compared with general population controls, both groups were significantly more likely to be convicted for all categories of criminal offending except sexual offences. Those with comorbid substance abuse accounted for a disproportionate amount of offending. The increased number of convictions in those with schizophrenia in the 1985 group compared with the 1975 group seemed to reflect a general increase in offending in those of a similar age, sex and place of residence. As such, the shift to community care was not marked by any significant change in relative rates of conviction in schizophrenia. The effect of community care on risk of violence in schizophrenia requires further study. One study examining homicide statistics in the UK has reported little fluctuation in the numbers of people with mental illness committing homicide between 1957 and 1995 and a 3% annual decline in their contribution to the official statistics (Taylor & Gunn, 1999).

Unselected birth cohort studies
Hodgins (1992), in a 30-year follow-up of an unselected Swedish birth cohort, studied the association between major mental disorder and criminality. Compared with those with no mental disorder, males with major mental disorder had a four-fold and women a 27.5-fold increased risk of violent offences. As the group with major mental disorder included a range of diagnostic entities, it was not possible to estimate the relative risk of violence for schizophrenia alone. A later study using the same methodology had similar findings (Hodgins et al., 1996).

Tiihonen et al. (1997), followed an unselected birth cohort of 12 058 individuals prospectively for 26 years. This was the first cohort study to demonstrate the quantitative risk of criminal and violent behaviour for specific psychotic categories (Table 17.2). The risk among males with schizophrenia for violent offences was 7 relative to controls without mental disorder. The risk of violent offences was highest among those with comorbid substance abuse.

Brennan et al. (2000) studied all subjects born in Denmark over a 4-year period and traced all arrests for violence and hospitalizations for mental illness that occurred for these individuals up to 44 years of age. Schizophrenia was the only major mental disorder associated with increased risks of violent crime among both men (odds ratio (OR) 2.0; 95% confidence interval (CI) 1.5–2.6) and women (OR 7.5; 95% CI 4.0–14.1) after adjusting for socioeconomic status, marital status and substance abuse (Table 17.2).

Table 17.2. *Associations between psychoses and violent convictions in studies of unselected birth cohorts*

Authors	Schizophrenia odds ratio (95% CI)	Affective psychosis odds ratio (95% CI)	Organic psychosis odds ratio (95% CI)
Tiihonen et al. (1997)[a]	M: 7.2 (3.6–16.6)	M: 10.4 (1.2–94)	
Brennan et al. (2000)[b]	M: 1.9 (1.4–2.6)	M: 0.8 (0.4–1.5)	M: 2.2 (1.4–3.5)
	F: 7.1 (3.3–15.3)	F: 1.4 (0.3–6.2)	F: 1.2 (0.1–10.8)
Arseneault et al. (2000)[c]	M + F: 2.45 (1.1–5.7)		

Notes:

CI, confidence interval; M, male; F, female.

[a] Results adjusted for social class of father at birth, residence in city and one parent background.

[b] Results adjusted for marital status, socioeconomic group, substance misuse and personality disorder.

[c] Results adjusted for sex, socioeconomic class and other concurrent disorders; schizophreniform disorder rather than schizophrenia assessed.

Arseneault et al. (2000) studied the past-year prevalence of violence in 961 young adults, who constituted 94% of a total city birth cohort. A combination of self-report and official violence records were used. Three axis I disorders were uniquely associated with violence after controlling for demographic risk factors and all other comorbid disorders: alcohol dependence, marijuana dependence and schizophrenia spectrum disorder. A diagnosis of schizophreniform disorder increased the risk of violence by more than twofold (Table 17.2) Ten per cent of violence risk was attributable to schizophrenia spectrum disorder. Comorbid substance misuse increased the risk associated with this disorder more than twofold.

Studies estimating the prevalence of schizophrenia in individuals who have committed violent acts

Numerous studies have estimated the prevalence of schizophrenia amongst prison inmates. Despite problems of unstandardized diagnoses and the frequent absence of comparison data among the general population, the evidence suggests an over-representation of those with schizophrenia among offender populations.

Taylor and Gunn (1984) using validated diagnoses studied the psychiatric status of male prisoners remanded to a prison in south London. Nine per cent of those subsequently convicted of nonfatal violence and 11% convicted of fatal violence had schizophrenia, a substantially higher prevalence than would have been expected in the general population for the same area (0.1–0.4%).

Teplin (1990) administered the Diagnostic Interview Schedule (DIS: Robins et al., 1981) to a stratified random sample of 728 male prisoners and compared the prevalence of schizophrenia among this group with that of the general population using Epidemiologic Catchment Area (ECA) study (Eaton and Kessler, 1985) data. The prevalence in the jail population (2.7%) was found to be three times higher than that of the general population (0.91%) after controlling for sociodemographic factors.

Eronen et al. (1996), in a study of 693 people convicted of homicide in Finland, investigated whether an association existed between specific DSM-III-R (American Psychiatric Association, 1987) disorders and homicide. Using the 1-month point prevalence estimates from the ECA study and indirect standardization to adjust for the confounding effect of age, schizophrenia was associated with an eightfold increase in homicide by men and 6.5-fold increase in women. This compares with even higher risks (>10) for those with substance abuse disorders.

Wallace et al. (1998), in a study of individuals convicted of serious offences in Victoria County, Australia, searched for evidence of a psychiatric contact on the county psychiatric register. Compared with the general population, those with schizophrenia were found to be over four times more likely to be convicted of interpersonal violence and 10 times more likely to be convicted of homicide.

Community prevalence studies

The above studies, although valuable in making inferences about the relationship between violence and schizophrenia, are subject to biases, which will be discussed below. Further data on unselected samples of people from the open community are needed to augment the findings. Probably the most influential study in the violence literature to date is that of Swanson et al. (1990). Using a representative weighted sample of 10059 adult residents from three of the five ECA study sites (Eaton and Kessler, 1985), the authors examined the relationship between violence and psychiatric disorder. The DIS incorporating questions relating to violence was administered. Violence was rated positive if the respondent admitted to any one of the following four behaviours: hitting or throwing things at one's partner; hitting one's child hard enough to cause bruises or injury; physical fighting; and using a weapon such as a stick, knife or gun. Violence was significantly related to younger age, male sex and lower socioecomomic status. Eight per cent of those with schizophrenia alone were violent compared with 2% of those without mental illness. Comorbidity with substance abuse increased this figure to 30%. Higher rates of violence were reported among individuals who had drug or alcohol abuse/dependence and no serious mental illness than among individuals with serious mental illness alone. Contrary to a number of studies of patient populations, violence was not significantly more prevalent among persons with schizophrenia than among those with other disorders.

Two other community epidemiological studies, finding increased risk of violence among psychiatric patients (Link et al., 1992) and those with major mental disorder (Stueve & Link, 1997), failed to provide data on schizophrenia as a separate diagnostic entity.

Methodological limitations of violence studies

The majority of studies since the late 1980s have demonstrated a statistical association between schizophrenia and violence. It can, therefore, be argued that the accumulated evidence from studies adopting different methodologies support a causal relationship because the consistency of findings across studies overshadows the methodological weaknesses of any one. Some have argued against this conclusion (Arboleda-Florez et al., 1998) suggesting that it overlooks the possibility of consistent design flaws including violence measurement, selection bias, confounding and poorly controlled comparisons, which may offer rival explanations for the current statistical associations. It is, therefore, important that the findings of each study be critically appraised in the light of the limitations inherent to research of this complexity.

A brief overview of these limitations from an epidemiological viewpoint are outlined below.

Definition and measurement of exposure (schizophrenia)

The use of unstandardized definitions of schizophrenia across studies limit consensus conclusions being drawn. Some studies include schizophrenia as part of a heterogeneous group of psychotic disorders, including affective diagnoses (Hodgins, 1992; Hodgins et al., 1996; Steadman et al., 1998) or do not give the diagnostic breakdown of subjects at all (Link et al., 1992). Fewer examine schizophrenia alone (Lindqvist and Allebeck, 1990; Wessely et al., 1994) and those that do use varying diagnostic techniques. Diagnoses are variously derived from case notes, psychiatric registers, clinical interviews or research interviews. Case note diagnoses are dependent on clinical judgements, leading to obvious differences in diagnostic practice. Those extracted from case registers are usually those made at discharge and are subject to the same limitations. These diagnoses may be more reliable, however, than those made at a single clinical interview because they are usually based on a period of observation in hospital, collateral information and previous history, which are likely to increase the validity of diagnoses. The use of one agreed diagnostic procedure in studies would allow comparisons of like with like. Additionally, illness duration should be measured, as it has been found that those at different stages of illness may have different propensities for violence (Modestin and Ammann, 1996).

Definition and measurement of outcome (violence)

The failure to detect significant episodes of violence, or the systematic skewing of data by using inappropriate measures, can lead to the wrong conclusion about the association between violence and schizophrenia. How violence is defined varies greatly. Little consistency exists as to what types of violence to measure and how to do this from study to study. In addition, most studies neglect the contextual and temporal aspects of violent acts.

Recorded prevalence rates differ depending on the levels of violence measured. Unsurprisingly, studies that include threats as well as physical contact record higher rates than those that include contact alone. It is virtually impossible to find violence defined the same way in any two studies by different researchers. This highlights the need for the development of a standardized, validated, reliable and acceptable rating instrument that could be adopted across studies.

Measurement of violence in studies has relied upon different single (self-report, informant, case notes, official records) or combined sources of information. All sources have inherent limitations. Self-report measures may under-report violence because of the desire for social acceptability or fear of adverse consequences of reporting. In case-control studies, bias may result if this reporting differs between cases and controls. Additionally, retrospective designs produce problems with recall of sometimes distant events. Informants, who are often nominated by patients, may not be the most suitable person to provide information or be aware of relevant incidents. Case notes are of limited usefulness as they are often incomplete. With regard to police contacts or arrest records, the proportion of violent acts that lead to arrest and prosecution vary as a function of the intensity and quality of policing, behaviour of the suspect, the availability of diversion to the mental health system and the severity of offence. It is also possible that offenders with major mental disorders are more easily detected than other offenders because they are more likely to stay at the scene of the crime and/or turn themselves into the police (Robertson, 1988).

Records of criminal convictions for all crimes and more specifically violent crime are a widely used data source across studies. Most violent individuals are not convicted (Elliott et al., 1986). The mentally ill tend to be diverted to the mental healthcare system at various stages from apprehension to conviction. As such, it is likely that only the more serious crimes will lead to conviction. For this reason, the association between schizophrenia and more minor forms of violence is impossible to estimate from this source. For more serious offending such as homicide, individuals are more likely to be brought to trial and convicted, and as such dependence on criminal registers is justified. Unfortunately, as with all such registers, they are prone to data errors, are not inclusive of all convictions and often relate to one geographical area taking no account of crimes committed outside that jurisdiction.

The more recent use of multiple combined measures for violence has highlighted the limitations of the majority of previous studies that relied on a single source. Steadman et al. (1998) used agency records, self-report and collateral informants to collect information on violent acts. The 1-year period prevalence for violence was 4.5% using agency records (arrest and rehospitalization records) alone, 23.7% adding patient self-reported acts that had not been in agency records, and 27.5% adding collateral informant-reported acts that had not been in either agency records or patient self-reports. Thus, the final prevalence was six times higher than it would have been if estimated from agency records alone. Mulvey et al. (1994a), specifically set out to compare the yield of violence when different sources were used. Results revealed a dramatically different picture of patient violence depending on the source of information used. Patient self-report revealed a violence prevalence of 37%, collateral informant 31%, medical records 9%, police 'rap' sheets 2% and records of involuntary commitments 1%. These results support the previous observation that self-report methods consistently produce a higher frequency of violence than official records (Elliot et al., 1986). Therefore, to provide accurate empirical data it is crucial that it be based on self-report in conjunction with collateral informant and official records. One problem inherent to the use of multiple measures is that judgements must be made about what constitutes a single episode of violence and how to handle the inconsistencies that may exist between reports.

Selection bias

Selection bias can occur whenever the identification of individual subjects for inclusion into a study on the basis of either exposure or outcome status depends in some way on the other axis of interest. This bias will result in an observed relationship between exposure (schizophrenia) and outcome (violence) that is different among those who are entered into the study than among those who would have been eligible but did not participate. For example, a psychotic individual's refusal to participate in a study or follow-up interviews might be related to his or her propensity for violence. If so, the rates of violence for those included in the samples may be lower than the true rates for individuals with schizophrenia.

Location of recruitment is, therefore, a crucial factor in interpreting any such association and in making judgements on generalizability of findings. Research on violence and mental illness is dominated by data on discharged patients, but most mentally disordered individuals are not hospitalized (Robins and Reiger, 1991).

Studies of acutely ill hospitalized patients are subject to selection bias, as those who are admitted are more likely than those who are not to be violent. Recently discharged patients have usually been judged not a risk at the time of discharge and may be less likely to be violent than when hospitalized. Cross-sectional prevalence studies in representative samples of community residents, with both treated and untreated mental disorders, largely overcome the problem of selection bias, although not completely. They frequently exclude those in jail (Steadman et al, 1998) and as such will underestimate any association.

It is not unusual to find high refusal and attrition rates in these studies, also leading to selection bias. In one study, only 50% of subjects completed all five follow-up interviews. These compliant subjects were found to be significantly less likely to have a history of previous violence, a major predictor of future violence, than those lost to follow-up (Steadman et al, 1998).

Another example is the Swedish cohort study (Hodgins, 1992). All those who died during the follow-up period were excluded. It has, however, been shown that a relationship exists between early death and violence. As such, the size of effect may be an underestimate of the true effect.

In analytic studies, the risk of violent offending in cases is expressed relative to the risk in controls. It is, therefore, important that the results be interpreted with specific reference to the control group chosen. If, for example, risk of offending in schizophrenia is estimated relative to nonpsychotic psychiatric controls (Wessely et al., 1994), the risk ratio will depend on whether or not that group contains an excess of patients with personality disorder and substance abuse disorders, which are both linked to violent behaviour. If national or population-based figures are used for comparison, they may not take into account the confounding effect of social class on violence (Wallace et al., 1998). Alternatively, if neighbourhood controls are chosen, the estimated risk may not be generalizable to the population at large (Steadman et al., 1998).

Other possible types of bias include interviewer bias and recall bias. On reading most violence studies, it is unclear whether interviewers were blind to subject status. If not, selective probing for symptoms of mental illness and/or violent episodes may result in interviewer bias. Recall bias may arise in comparing the mentally ill with normal controls if patients and their relatives, for example, are more sensitive to deviant behaviours and hence more likely to report them.

Confounding

A confounder is a factor that is associated with the exposure (schizophrenia) and independent of this exposure is a risk factor for outcome (violence). Additionally, it should not be on the causal pathway between exposure and outcome. Statistical relationships observed between schizophrenia and violence in any particular study will hinge on the investigator's understanding and statistical treatment of confounding factors (Arboleda-Florez et al., 1998). Because of the uncertainty of the causal pathway between schizophrenia and violence, it is unclear what variables to consider as confounders. Gender, age and race are likely candidates. In fact, most population-based studies comprise primarily young adults and as such may overestimate the relationship. Controversy exists regarding social class (Monahan, 1993) because it can be hypothesized that the social drift in schizophrenia that leads to lower social class is on the pathway to violence. The more robust studies do control for a range of possible confounding factors, but these are by no means uniform. The relationship is, however, even more complex than this, with a wide range of personal and situational factors that must be important in the mediation of violence being impossible to measure.

Predictors of violent behaviour in schizophrenia

Despite the limitation of violence studies, most conclude that the association between schizophrenia and violence is probably significant even when demographic factors are taken into account. Risk factors for violence that operate in those without mental illness operate in schizophrenia, with strong predictors including a history of previous violence and substance abuse. No sizeable body of evidence, however, clearly indicates the relative strength of schizophrenia or mental illness in general as a risk factor for violence compared with other risk factors (Mulvey et al., 1994b). Indeed, compared with the magnitude of risk associated with the combination of male gender, young age and lower socioeconomic status, the risk of violence presented by mental disorder is modest (Monahan, 1997).

Two factors appear to discriminate those with schizophrenia at increased risk of committing violent acts: comorbid substance abuse and acute psychotic symptoms. Substance abuse and antisocial personality disorder are much more strongly associated with violent behaviour than schizophrenia (Swanson et al., 1990). It has been repeatedly demonstrated that schizophrenia with comorbid substance abuse increases the risk of violence considerably compared with schizophrenia without comorbidity (Swanson et al., 1990; Cuffel et al., 1994; Tiihonen et al., 1997, Wallace et al., 1998; Rasanen et al., 1998). For example, in an Australian study, those with schizophrenia were found to be over four times more likely to be convicted of interpersonal violence and 10 times more likely to be convicted of homicide than members of the general population (Wallace et al, 1998). Those with schizophrenia and comorbid substance abuse were over eight times more likely to be convicted of interpersonal violence and four times more likely to be convicted of homicide than those with schizophrenia alone. It is important to note that, because there is an increase in violence risk in those without comorbidity, substance abuse merely increases the level of risk rather than causes it (Brennan et al., 2000; Arsenault et al., 2000). Hence the risk from substance abuse appears to be additive.

With regard to acute symptomatology, Taylor and Gunn (1984) noted that only 9 of 121 psychotic offenders were without acute psychotic symptoms at the time of their offence. In a subsequent analysis, Taylor estimated that 46% were definitely or probably driven by delusions (Taylor, 1985). But delusions are an extremely common psychopathological phenomenon in psychosis and serious violence is not. Other factors must be operating (Taylor, 1998).

In a methodologically robust study, Link et al. (1992) compared arrest rates and self-reported violence in a sample of approximately 400 New York residents with no history of psychiatric contact with those for current and former patients with heterogeneous diagnoses from the same area. Former patients were invariably more violent than the never-treated community sample and almost all the difference between the groups could be accounted for by active symptoms. A further study revealed that specific threat/control override symptoms largely explained the relationship. These threat/control override symptoms represent experiences of patients feeling that people are trying to harm them, and experiences of their minds being dominated by forces outside of their control. These symptoms significantly increased the risk of violence not only in patients but also in the never-treated community controls. These results have subsequently been replicated (Swanson et al., 1990, 1996, 1997; Link et al., 1998). If true, these findings about threat/control override delusions could have important implications for the prediction and management of violent behaviour in delusional patients. The data in these studies have, however, been criticized for being retrospective, having been gathered for other purposes and having weak measures of delusions and violence (e.g. data often based exclusively on self-report). Recent evidence from the MacArthur Violence Risk Assessment Study, a prospective, multisite study of violent behaviour in recently discharged patients, have largely overcome these methodological limitations and cast doubt on the importance of threat/control override delusions as mediators for violence (Appelbaum et al 2000). Neither delusions in general nor threat/control override delusions in particular were found to be associated with an increased risk of violence in this study. The authors suggest that the reliance on self-report in previous studies may have resulted in the mislabelling as delusions of other phenomena that can contribute to violence.

Risk of violence in society attributable to schizophrenia

Most research to date has examined the association between violence and schizophrenia in terms of relative risk, that is, the amount of risk posed by those with schizophrenia relative to others. Surprisingly, little work has focused on the more important public health issue of population attributable-risk percentage (PAR%), that is, the percentage of violence in the population that can be ascribed to schizophrenia and could thus be eliminated if schizophrenia was eliminated from the population. It is possible to perform some approximate calculations of the PAR% on data reported from some population-based studies measuring different aspects of violent behaviour. To calculate this figure, we first calculate the rate of violence in the total study population; we then subtract the rate of violence in the population removing all those with schizophrenia. This figure is then divided by the rate in the total population and multiplied by 100. In the ECA study in America, 2.7% of individuals who reported community violence over 1 year had schizophrenia (Swanson et al., 1990). Only 8% of those with schizophrenia were violent. In an unselected Finnish birth cohort followed to age 25, those with schizophrenia accounted for 4% of those registered for at least one violent crime (Tiihonen et al., 1997). In a Danish birth cohort followed to age 44, 2% of all males with lifetime arrests for violence and 9% of all females had schizophrenia. When we exclude those with comorbid substance misuse, these figures fall to 0.8% for males and 6% for females (Brennan et al., 2000). In Dunedin, New Zealand, 94% of a total city birth cohort were followed up at age 21. Without considering comorbidity, just over 10% of past-year violence committed by these young adults (based on a combination of self-report and criminal convictions) was attributable to schizophrenic spectrum disorders. Having comorbid substance abuse with either alcohol or marijuana was found to double the violence risk in this disorder (Arseneault et al., 2000).

Most of the above figures represent a fairly small percentage of the total violence in these populations. The problem is that the PAR% assumes that causality has been established. It, therefore, fails to take into account other risk factors or confounding factors that may be operating in the association between a particular risk factor and disease. As we have previously seen, for example, comorbidity substantially increases the risk of violence in schizophrenia and it is possible that were substance abuse to be eliminated from the population the contribution to violence made by schizophrenia alone could be much less.

To prevent unnecessary stigmatization of the seriously mentally ill, with all the attendant difficulties, it is the duty of researchers to present a balanced picture. By neglecting to report measures of both relative and absolute risk a skewed picture may emerge. An example of a balanced report found that men with schizophrenia were up to five times more likely to be convicted of serious violence than the general population (Wallace et al., 1998). Results also presented indicated that 99.97% of those with schizophrenia would not be convicted of serious violence in a given year and that the probability that any given patient with schizophrenia will commit homicide is tiny (approximate annual risk 1:3000 for men and 1:33000 for women).

Risk is generally presented in terms of odds ratios, yet research has shown that people find it difficult to digest such measures. Better ways are required for presenting risk magnitudes in a digestible form, and a logarithmic scale provides the basis for a common language for describing risk (Calman & Royston, 1997). It has been suggested that community risk scales that describe the magnitude of risk in relation to an individual's community may be most useful. If communities are grouped into roughly logarithmic clusters – individual (1), family (10), village (1000) etc. – such a classification allows individuals to think in terms of level of risk to themselves, their family, their town and so forth. This system also allows a consideration of how the risk of violence by people with schizophrenia compares with other risks, if these are also presented in the same way.

Directions for future research

The weight of the evidence to date is that, although a statistical relationship does exist, only a small proportion of the violence in our society can be attributed to persons with schizophrenia. Future research on the relationship between schizophrenia and violence is likely to focus not on whether such a relationship exists but on the precise form that the relationship takes. We lack clear information about causal pathways, and further inquiries regarding the interplay of various factors affecting the relationship are required. We have already seen this shift with the recent focus on threat/control override symptoms. More attention must be paid to the temporal and contextual settings of violent acts. It is essential that these risk factor studies be conducted in the most methodological robust manner, that is, with clear definitions of illness, multiple measurements of violence and avoidance of bias.

REFERENCES

American Psychiatric Association (1987) Diagnostic and Statistical Manual of Mental Disorders, III–Revised. Washington, DC: American Psychiatric Press.

Appelbaum PS, Robbins PC, Monahan J (2000) Violence and delusions: data from the MacArthur Violence Risk Assessment Study. American Journal of Psychiatry 157, 566–572.

Arboleda-Florez J, Holley H, Crisanti A (1998) Understanding causal paths between mental illness and violence. Social Psychiatry and Psychiatric Epidemiology 33, S38–S46.

Arseneault L, Moffitt TE, Caspi A et al. (2000) Mental disorders and violence in a total birth cohort: results from the Dunedin Study. Archives of General Psychiatry 57, 979–968.

Brennan PA, Mednick SA, Hodgins S (2000) Major mental disorders and criminal violence in a Danish birth cohort. Archives of General Psychiatry 57, 494–500.

Calman KC, Royston GH (1997) Risk language and dialects. British Medical Journal 315, 939–942.

Cuffel BJ, Shumway M, Choujian TL et al. (1994) A longitudinal study of substance use and community violence in schizophrenia. Journal of Nervous and Mental Disease 182, 704–708.

Eaton WW, Kessler LG (1985) The NIMH Epidemiologic Catchment Area Study. In: Epidemiological Field Methods in Psychiatry. New York: Academic Press.

Elliot D, Huizinga D (1986) Self-reported violent offending: a descriptive analysis of juvenile violent offenders and their offending careers. Journal of Interpersonal Violence 1, 472–513.

Eronen M, Hakola P, Tiihonen J (1996) Mental disorders and homicidal behaviour in Finland. Archives of General Psychiatry 53, 497–501.

Harris G, Rice M, Quinsey V (1993) Violent recidivism of mentally disordered offenders: the development of a statistical prediction instrument. Criminal Justice and Behavior 20, 315–335.

Hodgins S (1992) Mental disorder, intellectual deficiency, and crime; evidence from a birth cohort. Archives of General Psychiatry 49, 476–483.

Hodgins S, Mednick SA, Brennan PA et al. (1996) Mental disorder and crime: evidence from a Danish birth cohort. Archives of General Psychiatry 53, 489–496.

Humphreys MS, Johnstone EC, MacMillan JF et al. (1992) Dangerous behaviour preceding first admissions for schizophrenia. British Journal of Psychiatry 161, 501–505.

Karson C, Bigelow LB (1987) Violent behaviour in schizophrenic patients. Journal of Nervous and Mental Diseases 175, 161–164.

Lindqvist P, Allebeck P (1990) Schizophrenia and crime. A longitudinal follow-up of 644 schizophrenics in Stockholm. British Journal of Psychiatry 157, 345–350.

Link BG, Andrews H, Cullen FT (1992) The violent and illegal behaviour of mental patients reconsidered. American Sociological Review 57, 275–292.

Link BG, Stueve A, Phelan J (1998) Psychotic symptoms and violent behaviors: probing the components of 'threat/control-override' symptoms. Social Psychiatry and Psychiatric Epidemiology 33, S55–S60.

Modestin J, Ammann R (1996) Mental disorder and criminality: male schizophrenia. Schizophrenia Bulletin 22, 69–82.

Monahan J (1993) Mental disorder and violence: another look. In: Mental Disorder and Crime, Hodgins S, ed. CA: Sage Publications, pp. 287–302.

Monahan J (1997) Clinical and Actuarial predictions of violence. In: Modern Scientific Evidence: The Law and Science of Expert Testimony, Vol. 1, Faigman D, Kaye D, Saks M. et al., eds. St Paul, MN: West Publishing Company, pp. 300–318.

Monahan J, Appelbaum P (2000) Reducing violence risk: diagnostically based clues from the MacArthur Violence Risk Assessment Study. In: Effective Prevention of Crime and Violence Among the Mentally Ill, Hodgins S, ed. Dordrecht, the Netherlands: Kluwer, pp. 19–34.

Mullen PE, Burgess P, Wallace C et al. (2000) Community care and criminal offending in schizophrenia. Lancet 355, 614–617.

Mulvey EP, Shaw E, Lidz CW (1994a) Why use multiple sources in research on patient violence in the community. Criminal Behaviour and Mental Health 4, 235–258.

Mulvey EP, Shaw E, Lidz CW (1994b) Assessing the evidence of a link between mental illness and violence. Hospital and Community Psychiatry 45, 663–668.

Räsänan P, Tiihonen J, Isohanni M, Rantakillio P, Lehtonen J, Moring T (1998) Schizophrenia, alcohol abuse and violent behaviour: a 26 year followup study of an unselected birth cohort. Schizophrenia Bulletin 24, 437–441.

Robins LN, Reiger DA (1991) Psychiatric Disorders in America. New York: Free Press.

Robins LN, Helzer JE, Croughan J et al. (1981) NIMH Diagnostic Interview Schedule: Version

III. Rockville, MD: National Institute of Mental Health, Division of Biometry and Epidemiology.

Robertson G (1988) Arrest patterns among mentally disordered offenders. British Journal of Psychiatry 153, 313–316.

Spitzer RL, Williams JBW, Gibbon M (1990) User's Guide for the Structured Clinical Interview for DSM-III-R (SCID) Washington, DC: American Psychiatric Press.

Steadman HJ, Mulvey EP, Monahan J et al. (1998) Violence by people discharged from acute psychiatric inpatient facilities and by others in the same neighborhoods. Archives of General Psychiatry 55, 1–9.

Stueve A, Link BG (1997) Violence and psychiatric disorders: results from an epidemiological study of young adults in Israel. Psychiatry Quarterly 68, 327–342.

Swanson JW, Holzer ChE, Ganju VK et al. (1990) Violence and psychiatric disorder in the community: evidence from the epidemiologic catchment area surveys. Hospital and Community Psychiatry 41, 761–770.

Swanson JW, Borum R, Swartz MS (1996) Psychotic symptoms and disorders and the risk of violent behaviour in the community. Criminal Behaviour and Mental Health 6, 309–329.

Swanson JW, Estroff S, Swartz M et al. (1997) Violence and severe mental disorder in clinical and community populations: the effects of psychotic symptoms, comorbidity, and lack of treatment. Psychiatry 60, 1–22.

Taylor PJ (1985) Motives for offending among violent and psychotic men. British Journal of Psychiatry 147, 491–498.

Taylor PJ (1998) When symptoms of psychosis drive serious violence. Social Psychiatry and Psychiatric Epidemiology 33, S47–S54.

Taylor PJ, Gunn J (1984) Violence and psychosis. I. Risk of violence among psychotic men. British Medical Journal 288, 1945–1949.

Taylor PJ, Gunn J (1999) Homicides by people with mental illness: myth and reality. British Journal of Psychiatry 174, 9–14.

Teplin LA (1990) The prevalence of severe mental disorder among urban jail detainees: comparison with the Epidemiologic Catchment Area Program. American Journal of Public Health 80, 663–669.

Tiihonen J, Isohanni M, Räsänen P et al. (1997) Specific major mental disorders and criminality: a 26-year prospective study of the 1966 northern Finland birth cohort. American Journal of Psychiatry 154, 840–845.

Volavka J, Laska E, Baker S et al. (1997) History of violent behaviour and schizophrenia in different cultures. Analyses based on the WHO study on determinants of outcome of severe mental disorders. British Journal of Psychiatry 163, 69–76.

Walker Z, Seifert R (1994) Violent incidents in a psychiatric intensive care unit. British Journal of Psychiatry 164, 826–828.

Wallace C, Mullen P, Burgess P et al. (1998) Serious criminal offending and mental disorder. Case linkage study. British Journal of Psychiatry 174, 477–484.

Wessely SC, Castle D, Douglas AJ et al. (1994) The criminal careers of incident cases of schizophrenia. Psychological Medicine 24, 483–502.

Wing JK, Cooper JE, Sartorius N (1974) The Description and Classification of Psychiatric Symptoms: An Instruction Manual for the PSE and CATEGO Systems. Cambridge: Cambridge University Press.

World Health Organization (1967) Manual of the International Statistical Classification of Diseases, Injuries, and Causes of Death, 8th edn. Vol. 1. Geneva: World Health Organization.

World Health Organization (1978) Mental Disorders. Glossary and Guide to their Classification in Accordance with the Ninth Revision of the International Classification of Diseases (ICD-9). Geneva: World Health Organization.

Part V

Future directions and emerging issues

Introduction

How can we be sure that the diagnosis of schizophrenia actually relates to a valid entity? In Chapter 18, van Os and Verdoux challenge the existing beliefs about schizophrenia as a discrete diagnostic category and consider the evidence that psychosis exists as a continuous and dimensional phenotype. There is accumulating evidence that psychosis exists in nature as a continuous distribution of symptoms rather than a discrete, dichotomous disorder. Large-scale national surveys have found that about one-quarter of individuals surveyed admit to experiencing psychotic symptoms and most had never sought any help for these. In addition, there is evidence that psychosis consists of many overlapping symptom dimensions that may each be the result of a range of underlying risk factors. Van Os and Verdoux argue that a combination of categorical, continuous and multidimensional representations of psychosis will offer important advantages both for clinical practice and research.

The final two chapters in the book demonstrate how epidemiology can be used to improve the treatment of schizophrenia and, perhaps, ultimately to prevent the disorder. In Chapter 19, Thornicroft and Tansella select epidemiological findings that have been discussed in earlier chapters and, using a 'matrix' model, they show how these data can be exploited to plan better services for people who suffer from schizophrenia. The authors also hope that psychiatric services will support the conduct of research, especially large-scale, collaborative epidemiological studies.

Will we ever be able to prevent schizophrenia? In Chapter 20, McGrath argues that 'a major factor that has eroded confidence in primary prevention of schizophrenia has been a perception that we have made little progress in our understanding of the aetiology of the disorder'. Drawing on evidence presented in earlier chapters, McGrath seeks to dispel this feeling of 'nihilistic despair' by pointing out that we have indeed identified many risk factors for schizophrenia and there is now an 'urgent need' for strategic research designed to test these risk factors in epidemiological samples. In addition, collaboration with basic neuroscience will refine our knowledge of the mechanisms of action of these risk factors. The chapter ends on an encouraging note. 'The dream of making the primary prevention of schizophrenia a reality may be quixotic, but it is certainly not impossible'.

18

Diagnosis and classification of schizophrenia: categories versus dimensions, distributions versus disease

Jim van Os[1] and Hélène Verdoux[2]

[1]Department of Psychiatry and Neuropsychology, Maastricht University, the Netherlands and Institute of Psychiatry, London, UK
[2]Service Universitaire de Psychiatrie, Bordeaux, France

Introduction

Let us compare a diagnosis of schizophrenia with a diagnosis of coronary heart disease. Few would disagree that their aetiologies, symptoms, clinical needs, treatments and outcomes are rather different; therefore, the diagnostic contrast they provide in the classification of medical disorders can be considered extremely useful, that is, has clinical validity (Kendell, 1989). The clinician will use the diagnosis to prescribe a particular treatment, the service provider will organize services around the specific treatment needs associated with each group, and the researcher will test specific hypotheses regarding different biological and psychosocial risk factors and mechanisms in each disorder.

The current systems of classification of mental disorders are based on the assumption that it is similarly useful to discriminate between, for example, schizophrenia, schizoaffective disorder, affective psychosis, delusional disorder and other psychosis. However, psychotic disorders may show considerable overlap in their aetiologies, risk mechanisms, manifestations, treatment needs and outcomes. The greater the degree of overlap, the less useful it becomes to discriminate between the various disorders, and the less likely it becomes that the different disorders exist as such in nature (that is, are valid entities). It is, therefore, important to investigate systematically the degree of overlap by sampling across conventional diagnostic categories. However, as the great majority of research effort has its focus specifically on an isolated diagnostic category, data regarding the relative validity of common diagnostic labels remain wanting. Most of the validity research to date has been concerned with the distinction between nonaffective psychosis and affective disorder (Kerr and McClelland, 1991). This remains an important and clinically relevant area of debate and some of the epidemiological issues to do with the diagnostic validity of schizophrenia will hereafter be illustrated using this distinction.

Diagnosis of schizophrenia: an epidemiological perspective

Several competing definitions of schizophrenia exist. The 'narrow' definitions such as those specified by the criteria in the Diagnostic and Statistical Manual, third version and beyond (DSM: American Psychiatric Association, 1987; American Psychiatric Association, 1994) are, in epidemiological terms, biased towards younger male patients with a more severe type of illness, whereas samples defined by 'broader' criteria such as those in the Research Diagnostic Criteria (RDC: Spitzer et al., 1990) and International Classification of Diseases (ICD), 10th version (ICD-10: World Health Organization, 1992), include more women with affective symptoms and have a more variable illness course (Copolov et al., 1990; Castle et al., 1993; Mason et al., 1997). The existence of several competing definitions suggests lack of agreement about how, or indeed if, schizophrenia exists as such in nature. If engineers used variable definitions of the same basic entity, few would care to argue that their constructs were safe. By analogy, the construct validity of the schizophrenia concept may be weak. Some propose that the nosological validity of schizophrenia is well established and that the diagnosis stands on solid ground (Andreasen, 1995). Others argue that, although the validity remains uncertain, current concepts will have to suffice until more details about heterogeneity, causes and fundamental mechanisms are discovered (Kendell, 1993). Yet others argue that the diagnosis is a convenience label with no base in ontological reality and that substantial improvement may be obtained by actively pursuing the use of alternative, more empirical, approaches towards phenotypic classification (Bentall et al., 1988; Costello, 1992). Although opinions appear to be divided, there is consensus that surprisingly few research efforts are dedicated to establish the validity of current nosological concepts (Kendell, 1993).

Levels of care

It is apparent that the definition of schizophrenia has its origins in the wards of Europe's 19th and early 20th century institutions for individuals with severe mental illness, and that the definitions which can be encountered in the current systems of classification of DSM and ICD are also largely based on what can be observed at the extreme end of the pathways to care for mental illness (level 5; see Fig. 18.1) (Goldberg and Huxley, 1980). At this level (the psychiatric hospital), the prevalence of psychotic disorder is around 20–40%, and the prevalence of psychotic symptoms may be as high as 50–70%, depending on country and setting (Jaffe, 1966; McCreadie et al., 1983; Barber et al., 1988; Robinson, 1988; O'Grady, 1990; Avasthi et al., 1991; Chiou et al., 1994). More recently, awareness has grown that individual symptoms such as delusions, hallucinations, restricted affect and lack of initiative are also prevalent at lower levels along the pathways to care, such as in the

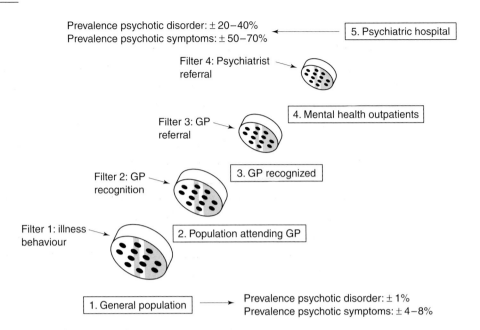

Prevalence psychotic disorder: ± 20−40%
Prevalence psychotic symptoms: ± 50−70%   ←   5. Psychiatric hospital

Filter 4: Psychiatrist
referral

4. Mental health outpatients

Filter 3: GP
referral

3. GP recognized

Filter 2: GP
recognition

2. Population attending GP

Filter 1: illness
behaviour

1. General population   →   Prevalence psychotic disorder: ± 1%
Prevalence psychotic symptoms: ± 4−8%

Fig. 18.1.   Filter model of psychotic symptoms and psychotic disorder. GP, general practitioner.

population attending general practitioners (GPs; level 2) (Verdoux et al., 1998a) and individuals in the general population who have not yet developed any illness behaviour (level 1) (Zukerman and Cohen, 1964; Cox and Cowling, 1989; Kendler et al., 1991; Peters et al., 1999a; Rosa et al., 2000). At these levels, the lifetime prevalence of even psychiatrist-rated psychotic symptoms may be as high as 4–8% (Eaton et al., 1991; Tien, 1991; van Os et al., 2000).

Two important questions flow from these observations. As the data suggest that positive and negative psychotic symptoms also have a distribution in nonpatients, the first question becomes to what degree this distribution at level 1 and level 2 is continuous with the clinical phenotype at the extreme of level 5. The second, related, question is to what degree our clinical phenotypes must be seen as mixtures of correlated but separable symptom dimensions instead of dichotomous disease entities with specific and unconfounded causes. We will refer to the first question as the continuity hypothesis and to the second question as the dimensional hypothesis.

The continuity hypothesis: diseases or distributions?

Anyone working in a clinical mental health setting, especially the psychiatric hospital, is naturally inclined to think that psychosis reveals itself as 'cases' in need of treatment. This clinical perspective has greatly influenced the conceptualization of the psychosis phenotype, as evidenced by current systems of classification such as

DSM-IV and ICD-10. The psychosis phenotype is generally thought of as a dichotomous entity, which can be identified by applying criteria that have been derived from clinical observations on individuals who managed to pass through the various filters of help-seeking behaviour and recognition that separate symptoms in the general population from treatment at the level of mental health services (Tien et al., 1992). From the epidemiological perspective, however, things look somewhat different. Rose and Barker (1978) cogently argued that, contrary to the situation in clinical practice, disease at the level of the general population usually exists as a continuum of severity rather than as an all-or-none phenomenon. For example, blood pressure and glucose tolerance are continuously distributed characteristics in the general population, but because the clinical decision to treat is dichotomous we use the terms hypertension and diabetes in medicine. This clinical perspective, however, cannot be equated with evidence that these conditions exist as such in nature: they are the extremes of a continuous characteristic.

Perceptions of the psychosis continuum

The hypothesis that psychosis exists in nature as a distribution of symptoms is not so bold as it may seem. For example, in the case of depression, both genetic and community studies suggest that the phenotype is more likely to exist as a continuous (albeit skewed (Weich, 1997)) distribution of symptoms rather than a true disease dichotomy (Anderson et al., 1993; Whittington and Huppert, 1996; Kendler and Gardner, 1998). Given the substantial degree of overlap in terms of psychopathology, outcome, risk factors and treatment between depression and psychosis, it is unlikely that psychosis, contrary to depression, would have a completely noncontinuous, dichotomous distribution. Although possibly more skewed because of their lower prevalence, a degree of continuity in the distribution of symptoms is to be expected. This altogether reasonable hypothesis, however, has attracted relatively little research effort, especially on the part of the psychiatric profession (Claridge, 1997; pp. 301–317).

The supposition of a psychosis continuum does not necessarily imply that there is a continuum of disorder. For example, in the US National Comorbidity Survey, around 28% of individuals endorsed psychosis-screening questions. However, when clinicians made diagnoses, the rate of even broadly defined psychosis was only 0.7% (Kendler et al., 1996). This suggests that the clinical definition of psychosis may represent only a minor and biased selection of the total (not necessarily clinical) phenotypic continuum.

Causal risk factors and distribution

The existence of lesser states on a distributed continuum in the population may perhaps be better thought of as a risk factor for what clinicians would call disorder,

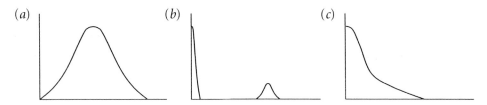

Fig. 18.2.   Possible degrees of continuity of psychosis distributions. (*a*) There is a continuous and normal distribution of psychotic traits in the general population, much as one would expect of, for example, weight or blood pressure. (*b*) There is a clear bimodal distribution, with the great majority of the population having negligible values of the psychosis trait, whereas a very small proportion has extremely high values. (*c*) There is a continuous but only half-normal distribution, with the majority of the population having very low values, but also a significant proportion with nonzero values.

rather than a forme fruste of disease (Claridge, 1994, 1997). In epidemiological terms, this argument can be explored by examining the possible combinations of underlying causes of the presumed psychosis continuum in relation to the predicted distribution of the trait. For example, if psychosis is the result of a single, unconfounded, fully penetrant cause, such as a single gene, the distribution would be truly dichotomous. However, it is very unlikely that psychosis is caused by a single factor, and a multifactorial aetiology, similar to that seen in other chronic disorders such as diabetes and cardiovascular disease, is more likely. If there are, for example, five or more different causal risk factors for psychosis, the observed distribution of the psychosis trait would be highly dependent on the degree to which these causal factors interact, their prevalence and the degree to which their effect sizes differ. If, on the one hand, the effects of each of the five causes are moderate, similar in magnitude and contribute additively and independently to the risk function, it can be shown that, according to what statisticians call the central limit theorem, psychosis would have to exist in nature as a quantitative trait, as depicted in Fig. 18.2*a* (Kendler and Kidd, 1986). If, on the other hand, the five different causes interact in such a way that expression of psychosis would only occur in the case of joint exposure to all five factors simultaneously (i.e. complete coparticipation of the causes), the distribution would more closely resemble a dichotomy as depicted in Fig.18.6*b*. If the five causes contributed independently to the risk of psychosis but also coparticipated to a degree, the distribution would lie somewhere between that of Fig. 18.2*a* and Fig. 18.2*b* (see Fig. 18.2*c*), depending on the degree of independent additive action and coparticipation of the causes. In the case of large differences in effect size, with one or two very rare but extremely potent causes overshadowing the effect of more prevalent but weak causes, the appearance of the distribution would also be less continuous and more quasicontinuous. In practice, therefore, always assuming that psychosis is subject to more than one causal influence, it is likely that the 'real' distribution of psychosis lies somewhere between the dichotomous one in Fig. 18.1*a* and the continuous one in Fig. 18.1*b*, depending on the degree of interaction between the different causes, and differences in their effect size.

Distributions of psychotic symptoms

Studying the distribution of psychosis may tell us something about the degree of continuity and underlying causation. However, the resulting distribution very much depends on how the trait is measured. Broadly two approaches can be distinguished.

The first approach is to measure in the general population the same symptoms that are seen in patients with psychotic disorders. The implicit assumption in this approach is that having symptoms of psychosis, such as delusions and hallucinations, cannot necessarily be equated with disorder, this being dependent on symptom factors, such as intrusiveness, frequency and comorbidity of symptoms, and personal and cultural factors, such as coping, illness behaviour, societal tolerance and the development of functional impairments. Consequently, even though the prevalence of clinical disorder is low, the prevalence of the symptoms can conceivably be much higher.

The second approach assumes that, in the subdisorder range along the continuum, the expression of the trait is attenuated and takes on the form of 'schizotypal' signs and symptoms. In this context, a range of different schizotypy instruments has been developed, some include items that are close to the 'pathological' experiences seen in psychosis (e.g. the Perceptual Aberration Scale (PAS; Chapman et al., 1978)); others are more 'normalized' (e.g. the Schizotypal Personality Scale; Claridge and Broks, 1984), and yet others are based on the signs and symptoms seen in the relatives of patients with schizophrenia, which are the main source for the DSM criteria for schizotypy (e.g. Schizotypal Personality Questionnaire (SPQ; Raine, 1991)). The choice of instruments greatly influences the resulting distribution in prevalence studies. For example, the distribution of the number of delusions and hallucinations per person will be very skewed compared with the sum score of a schizotypy instrument with normalized items, whereas an instrument like the PAS will be somewhere in between that of a dichotomous and a truly continuous one. The distribution will also be influenced by the symptom dimension that the instrument is aiming to capture, for example positive or negative dimensions (Chapman et al., 1976).

Prevalence of symptoms of psychosis

The finding that the signs and symptoms of the clinical disorder, irrespective of the presence of need for care or illness behaviour, have a more continuous distribution

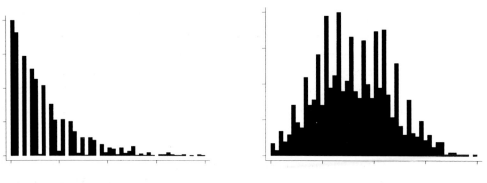

| Perceptual aberration scale | Schizotypal personality questionnaire |

Fig. 18.3.   Distributions of schizotypy according to the instrument used. (Based on data from Stefanis et al., 2002.)

than the dichotomously defined disorder would suggest that the phenotype in question is more continuous. In schizotypy research, the distribution is highly dependent on the instrument used. For example, in a study on a representative sample of around 2000 young men in Greece, Stefanis and colleagues (2002) found that the distribution of the PAS (more clinical in its approach to schizotypy) was half normal, whereas the distribution of the SPQ total score (more normalized in its approach to schizotypy) was approximately normal (Fig. 18.3). These distributions of variably defined schizotypy variables are, in the absence of associations with third variables, in themselves difficult to interpret. Therefore, studies assessing the prevalence of psychotic symptoms themselves, rather than variably defined attenuated experiences, may be more useful.

Hallucinations

There are normal individuals who experience hallucinations under no special circumstances, and surveys have shown that more people experience hallucinations than come into contact with medical or psychiatric services. For example, Romme et al. (1992) conducted a self-selecting survey of auditory verbal hallucinations in 450 people who had responded to a request on television. Of the 173 subjects who responded to the questionnaire, 76 were not in psychiatric care.

A number of studies have assessed hallucinatory experiences in samples of healthy college students using questionnaire measures. These studies have yielded consistent findings, showing that a considerable proportion of individuals experience hallucinations at some time in their lives. Posey and Losch (1983) questioned a sample of 375 college students. Among this sample, 71% reported some experience of at least brief, occasional hallucinated voices during periods of wakefulness and 39% reported hearing their thoughts spoken aloud. Barrett and Etheridge (1992) found that 30–40% of a sample of 586 college students reported the experience of hearing voices, and almost half of these indicated that the experience occurred at least once a month. Reports of verbal hallucinations were not related to measures of overt or incipient psychopathology. The Launay–Slade Hallucination Scale measures predisposition towards experiencing hallucinations (Launay and Slade, 1981).

A few studies have attempted to estimate the prevalence of hallucinatory experiences in the general adult population. The earliest study was carried out in 1894 by Sidgewick and colleagues, of the Society for Psychical Research. They interviewed 17 000 adults, excluding people with obvious psychiatric or physical illness, using a standard interview schedule. Nearly 8% of men and 12% of women in the sample reported at least one hallucinatory experience in their lifetime (Sidgewick et al., 1894). In the first modern survey of hallucinations, McKellar (1968) questioned a group of 500 'normal' people, and 125 (25%) of these reported at least one hallucinatory experience. Tien reported data from the National Institute of Mental Health (NIMH) Epidemiologic Catchment Area (ECA) study carried out in the USA between 1980 and 1984. The study interviewed 18 572 community residents using the NIMH Diagnostic Interview Schedule (DIS; Robins et al., 1981). The lifetime prevalence of hallucinations (not related to drugs or medical problems) in this sample was 10% for men and 15% for women, and the overall rates were similar for visual, auditory and tactile hallucinations. Furthermore, the proportions of hallucinations causing no distress or impairment of function were much higher than those associated with distress or impairment (Tien, 1991). Johns and colleagues analysed responses on the Psychosis Screening Questionnaire (PSQ) collected as part of the Fourth National Survey of Ethnic Minorities. The annual prevalence of hallucinatory experiences (hearing or seeing things that other people could not) was 4% in the sample of 2800 White respondents (Johns et al., 2002).

Delusions

Normal individuals can hold overvalued and delusional ideas. In a survey of 60 000 British adults, Cox and Cowling (1989) found that beliefs in unscientific or parapsychological phenomena were commonly held. For example, 50% of the sample expressed a belief in thought transference between two people, 25% believed in ghosts and 25% in reincarnation (Cox and Cowling, 1989). Using a formal diagnostic interview in a general population sample, Eaton and colleagues (1991) found that bizarre delusions were reported by around 2% of the general population. Paranoid delusions and delusions of having special powers had prevalence rates of 4–8% (Eaton et al., 1991).

To measure delusional ideation in the normal population, Peters et al. (1999a) developed the Peters Delusions Inventory (PDI), using the Present State Examination (PSE; Wing et al., 1974) as a template. The 40 items selected covered a wide range of delusional beliefs, and the original PSE questions were toned down to measure attenuated rather than florid psychotic symptoms. For each delusional belief endorsed, questions also assessed associated distress, preoccupation and conviction. Peters et al. (1999a) administered the PDI to 272 healthy adults and 20 psychotic inpatients. Although the psychotic patients had significantly higher mean PDI scores, the ranges of scores were almost identical between the healthy and deluded groups. Thus, nearly 10% of the healthy sample scored above the mean of the deluded group. These overlapping distributions between the two groups provide further support for the notion of a continuum between normality and psychotic symptoms (Peters et al., 1999a). Verdoux and colleagues used the 21-item version of the PDI (Peters et al., 1996) to assess the prevalence of delusional ideation in 790 primary care patients in southwest France. The sample comprised individuals aged over 18 years who attended their GP, for a variety of reasons, on 4 half-days over a 2-week period. Individual PDI item endorsement by subjects with no history of psychiatric disorder ranged from 5 to 70%. Psychotic patients endorsed nearly all the PDI items more frequently, and the main discriminative items between psychotic and nonpsychotic patient groups were delusional ideas with persecutory, religious and guilt themes (Verdoux et al., 1998a).

People with intense spiritual or religious beliefs can have experiences similar to the positive symptoms of schizophrenia (Jackson, 1997). Peters et al. (1999b) explored the prevalence of delusional ideation in members of new religious movements (Hare Krishnas and Druids) compared with two control groups (nonreligious and Christian) and a group of deluded psychotic inpatients, using two delusion inventories. Individuals from the new religious movements scored significantly higher than the control groups on all the delusional measures apart from levels of distress. They could not be differentiated from psychotic patients on the number of delusional items endorsed on the PDI or on levels of conviction, but they were significantly less distressed and preoccupied by their experiences (Peters et al., 1999b).

Cooccurrence of delusions and hallucinations

The studies reviewed above provide evidence for the continuity of the individual phenomena of hallucinations and delusions. However, in patients with psychotic disorder, the positive symptoms of hallucinations and delusions typically occur together (Bilder et al., 1985; Liddle, 1987a; Peralta et al., 1992), and this clinical observation is compatible with the theory proposed by Maher that some delusions arise secondarily in an attempt to explain abnormal perceptions (Maher, 1974, 1988). Observational studies suggest that there is also an association between the presence of these psychotic experiences in nonclinical samples. In the study by Verdoux and colleagues (1998a), 16% of subjects with no history of psychiatric disorder reported that they had experienced auditory hallucinations during their lifetime, in addition to endorsing delusional items on the PDI. In the Johns et al. (1998) study, there was an association between reports on the PSQ of hallucinations and other psychotic experiences.

Data on psychotic symptoms collected as part of the Dutch NEMESIS study (Bijl et al., 1998) suggest a psychosis continuum in the general population. In this study, a representative general population sample of 7076 men and women was interviewed using the Composite International Diagnostic Interview (CIDI). For the 17 CIDI core positive psychosis items, the authors studied the four possible ratings on each of these 17 items: (i) a rating of 'true', psychiatrist-verified presence of hallucinations and/or delusions; (ii) a rating indicating that the symptom was present but the subject did not appear to be bothered by it; (iii) a rating indicating that the symptom was the result of drugs or physical disorder; and (iv) a rating indicating that the symptom appeared to be present but the interviewer was uncertain because there could have been a plausible explanation. Although all symptom ratings were strongly and independently associated with the presence of DSM-III-R psychotic disorder in terms of relative risk, the authors found that, of the 1237 individuals with any type of positive psychosis rating (17.5%), only 26 (2.1%) had a DSM-III-R diagnosis of nonaffective psychosis. In addition, they reported that the prevalences of all four positive symptom ratings were elevated in both those with and those without any DSM-III-R psychiatric disorder, although more so in the former (odds ratio (OR) 3.2; 95% confidence interval (CI) 2.8–3.7). The presence of any rating of hallucinations was strongly associated with the presence of any rating of delusion, supporting Maher's hypothesis of psychological mechanisms of delusion formation. Associations between hallucinatory and delusional experiences were apparent not only in individuals with any CIDI DSM-III-R lifetime diagnosis (OR 5.5; 95% CI 4.4–6.9) but also in individuals without a CIDI lifetime diagnosis (OR 4.3; 95% CI 2.9–6.3), suggesting continuity of psychological mechanisms of delusion formation across patient and nonpatient groups. Although psychotic symptoms in this sample were much more common than psychotic disorders, the distribution of individual total psychotic symptom scores in the sample was very skewed. These findings, therefore, suggest that both symptoms and underlying psychological mechanisms of psychosis occur as part of a continuous, albeit very skewed, distribution that shows only very partial overlap with clinical disorder.

Similarity in underlying dimensional representation

The above findings suggest that the positive symptoms of psychosis are prevalent in the general population but give little information about other symptoms and how different symptoms might cluster together. One way to test further the hypothesis of a psychosis continuum would be to investigate whether nonclinical or attenuated 'schizotypal' phenomena show a similar pattern of clustering into different symptom dimensions as their equivalents do in clinical psychotic disorders such as schizophrenia. Schizotypy refers to the personality trait of experiencing 'psychotic' symptoms, and psychometric identification of nonclinical schizotypal traits in the normal population provides further evidence for a continuum model of psychosis (Claridge, 1997; pp. 3–19). Schizotypy, or 'psychosis-proneness', may be a quantitative rather than a qualitative trait, ranging from normality at one end, through eccentricity and different combinations of schizotypal characteristics to florid psychosis at the other.

There is growing evidence from factor analytical studies that schizotypy is a multidimensional construct composed of three and possibly four dimensions: a positive dimension (aberrant perceptions and beliefs), a negative dimension (introvertive anhedonia), a conceptual disorganization dimension and an asocial/nonconformity dimension (Vollema and van den Bosch, 1995). Although the nonconformity dimension has been fairly consistently replicated, its presence may reflect a covarying normal personality trait resembling Eysenck's 'toughmindedness' (Eysenck and Eysenck (1973) The Manual of the Personality Questionnaire; unpublished manuscript), rather than a core component of schizotypy itself (Vollema, 1999). Other authors have proposed a slightly different three-factor model with a third factor of social impairment (Lenzenweger, 1991; Venables and Rector, 2000). Several authors have drawn attention to the striking resemblance between the exploratory and confirmatory factorial solutions of the signs and symptoms of schizotypy and those observed in schizophrenia. For example, the dimensions of positive, negative and disorganization symptoms reported in schizophrenia (Bilder et al., 1985; Liddle, 1987a; Peralta et al., 1992) resemble the dimensions reported in schizotypy (Bentall et al., 1989; Claridge, 1990; Raine et al., 1994; Vollema and van den Bosch, 1995; Gruzelier, 1996; Vollema and Hoijtink, 2000). These findings, therefore, suggest that psychosis may exist as a continuum of variation along various comorbid symptom dimensions (van Os et al., 1999c).

Familial clustering and longitudinal associations

If there is variation on a continuum, one would expect that lesser states on the continuum would show familial and longitudinal continuity. In other words, one would expect that (i) the families of probands with clinical psychotic disorder have higher rates of psychosis-like symptoms and/or schizotypy and vice versa and (ii) that individuals with high levels of psychosis-like symptoms and/or schizotypy have a higher risk of developing clinical psychotic disorder. Family studies have shown that schizotypy cooccurs with schizophrenia in the same family more often than would be expected by chance (Kendler et al., 1993b, 1995; Kendler and Walsh, 1995). This suggests that the same social and/or genetic factors that contribute to schizophrenia also contribute to schizotypy, i.e. that the two conditions are at least in part aetiologically continuous.

Similarly, follow-up studies of subjects with elevated schizotypy scores have demonstrated high rates of clinical psychosis and related disorders (Chapman et al., 1994; Kwapil et al., 1997). In a New Zealand birth cohort of 1000 children aged 11 years, presence of self-reported psychotic symptoms increased the risk for schizophreniform disorder at age 26 years more than 16 times (Poulton et al., 2000). This suggests that lower states on the continuum are a risk factor for more elevated states, and that transitions over the continuum occur with time.

Associations with demographic risk factors

Those with incident (or first-onset) disease show, as a group, a characteristic pattern of associations with a range of demographic variables. They are more likely to be young, single and unemployed. They also have a lower mean level of education and are more likely to reside in urban environments (Galdos et al., 1993; Kendler et al., 1996; Marcelis et al., 1998). The characteristic age-related variation in the incidence of schizophrenia is mirrored in a similar age-related expression of schizotypy (Rust, 1988; Claridge et al., 1996), delusional ideation measured with the PDI (Peters et al., 1999a) and delusions and hallucinations in the absence of a clinical psychotic disorder (van Os et al., 2000). Verdoux and colleagues (1998b) speculated that early adulthood, when levels of psychosis-like experiences are highest, may be a critical developmental phase for the expression of the trait psychosis, other factors determining at what level of the continuum the expression will occur. With regard to the other demographic factors that are associated with schizophrenia, similar associations have been reported for nonclinical psychotic and psychosis-like symptoms (van Os et al., 2000). Although it is not known whether, for example, single marital status and urban residence are causally related to the incidence of psychotic disorder or the result of premorbid drift, the similarity of the pattern of associations between psychotic disorder and mental states that occupy a lower position in the distribution is again suggestive of a continuum of psychotic experiences.

Psychosis 'transitions'

There is a great deal of current interest in preventing individuals from making 'transitions' from nonclinical to clinical psychotic states (Ch. 7). It then becomes important to understand what causes individuals on some position at the hypothesized continuum to become a clinical 'case'. It is important to distinguish between a truly continuous and a quasicontinuous relationship between symptoms and

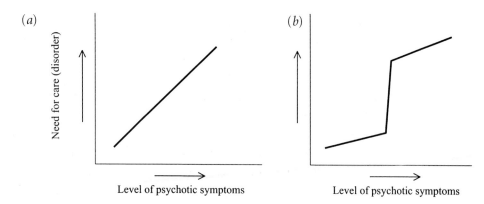

Fig. 18.4.   Relationship between psychotic symptoms and psychotic disorder. (*a*) Continuity, where there is a continuous relationship between level of psychotic symptoms and the need for care. (*b*) Discontinuity, where the initial increase is linear, but after a certain threshold the risk increases disproportionally.

disorder (Claridge, 1994). For example, with regard to the transition from having one or more psychotic symptoms to becoming a patient with a psychotic disorder, there may be a true linear relationship between symptoms and disorder without major discontinuity (Fig. 18.4*a*). However, another possibility is that psychotic symptoms behave like hypertension, which is on a direct continuum with continuous normal variation in blood pressure and in itself is not symptomatic, but beyond a certain threshold the risk of somatic complications involving other organs increases exponentially (Fig. 18.4*b*). This latter possibility, the most likely one according to some (Häfner, 1988, 1989), corresponds to a continuum–threshold relationship between psychosis proneness in the form of psychotic symptoms and the clinical disorder. For example, it may be that above a 'critical' value of psychosis an individual becomes much more likely to develop need for care caused by the psychotic symptoms themselves. Alternatively, an individual exposed to a number of independent risk factors with small effect sizes and a certain level of psychosis may develop an abrupt, nonlinear increase in need for care after exposure to additional, interacting risk factors with possibly larger effect sizes, resulting in overt disorder.

    If there is a discontinuous relationship, what are the factors that are additionally important in bringing about an abrupt change? A full consideration of the range of possible biological and social factors is beyond the scope of this chapter, but some psychological aspects of the transition from having symptoms to becoming a patient will be considered here. Psychotic or psychotic-like symptoms vary in terms of frequency, degree of conviction, preoccupation, implausibility, influence on behaviour, distress and secondary attributions, all of which may be of crucial importance in producing illness and help-seeking behaviour. The evidence suggests that the implausibility of experiences and degree of conviction may not be related to illness status (Garety and Hemsley, 1994). However, there do seem to be some other qualitative differences in psychotic experiences between psychiatric patients and nonpatients, such as the cultural context and degree of preoccupation and distress (Peters et al., 1999a,b). For example, in studies of predisposition to hallucinations in student samples (Bentall and Slade, 1985; Young et al., 1986), hardly any subjects reported that they had been troubled by hearing voices, whereas patients with schizophrenia most commonly experience stressful auditory verbal hallucinations (Kendell, 1985). Peters et al. (1999b) found that individuals from new religious movements were similar to psychotic patients in terms of number of delusional items endorsed on the PDI and levels of conviction, but were similar to controls in terms of levels of distress. Therefore, as far as the distinction patient/nonpatient is concerned, it may be important to consider two interacting risks: one that determines which position a person is going to occupy along the psychosis continuum, and one that determines whether a person at a certain point on the continuum is going to develop illness behaviour. Thus, two persons at different positions on the continuum may experience differences in the number, intrusiveness or frequency of symptoms, or the degree of other comorbid symptom dimensions such as negative symptoms, thought disorder or cognitive impairment (Kendler et al., 1996). Because of this, the person in the higher position may have a higher risk of becoming a mental health patient. Conversely, however, at each point of the continuum two persons with the same level of psychotic symptoms may differ in that one copes well and does not develop illness behaviour, whereas the other may develop functional impairments and need for care (Claridge, 1997; pp. 301–317). Further research is needed to clarify these relationships.

The dimensional hypothesis: categories versus dimensions

What should be grouped: individuals or symptoms?
Grouping symptoms

The usual way to diagnose mental illness is to group individuals according to certain symptom characteristics. An example is given in Fig. 18.5, in which the criteria for schizophrenia according to DSM-IV are depicted. According to the first criterion, at least two symptoms out of five must be present, yielding 19 possible combinations. According to the second criterion, at least one out of three symptoms must be present, yielding another six combinations. The total possible number of combinations of symptoms is, therefore, $19 \times 6 = 114$. In other words, somebody with disorganized speech and grossly disorganized behaviour fulfils the criteria for schizophrenia as much as somebody who hears a voice giving a running commentary on his behaviour. The implicit assumption in this type of categorization is that

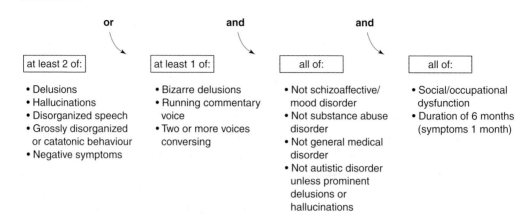

Fig. 18.5.   DSM-IV criteria for schizophrenia.

all the 114 different combinations of symptoms are associated with the same aetiologies and treatment needs: if they all had different causes and needed different treatments there would be little point in clustering them together. There have, therefore, been attempts to examine to what degree the symptoms in these 114 combinations show a natural tendency to occur together. This can be done by collecting detailed psychopathological information in groups of patients with a diagnosis of schizophrenia and conducting analyses to determine which symptoms tend to occur together and which symptoms do not. Symptoms that tend to cluster together within patients (in statistical terms are correlated with each other) can, thus, be identified and grouped into different symptom dimensions. Each patient can be characterized by how high or how low he or she scores on a number of different symptom dimensions (for example, positive and negative symptom dimensions; see below). This is the dimensional representation of psychopathology, which contrasts with, but can be used in combination with, the traditional categorical representation. The advantages of the dimensional representation, listed by Kendell (1993), are that they provide more information (each patient can have a unique mix of scores on different dimensions), do not impose boundaries where none may exist (avoiding the need to label patients as 'atypical'), can be flexibly transformed into categories, and back again if needed, and avoid patients being equated with their diagnostic category (as indicated by the frequent use of the term 'schizophrenics' or 'schizophrenic patients'). The disadvantages are that it is difficult to determine the number of dimensions needed to summarize symptoms, that scales are needed to measure symptoms and that more information needs to be managed diagnostically.

Grouping individuals

The advantage of the categorical representation is that categories are familiar, easy to understand for those who underwent medical training and conceptually much closer to the dichotomous decision to treat in clinical practice. A disadvantage, however, of the categorical representations in DSM and ICD is that they are not the product of empirical investigation but instead tend to reflect historical notions and agreement among the members of expert committees of a certain profession. In other words, they are mostly concept driven and only partly data driven. The same holds for the search for so-called subtypes of schizophrenia, in which subtypes are mostly proposed on the basis of a single operationalized concept, for example 'neurodevelopmental schizophrenia' (Murray, 1994), 'type I versus type II schizophrenia' (Crow, 1985), 'disorganized schizophrenia' (American Psychiatric Association, 1994) and 'deficit syndrome schizophrenia' (Carpenter, 1994). Although many mean differences between diagnostic categories or between subtypes can usually be shown, the weakness of this approach is that it is focused entirely on a single operationalized concept and, therefore, ignores other sources of multivariate heterogeneity in the data (Sham et al., 1996). Any mean differences between groups may be driven by a large amount of underlying, unexplained, multivariate heterogeneity and may, therefore, be wrongly attributed to the observed single concept distinction (e.g. affective psychosis versus schizophrenia, neurodevelopmental versus adult-onset psychosis, deficit syndrome versus non-deficit syndrome) (van Os et al., 2000). One way to overcome the limitations of this a priori single-concept approach is to group individuals using data-driven, multivariate empirical methods. Thus, in the method of factor analysis described above, the investigator determines whether different symptoms can be grouped together. Similarly, cluster analysis and the related method of latent class analysis is used to determine whether individuals can be grouped on the basis of their similarities on a number of, for example, psychopathological variables.

Validity of dimensional and categorical representations

As discussed above, the relative validity of a diagnostic system can be determined by examining to what degree the system can provide a contrast with regard to aetiology, psychopathology, treatment and outcome (Robins and Guze, 1970; Carpenter et al., 1980). In the context of a categorical representation of psychopathology (traditional diagnostic categories or latent classes), this would mean that individuals falling into two diagnostic categories (or latent classes) A and B would have been exposed differentially to risk factors, had different treatment needs, different symptoms and different outcomes. In addition, one would expect the two categories to provide a reasonably sharp symptomatic contrast.

In the context of a dimensional representation, however, validation would be assessed by demonstrating that the scores on dimensions A and B would be differentially associated with the presence of a particular risk factor, a particular treatment need or a particular outcome. In addition, one would expect that certain symptoms would occur together much more often than they would with other

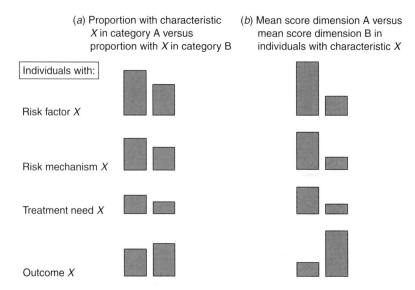

(a) Proportion with characteristic   (b) Mean score dimension A versus
X in category A versus   mean score dimension B in
proportion with X in category B   individuals with characteristic X

Individuals with:

Risk factor X

Risk mechanism X

Treatment need X

Outcome X

Fig. 18.6.   Diagnostic validation in categorical (a) and dimensional context (b) (right). Hypothetical example comparing the degree of contrast provided by categorical and dimensional representations of psychopathology. The degree of contrast provided in each domain is greater for the dimensional representation on the right than for the categorical representation on the left, suggesting that the dimensional representation has greater validity.

symptoms and that they would do so consistently across different investigations. If it can be shown that the dimensional representation provides greater contrast than the categorical representation on the domains of risk, treatment and outcome, the dimensional representation can be considered more useful (Fig. 18.6).

Discontinuity

The method of validation discussed above essentially investigates mean differences between groups or dimensions. However, mean differences do not necessarily validate a concept. For example, there may be mean differences in height and proficiency in Spanish between men living in Spain and men living in Norway, but this does not mean that two separate human species have been validated. A more rigorous strategy to examine the validity of diagnostic distinctions is the search for discontinuity (Kendell and Brockington, 1980). For example, in a mixed group of patients with diagnoses of affective psychosis and schizophrenia, each patient may be allocated a psychopathological score indicating to what degree his/her symptoms are typically affective or typically schizophrenic. Such a score indicating the difference in psychopathology between two groups can be calculated with the help of, for example, a discriminant function analysis. This discriminant psychopathological score can subsequently be plotted against some continuous third variable used in

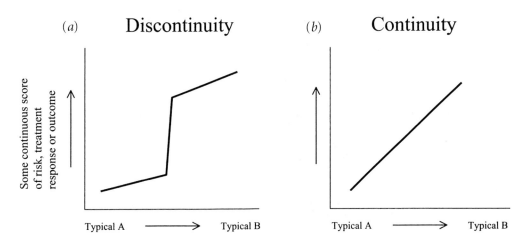

Psychopathological score discriminating between disorder A and disorder B

Fig. 18.7.   The search for discontinuity (see text for explanation).

the validation procedure, such as cerebral ventricle size, response to lithium treatment or outcome score. If the mean risk, treatment response or outcome score varies in a linear, dose–response manner with the discriminant psychopathological score, there is no evidence for discontinuity. However, if it can be shown that at some point of the discriminant psychopathological score, a small change in psychopathology leads to a large 'jump' in the value of risk, treatment response or outcome, the data are compatible with discontinuity between affective psychosis and schizophrenia, as it suggests that there is a point where one disorder 'begins' and the other 'ends' (Fig. 18.7). A limitation of this method is that absence of discontinuity is no proof of continuity, and that other, more difficult to interpret, nonlinear relationships may transpire. However, it remains a powerful method, as shown by recent work, albeit outside the realm of psychosis (Kendler and Gardner, 1998).

Evidence for the validity of the dimensional versus categorical approach

Given the alternative ways in which symptoms may be represented (a priori diagnostic categories, latent classes, symptom dimensions), what is the evidence about the degree of contrast these representations provide in the domains of psychopathology, aetiology, treatment and outcome?

Traditional categories

Psychopathological contrast

In a categorical representation of psychopathology, the degree of useful psychopathological contrast that the categories provide can be illustrated by quantifying how likely it is that a patient with a high level of positive or negative symptoms has a diagnosis of schizophrenia compared with a patient with a low level of positive or

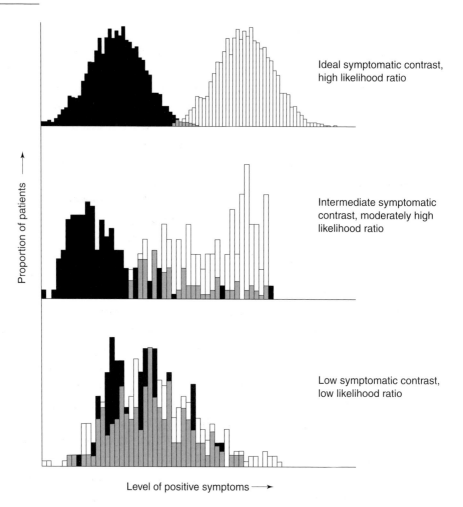

Fig. 18.8.   Distribution of, for example, individual scores on the positive symptom dimension in psychotic patients with (□) and without (■) a diagnosis of schizophrenia. Areas in grey indicate overlap in the distribution of scores. The diagnosis of schizophrenia is used as a test to predict the likelihood of high levels of positive symptoms.

negative symptoms. If the patient with a high level of positive or negative symptoms is 10 times more likely to have a diagnosis of schizophrenia than a patient with low levels of these symptoms, it may be argued that the diagnostic likelihood ratio is high enough to provide a reasonable diagnostic contrast (Fig. 18.8).

Although the diagnostic likelihood ratio is the traditional epidemiological measure of diagnostic value (Sackett et al., 1997), very few investigations have been carried out in relation to the diagnosis of schizophrenia. The early studies using different, though related, approaches did not find evidence that traditional diagnostic categories provided much diagnostic contrast (Pope and Lipinski, 1978) or psychopathological discontinuity between them (Kendell and Gourlay, 1970). Only one study claimed to have identified a discriminate function to distinguish schizophrenia, but this concerned a distinction from a combination of all other mental disorders and the absence of any disorder (Cloninger et al., 1985). More recent studies also provide little evidence for high levels of diagnostic contrast between diagnostic categories in the functional psychoses. In one study involving more than 700 patients with chronic psychotic illness, the diagnostic likelihood ratio for high levels of positive, negative and disorganization symptoms did not exceed 2 in comparisons between patients with schizophrenia and patients with affective and schizoaffective psychosis (UK700 Group, 2000). The likelihood ratios for high levels of depressive and manic symptoms were better, although there was still considerable overlap in the distributions of these symptoms between affective and nonaffective psychotic categories. In another study of 660 inpatients with a range of psychotic illnesses, the diagnostic value of the presence of so-called first-rank symptoms (FRS: of which a single one is enough to fulfil the diagnostic criterion for DSM-IV schizophrenia) was examined. The presence of FRS did not substantially increase the likelihood of having schizophrenia, with the value of likelihood ratios not exceeding 3 (Peralta and Cuesta, 1999a). Although some individual symptoms may have better discriminating properties in assigning a cross-sectional diagnosis (Cuesta and Peralta, 1995), these results suggest that the diagnostic value of the distinction between affective and nonaffective psychosis is rather weak, at least as far as the typical nonaffective dimensions of positive, negative and disorganization symptoms are concerned. The diagnostic contrast provided for affective symptoms seems rather better, which led Bell and colleagues (1998) to conclude that constructs like DSM-III-R schizophrenia are more clearly specified by what they are not (i.e. the absence of affective symptoms) rather than by what they actually are (the presence of characteristic psychotic symptoms).

Contrast in aetiology

Kendell wrote in 1991 that 'time after time research workers have compared groups of schizophrenics and normal controls and found some difference between the two which they assumed to be a clue to the aetiology of schizophrenia, only for someone else, years later, to find the same abnormality in patients with affective psychoses'. It is safe to say that there is little in terms of specificity with regard to risk factors, treatment and outcome. However, there are many mean differences between groups. For example, exposure to life events may precipitate both a depressive and a schizophrenia episode, but the risk of onset of depression is greater than the onset of schizophrenia. In other words, although there may be no qualitative differences between diagnostic groups such as schizophrenia and the affective psychoses, there do appear to be quantitative differences in terms of the effect size of the risk factor (or, in some instances, the timing of the exposure). A summary of influential studies is given in Table 18.1. What transpires is that the effect size of developmental, perinatal and

Table 18.1. Pattern of differences in effect size for affective disorder and schizophrenia

Risk factor	Group	Comparisons	Relative risk[a]
Life events	Bebbington et al. (1993)	Psychotic depression versus controls	6.9
		Mania versus controls	3.6
		Schizophrenia versus controls	4.8
	Paykel (1978)[b]	Nonpsychotic depression versus controls	2–5
		Schizophrenia versus controls	2–3
	Dohrenwend et al. (1995)	Major depression versus controls	Both elevated risk, but significantly
		Nonaffective psychosis versus controls	higher event rate in depressives
Expressed emotion	Butzlaff and Hooley (1998)[b]	Relapse versus nonrelapse mood disorder	0.45[c]
		Relapse versus nonrelapse schizophrenia	0.30[c]
Urban birth	Marcelis et al. (1998)	Incidence rate affective disorder in urban versus rural born	1.4
		Incidence rate schizophrenia in urban versus rural born	2.0
Lower cognitive ability of age 15 years	Jones et al. (1994)	Nonpsychotic depression versus controls	1.5
	van Os et al. (1997b)	Schizophrenia versus controls	2
Cerebral ventricle size	Elkis et al. (1995)[b]	Nonpsychotic mood disorder versus controls	0.44[c]
		Nonpsychotic mood disorder versus schizophrenia	−0.20[d]
Early gestational famine exposure	Brown et al. (1989)	Risk affective disorder in exposed versus nonexposed	1.09[e]
		Risk schizophrenia in exposed versus nonexposed	1.73
Later gestational famine exposure	Brown et al. (1999)	Risk affective disorder in exposed versus nonexposed	1.36
		Risk schizophrenia in exposed versus nonexposed	1.05[e]
One relative with schizophrenia	Kendler et al. (1993a)	Affective psychosis probands versus controls	3.9
		Nonpsychotic affective illness probands versus controls	1.0[e]
		Schizophrenia probands versus controls	6.5

Depression in relative	Maier et al. (1993)	Unipolar depression probands versus controls	2.0
		Schizophrenia probands versus controls	1.9
Parent with affective disorder	Erlenmeyer-Kimling et al. (1997)	Risk affective psychosis versus controls	7.5/0
		Risk schizophrenia-related psychoses[f] versus controls	8.6
Parent with schizophrenia	Erlenmeyer-Kimling et al. (1997)	Risk affective psychosis versus controls	6/0
		Risk nonpsychotic bipolar disorder versus controls	1.4[e]
		Risk schizophrenia-related psychoses[f] versus controls	25.6

Notes:

[a] All relative risk values were reported as statistically different with the exception of those marked [e].

[b] Review article.

[c] Not a relative risk but a standardized effect size.

[d] Standardized effect size indicating that schizophrenia patients had larger ventricle size.

[e] Not statistically different.

[f] Schizophrenia; schizoaffective disorder, mainly schizophrenia; unspecified psychosis.

neuroradiological risk factors is greater (or earlier, in the case of prenatal famine) for schizophrenia than for affective disorder, whereas the effect size of social adversity in the form of life events or expressed emotions is greater for affective disorder. In addition, the rate of schizophrenia is increased in probands with affective psychosis, but less so than in probands with schizophrenia. The rate of nonpsychotic unipolar depression may be increased in relatives of those with schizophrenia, but not the rate of nonpsychotic bipolar disorder. Therefore, an interpretable pattern of quantitative differences rather than qualitative differences is seen between categories, with the possible exception of familial morbid risk of bipolar illness, which may be specific for affective psychosis. These data, therefore, suggest that a dimensional representation may be useful.

Contrast in treatment and outcome

The contrast in terms of treatment and outcome has been reviewed extensively elsewhere (Kerr and McClelland, 1991). The evidence here also cannot be taken as a straightforward validition of traditional categories of psychotic illness. Although mean differences exist between groups, no outcome discontinuities or treatment specificity has been demonstrated. For example, it has been shown repeatedly that patients with a diagnosis of schizophrenia have the poorest outcome, with schizoaffective patients occupying an intermediate position between schizophrenia and affective psychosis (Tsuang and Dempsey, 1979; Brockington et al., 1980a,b; Harrow and Grossman, 1984; Samson et al., 1988; Marneros et al., 1989, 1990; Coryell et al., 1990a,b; Maj and Perris, 1990; Grossman et al., 1991). Therefore, rather than discrete qualitative differences in outcome, there appears to be a 'dose–response' relationship between degree of affective symptomatology and outcome. Kendell and Brockington (1980) specifically tried to disprove the existence of such a linear relationship but failed. Similarly, associations with treatment do not support straightforward validation of the categories of psychotic illness. For example, antipsychotic drugs are effective against psychotic symptoms in both affective and nonaffective illness, and lithium relieves elevation of mood equally well in both mania and schizophrenia (Johnstone et al., 1988). Antidepressant treatment has been shown not only to alleviate depressive symptoms in schizophrenia (Siris et al., 1987), but also to reduce the rate of psychotic relapse (Siris et al., 1994).

Latent classes

Psychopathological contrast

Latent class and cluster analyses have been carried out in different ways. Some researchers accept the validity of the variably defined schizophrenia diagnosis and search for subtypes within this diagnostic construct (Carpenter et al., 1976; Farmer et al., 1983; Goldstein et al., 1990). However, this approach is somewhat contradictory, as the data-driven method is limited to a sample within an unproven, concept-driven diagnostic category. Others have, therefore, extended their samples to include all nonaffective psychosis (Castle et al., 1994) and, even better, all affective and nonaffective psychosis (Kendler et al., 1998). The results of these latter two investigations show that the results are highly dependent on (i) the sample included (with or without inclusion of affective psychosis), and (ii) the type of variables that are used in the multivariate analyses (Table 18.2). The investigation by Kendler and coworkers (1998) resulted in more classes (six), possibly because more symptomatology and course variables were included in the analyses, especially with regard to affective symptoms. By comparison, the study by Castle et al. (1994) included two aetiological variables and produced three classes. Both investigations concurred in that both identified a more or less 'classic' schizophrenia syndrome. However, the identification of this syndrome cannot be considered as a validation of DSM or ICD schizophrenia as such. In the study by Kendler and colleagues (1998), the DSM-III-R diagnoses allocated to the individuals in the different classes were investigated (Table 18.2). DSM-III-R schizophrenia formed a substantial part of three of the six classes and the same held for DSM-III-R schizoaffective psychosis. Although the data-driven classes were significantly associated with the concept-driven DSM-III-R diagnoses and the classes bore a substantial resemblance to historical notions of diagnosis, there was no one-to-one relationship between classes and DSM-III-R diagnoses.

In another study of 785 individuals with any nonaffective psychosis, five classes were reported; however, the details provided in the paper were insufficient to be included in Table 18.2 (Kendler et al., 1997). These five classes were, approximately (i) a class characterized by good outcome, later onset, moderate levels of positive, high levels of affective (manic) symptoms and low levels of negative symptoms; (ii) a class characterized by high levels of negative symptoms and low levels of positive and affective symptoms and poor outcome; (iii) a class characterized by high levels of both positive and negative symptoms, early age of onset and (moderately) poor outcome; (iv) a class with intermediate levels of positive, negative and affective symptoms; and (v) a class with very low levels of positive symptoms and pronounced catatonic symptoms, certain negative symptoms and a relapsing–remitting illness course. As these classes were largely defined in terms of quantitative variation of negative, positive and affective symptoms, the classification is in fact quite close to a dimensional representation of psychopathology (see below).

Contrast in aetiology, treatment and outcome
Castle and colleagues (1994) and Kendler and colleagues (1998) both tried to validate their findings by examining to what degree the different classes showed different associations with aetiological and treatment response variables. In the first

Table 18.2. Outcomes of two latent class analyses of psychosis

Sample	Variables used	Classes	Corresponding DSM-III-R category
Epidemiological sample of nonaffective psychosis (but including schizoaffective psychosis) ($n = 447$): Castle et al. (1994)	Family history of schizophrenia Restricted affect Persecutory delusions Poor premorbid adjustment Dysphoria Early onset Winter birth Male sex	1. Neurodevelopmental (early onset, poor premorbid adjustment, restricted affect, male preponderance) 2. Paranoid (later onset, persecutory delusions, equal sex ratio) 3. Schizoaffective (preponderance females, dysphoria, persecutory delusions)	– – –
Epidemiological sample major affective illness and nonaffective psychosis ($n = 343$): Kendler et al. (1998)	Illness >6 months Positive thought disorder Negative thought disorder Affective symptoms predominate Restricted affect Persecutory delusions Schneiderian delusions Schneiderian hallucinations Other auditory hallucinations Deterioration form premorbid functioning Elevated mood Excessive activity	1. Classic schizophrenia (delusions, hallucinations, negative symptoms, low levels affective symptoms, chronic course, poor outcome) 2. Major depression (rarely psychotic and negative symptoms, benign course, good outcome, no manic symptoms, common and prominent depressive symptoms) 3. Schizophreniform disorder (delusions, hallucinations, sometimes manic symptoms); compared with classic schizophrenia: less-prominent negative symptoms, more benign illness course, much better outcome, short episodes of illness 4. Bipolar schizomania (prominent psychotic, manic and depressive symptoms); affective symptoms predominant; intermediate levels with negative symptoms, benign course/outcome	1. Schizophrenia (85%) 2. Major depression (95%) 3. Other nonaffective psychoses (54%), schizophrenia (21%), bipolar illness (15%) 4. Bipolar illness (57%), schizoaffective disorder (32%)

Reckless acts		
Pressured speech		
Dysphoria		
Psychomotor change		
Tired		
Excessive self-reproach		
Reduction in weight/appetite		
Chronic course		
Poor outcome		
	5. Schizodepression (prominent depressive symptoms, outcome between classic schizophrenia and major depression); compared with classic schizophrenia: more-prominent psychotic symptoms, similar level negative symptoms. Affective symptoms not usually predominant	5. Schizophrenia (58%), schizoaffective disorder (26%)
	6. Hebephrenia (like classic schizophrenia but much more likely to be thought-disordered and with manic, excited or disinhibited symptoms)	6. Schizophrenia (60%), schizoaffective disorder

Notes:

DSM-III-R, see American Psychiatric Association (1987).

study, a partial separation between the first two classes was achieved on the basis of premorbid and treatment response variables, but the third class was less distinct (Sham et al., 1996). The study by Kendler and colleagues (1998) was interesting in that associations between the classes on the one hand, and familial risk for psychiatric disorders on the other, based on detailed family interview data, were assessed. This revealed that the familial risk of schizophrenia and schizophrenia spectrum disorders were significantly increased in the probands of all classes, whereas an increase in familial risk for mood disorders was more specific (although far from entirely specific) for the proband classes characterized by mood symptoms. Therefore, in terms of familial morbid risk, the nonaffective classes were better validated by what they were not than by what they were, which is reminiscent of the findings on psychopathological contrast reported by Bell and colleagues (1998). One of the classes reported by Kendler and colleagues was a schizophreniform disorder class, which was characterized by short episodes of illness, a benign course and good outcome. A previous study based on a large epidemiological sample had commented on the geographical variation of this type of nonaffective acute remitting psychosis, rates being about ten times higher in developing countries and in women (Susser and Wanderling, 1994).

Symptom dimensions

Psychopathological contrast

The dimensional approach identifies, with the help of statistical procedures, groups of symptoms that occur together more often than would be expected by chance alone. These empirically derived groups of symptoms are usually called dimensions or syndromes. After the pioneering early work of researchers in the 1960s and 1970s (Overall and Gorham, 1962; Everitt et al., 1971; Fleiss et al., 1971), the existence of three syndromes in the diagnostic category of schizophrenia was reported in the 1980s (Bilder et al., 1985; Liddle, 1987b; Peralta et al., 1992). Apart from the positive and the negative syndromes, a syndrome of disorganization (characterized by thought disorder, inappropriate affect and bizarre behaviour) is often identified. Although the disorganization syndrome is the least replicable of the three syndromes, latent structure modelling of schizophrenia symptomatology strongly suggests that the two-factor solution of positive and negative symptoms is a very poor representation of the data (Peralta et al., 1994), and meta-analytic work supports the existence of a third 'conceptual disorganization' factor (Grube et al., 1998). The three schizophrenia syndromes themselves appear to be an 'oversimplification', in that they may be the higher-order factors of many more first-order dimensions (Peralta and Cuesta, 1999b).

It has been pointed out, however, that the schizophrenia syndrome studies, just as the early latent class studies, suffer from the fact that data-driven methods were

Table 18.3. Dimensions of psychosis in three studies

Study	No.	Dimensions
Kitamura et al. (1995)	584	1. Depressive
		2. Manic
		3. Positive
		4. Negative
		5. Catatonic
McGorry et al. (1998)	509	1. Depressive
		2. Manic
		3. Positive
		4. Negative/catatonic/disorganization
van Os et al. (1999a)	708	1. Depressive
		2. Manic
		3. Positive
		4. Negative

used in samples that were restricted by concept-driven nosological boundaries (McGorry et al., 1998). These comments were confirmed by studies showing that the same three syndromes also occur in the affective psychoses (Maziade et al., 1995; Peralta et al., 1997; Ratakonda et al., 1998). Other studies, therefore, have attempted to identify symptom dimensions in samples including the whole range of traditional psychotic disorders and have also included measures of affective symptomatology, which had been largely ignored in earlier studies (Soni et al., 1992). These studies have been fairly consistent (although using quite different samples) in showing dimensions of positive, negative, depressive and manic symptoms and a more variable dimension of catatonic and/or disorganization symptoms (Table 18.3). Interestingly, multivariate symptom dimensions studies in samples restricted to patients with schizophrenia also yield a rather similar five-factor solution if some measures of affective symptoms are included (Lindenmeyer et al., 1995a,b). Most studies of symptom dimensions in psychosis used multivariate techniques where orthogonality was imposed on the factorial solutions, producing uncorrelated symptom dimensions. However, zero-correlation of symptom dimensions strains reality (for example, positive and negative symptoms tend to occur together), and studies using statistical techniques that allowed for correlation between factors did find that the various symptom dimensions covary with each other (Peralta et al., 1997; McGorry et al., 1998). The dimensional representation of the psychosis phenotype, therefore, suggests that psychosis is the simultaneous variation of up to five distinct, albeit correlated, symptom dimensions.

Contrast in aetiology and familial morbid risk

With regard to aetiological contrast, much work in the area of dimensions of psychosis has been done in relation to familial morbid risk. In general, three different, though related, methods have been applied. In the first, sibling pairs concordant for psychotic illness are examined in order to establish to what degree levels of positive, negative and other symptom dimensions in one sibling correlate with the same symptom dimension in the other. A differential and independent pattern of correlations across the different dimensions would support their validity. The results of this type of study to date are summarized in Table 18.4.

A related method is to examine, in pairs of twins concordant and discordant for psychosis, which symptoms in the proband-twin predict presence of psychotic illness in the co-twin. Differential predictive power for the various symptom dimensions would suggest different degrees of genetic influence and thus support their validity. Dworkin and colleagues (Dworkin and Lenzenweg, 1984) examined 151 pairs, derived from five different twin studies, of genetically identical (monozygotic, MZ) twins concordant and discordant for psychosis. The greater the number of negative symptoms in a twin with schizophrenia, the greater the likelihood that the other twin was affected as well. However, no such relationship was found for positive symptoms. In this study, no measure of affective symptoms was included. Farmer and colleagues (1983) examined the concordance ratio of MZ/dizygotic (DZ) twins (a measure that is strongly positively correlated with the heritability estimate of a disorder) as a function of probands and co-twin diagnosis. The addition of affective disorder with mood-incongruent delusions to the schizophrenia spectrum brought about a marked increase in the MZ/DZ concordance ratio and identified, by implication, a 'more genetic' combination than schizophrenia alone. However, the addition of any affective diagnosis category to the phenotype reduced the MZ/DZ concordance ratio.

The third, related method used in the literature is to try to predict, in probands with psychotic illness, the degree of familial psychopathology on the basis of the proband's scores on symptom dimensions (Ch. 10). In a study of 66 patients with RDC schizophrenia, it was reported that a history of schizophrenia and other non-affective psychoses was best predicted by probands' scores on subsyndromes derived from the inappropriate affect/bizarre behaviour and positive formal thought disorder factors (Cardno et al., 1997). In a study of 150 psychotic patients and 548 of their first-degree relatives, the negative syndrome was found to predict psychosis in the first-degree relatives, and the manic syndrome predicted mania in the relatives. The disorganization syndrome predicted psychotic illness in first-degree relatives, but only in patients with a diagnosis of schizophrenia (van Os et al., 1997a).

Can we conclude, therefore, that the different symptom dimensions show typical and/or contrasting patterns of correlations with various measures of familial morbid risk? The studies that looked at concordance of dichotomously defined syndromal measures (e.g. absence or presence of a negative symptom syndrome instead of a continuous negative symptom score) and the studies that were confined to formally defined (DSM, ICD or RDC) schizophrenia are weaker methodologically. This is because in these studies a situation may easily arise where 99% of both probands and co-siblings have evidence of the same positive symptom syndrome (as this is per definition required for a psychotic diagnosis), in which case it is impossible to show meaningful covariance. A limitation of all the sibling-pair studies (at least as far as the issue of validation is concerned) is that none attempted to assess the degree of correlation or concordance across dimensions, instead of just within dimensions. If negative symptoms in the proband sibling consistently correlated higher with negative symptoms in the co-sibling than with positive symptoms, a degree of familial specificity would have been established for the various dimensions. Such bivariate syndromal analyses will hopefully soon follow. In the meantime, several trends are apparent. All correlations and other measures of association are small, suggesting that all variation in symptom dimensions is to a large degree random rather than the result of some systematic familial effect. It appears that, of the various symptom measures, positive symptoms may have lower predictive power of symptoms or illness in the relatives than the disorganization and negative symptoms. The study by Loftus and colleagues (2000), however, suggested that the correlation is much higher for first-rank symptoms that are not some type of auditory hallucination, whereas the study by Hwu and colleagues (1997) suggested that concordance for positive symptoms may be much higher in sibling pairs who do not have negative symptoms. The disorganization syndrome was not only found to be associated with similar symptoms in the co-sibling in a number of sibling-pair studies but also found to predict psychosis in the first-degree relatives of patients with schizophrenia. The negative syndrome also predicts negative symptoms/psychotic illness in the relatives, though somewhat less consistently; where they were examined specifically, affective symptoms mostly predicted similar symptoms in the relatives.

Contrast in course and outcome
Other important contrasts in studies of symptom dimensions have included contrasts in prognosis, neuropsychological parameters and neuroimaging. Although effect sizes and methodologies vary considerably between studies, a persistent finding has been that negative symptoms predict poor course and outcome, whereas positive symptoms appear to have less impact on course and outcome variables (Pogue Geile, 1989). It has been suggested that, in particular, increases in the level of negative symptoms early on in the illness course indicate poorer prognosis

Table 18.4. Sib-pair concordance of symptom dimensions

Sample	Design	Factor solution	Correlation	
			Method 1[a]	Method 2[a]
457 sib-pairs with any nonaffective psychosis (Kendler et al., 1997)	Correlation within sib-pairs	Negative symptoms	0.16*	
		Positive symptoms	0.14*	
		Affective symptoms	0.27*	
80 sibships (n = 169) with DSM-III-R schizophrenia (Burke et al., 1996)	Intrapair correlations	Negative	0.23*	0.26*
		Positive	0.45*	0.08
		Disorganization	0.28*	0.15
		Depressive[b]	0.13	0.10
		Manic[b]	0.23*	−0.01
			Method 1[c]	Method 2[c]
109 sib-pairs with DSM-IV schizophrenia or schizo-affective psychosis (Cardno et al., 1999)	Within-pair correlations	Negative[b]	0.16	0.11
		Positive[b]	0.18	0.11
		Disorganization	0.32*	0.20*
		First-rank delusions	0.11	–
151 monozygotic twins with at least one patient with DSM-III schizophrenia (Dworkin and Lenzenweger, 1984)	Within-pair correlations	Negative[b]	0.26*	
		Positive[b]	0.03	
103 sib-pairs with DSM-III-R schizophrenia or schizo-affective disorder (Loftus et al., 2000)	Correlation within sib-pairs	First-rank symptom I (thought withdrawal, insertion, broadcasting, delusions of control)	0.21*	
		First-rank symptom II (third-person voices, thought echo, running commentary voices)	0.04	

			Observed/expected	All pairs	No negative symptoms
114 sib-pairs with DSM-III-R schizophrenia or schizoaffective disorder (Loftus et al., 1998)	Assessment of observed versus expected concordance of dichotomously defined syndrome measure	Positive syndrome	9.0/89.5[d]		
		Negative syndrome	18.0/15.5[d]		
		Disorganized syndrome	42.0/34.0[d*]		
		Affective syndrome	5.0/3.0[d]		
		First rank syndrome	68.0/68.0[d]		
53 sibships with schizophrenia or schizoaffective disorder (DeLisi et al., 1987)	Assessment of observed versus expected concordance of dichotomously defined symptom measure	Auditory hallucinations	30.0/29.8[d]		
		Visual hallucinations	20.0/15.9[d*]		
		Paranoid delusions	35.0/36.7[d]		
		Thought disorder	24.0/22.7[d]		
		Major depressive episode	17.0/11.8[d*]		
		Negative symptoms	11.0/10.0[d]		
46 sib-pairs with clinical diagnosis of schizophrenia (Hwu et al., 1997)	Kappa statistic of dichotomously defined syndromal measure[e]	Delusion-hallucination syndrome		0.3	0.55
		Thought disorganization syndrome			1.00
		Negative syndrome		0.21	–
		Severe negative syndrome			–

sib, sibling.

[a] Method 1 case-note and Method 2 interview material.

[b] Composite variable not identified through multivariate factor analysis.

[c] Method 1 SANS-SAPS and Method 2 OPCRIT material.

[d] Observed/expected.

[e] Kappa statistic was calculated for the four single symptom dimensions in the third column.

* Statistically significant in study sample.

(Fenton and McGlashan, 1991). One prospective study on the level of community functioning in schizophrenia found that the disorganization syndrome was more predictive of community functioning than the positive or negative symptom dimensions (Norman et al., 1999). Two studies that prospectively related course and outcome to baseline symptom dimensions defined multivariately in patients with broadly defined psychotic illness found poorer prognosis associated with negative and disorganization syndromes, and better prognosis associated with affective syndromes (van Os et al., 1996; Hollis, 2000). In addition, these and related studies found that the dimensional representation of psychopathology was a better predictor of both need for care and outcome in psychotic patients than formal diagnosis, and that changes in the various symptom dimensions differentially predict changes in important patient outcomes (Johnstone et al., 1992; van Os et al., 1999a,b). It is not known whether negative associations between outcome on the one hand and the disorganization and negative syndromes on the other are mediated by different mechanisms. Both appear to be associated with prognostically unfavourable variables such as single marital status, poor premorbid adjustment, impairment of interpersonal relationships and impersistence at work (Liddle, 1987a; Gureje et al., 1994; van Os et al., 1996; Salokangas, 1997; Cuesta et al., 1999).

Contrast in neuropsychology

Many studies have examined differential associations between symptom dimensions and neuropsychological variables, but unfortunately, at least for the purposes of validation, most were confined to narrowly defined diagnostic categories of schizophrenia with a chronic illness course and most excluded affective symptoms from the analysis. Given the fact that depressive symptoms are strongly associated with experience of psychological deficits, their inclusion seems necessary (Liddle et al., 1993). In spite of these shortcomings, the results seem to be consistent in some regard (Table 18.5) in that the disorganization and negative syndromes are consistently associated with neuropsychological measures of executive functioning, memory, language and other test variables, whereas associations with the positive syndrome have only been rarely reported. Interestingly, only one study included depressive symptoms; this study found that this symptom dimension had the strongest association with cognitive measures (Holthausen et al., 1999). Although some authors have proposed that the disorganization and negative syndrome dimensions show a differential pattern of neuropsychological associations, this is not readily appreciated from the qualitative review in Table 18.5. What seems to be apparent is that measures of verbal fluency and memory are more consistently associated with the negative symptom dimension than with symptoms of disorganization. One study suggested that the apparent lack of difference between the

Table 18.5. Symptom dimensions and cognitive performance

Disorganization	
Negative	Distractibility (Holthausen et al., 1999)
	Digit vigilance (Eckman and Shean, 2000)
	Finger tapping (Holthausen et al., 1999)
	Cognitive flexibility (Mahurin et al., 1998)
	Trails A (Liddle and Morris, 1991; Brown and White, 1992; Basso et al., 1998)
	Trails B (Brown and White, 1992; Basso et al., 1998)
	Psychomotor speed (Mahurin et al., 1998)
	Verbal fluency (Liddle and Morris, 1991; Brown and White, 1992; Norman et al., 1997; Basso et al., 1998; Mahurin et al., 1998)
	Wisconsin/modified card sorting test (Brown and White, 1992; Norman et al., 1997; Basso et al., 1998)
	Wechsler Memory Scale-R (Norman et al., 1997; Basso et al., 1998)
	Wechsler Memory Scale-R attention (Basso et al., 1998)
	Wechsler Memory Scale-R visual memory (Basso et al., 1998)
	Logical memory (Eckman and Shean, 2000)
	Long-term memory (Liddle 1987a)
	Working memory (Mahurin et al., 1998)
	Object naming (Liddle 1987a)
	Similarities (Liddle 1987a)
	Object classification (Liddle 1987a)
	Stroop interference (Liddle and Morris, 1991)
	Continuous performance test (Liu et al., 1997)
	WAIS-R IQ (Basso et al., 1998)
	Visual search (Mahurin et al., 1998)
Positive	Trails A (Basso et al., 1998)
	Trails B (Holthausen et al., 1999)
	Wechsler Memory Scale Revised (Norman et al., 1997)
	Ray Auditory Verbal Learning Test (Norman et al., 1997)
	Verbal memory (Mahurin et al., 1998)
	Selective attention (van der Does et al., 1996)
Depressive	Stroop colours (Holthausen et al., 1999)
	Trail making A (Holthausen et al., 1999)
	Trail making B (Holthausen et al., 1999)
	Fingertapping (Holthausen et al., 1999)
	Wisconsin/modified card sorting test (van der Does et al., 1993)
Excitement	Continuous performance test (Liu et al., 1997)

disorganization and negative symptom dimensions is an artifact, and that real differences between the two only become apparent if patients are being coached and receive incentives (Rowe and Shean, 1997). Another study suggested that subtle differences between the two syndromes become apparent if a distinction is being made between patients with persisting and remitting illness (Baxter and Liddle, 1998). There have also been reports of differential patterns of cerebral blood flow associated with dimensions of positive, negative and disorganization symptoms (Liddle et al., 1992; Ebmeier et al., 1993; Yuasa et al., 1995; Erkwoh et al., 1997), and of differential association patterns between symptom dimensions and structural magnetic resonance data (Chua et al., 1997).

Conclusions

DSM and ICD diagnostic categories in the functional psychoses reflect historical notions of severe mental illness in clinical settings. There are many mean differences between the different categories, but separation with regard to psychopathology, aetiology, treatment and outcome cannot be obtained. Empirically derived latent classes of psychotic illness on the whole resemble DSM diagnostic categories and selected subtypes, suggesting a degree of internal validity of DSM categories of psychosis. However, individual patients are frequently grouped in a class that is distinct from the DSM category to which they had been allocated, which tends to weaken the internal validity. For both the DSM/ICD categories and the empirical latent classes, the pattern of differences with regard to aetiology, treatment and outcome is mainly quantitative rather than qualitative, suggesting that what are presented as heterogeneous disorders may be better thought of as an illness continuum with various overlapping symptom dimensions (Griesinger, 1845; Menninger et al., 1958; Crow, 1986). For example, the fact that the familial morbid risk of DSM schizophrenia is nonspecifically increased in all diagnostic categories of psychotic illness suggests that some common risk factor may underlie all DSM psychotic illness categories. The fact that the familial morbid risk of schizophrenia is greater in the relatives of DSM schizophrenia probands than it is in DSM affective psychosis probands suggests that the 'dose' of the risk factor has some pathoplastic effect on illness presentation and outcome, greater dose resulting in an illness with more negative symptoms and poorer outcome. The reverse may hold for other risk factors. For example, the fact that exposure to stressful life events is more likely to result in depression than in schizophrenia (as indicated by greater effect sizes in case-control studies, as shown above) suggests that a greater 'dose' of social precipitants results in more affective, especially depressive, symptoms and better outcome (van Os et al., 1998; Ventura et al., 2000).

If the psychosis phenotype is indeed characterized by variation in several symptom dimensions that are each the result of the pathoplastic effects of a range of underlying risk factors, it may be useful to identify the dimensions of psychosis. Unfortunately, some confusion is apparent in that two parallel efforts appear to be underway: one in which dimensions are identified across the range of diagnostic categories of psychosis, and one in which researchers accept the validity of the DSM or ICD diagnosis of schizophrenia to the exclusion of all other diagnostic categories. Nevertheless, the solutions of multivariate exploratory and confirmatory factor analyses of the symptoms of psychosis and DSM/ICD schizophrenia appear to be reasonably replicable in a variety of settings, diagnostic groups and patient samples, suggesting acceptable internal validity. The external validity of these symptom dimensions, however, appears weaker. There is a consistent degree of aetiological and outcome contrast apparent between positive and affective symptom dimensions on the one hand and the other symptom dimensions on the other, but there is less evidence of 'separability' of the negative and disorganization dimensions. Although it is possible that the measures of aetiology, treatment and outcome used were not sensitive enough to detect real differences between the various symptom dimensions, the external validity remains, for the time being, incomplete.

In the few studies that directly compared dimensional and categorical representations of psychopathology, the former appeared to be more useful in terms of yielding information on patients' needs and outcome, although this may not hold for all needs and all outcomes. Until further progress is made, it seems unwise to continue to rely on traditional diagnostic categories alone. Instead, the use of a combination of (polydiagnostic) categorical and (multi-) dimensional representations of psychosis may offer important advantages, both in clinical practice and research (Strauss, 1973).

Acknowledgements

We thank Nick Stefanis and his team for kindly providing us with the distributions of the schizotypy data, and Louise Johns for help in constructing the section on continuity.

REFERENCES

American Psychiatric Association (1987) Diagnostic Criteria from DSM-III-R. Washington, DC: American Psychiatric Association.

American Psychiatric Association (1994) Diagnostic Criteria from the DSM-IV. Washington, DC: American Psychiatric Association.

Anderson J, Huppert F, Rose G (1993) Normality, deviance and minor psychiatric morbidity in the community. Psychological Medicine 23, 475–485.

Andreasen NC (1995) Symptoms, signs, and diagnosis of schizophrenia. Lancet 346, 477–481.

Avasthi A, Khan MK, Elroey AM (1991) Inpatient sociodemographic and diagnostic study from a psychiatric hospital in Libya. International Journal of Social Psychiatry 37, 267–279.

Barber JW, Kerler R, Kellogg EJ et al. (1988) Clinical and demographic characteristics of chronic inpatients: implication for treatment and research. Psychiatric Quarterly 59, 257–270.

Barrett TR, Etheridge JB (1992) Verbal hallucinations in normals, I: people who hear voices. Applied Cognitive Psychology, 6, 379–387.

Basso MR, Nasrallah HA, Olson SC, Bornstein RA (1998) Neuropsychological correlates of negative, disorganized and psychotic symptoms in schizophrenia. Schizophrenia Research 31, 99–111.

Baxter RD, Liddle PF (1998) Neuropsychological deficits associated with schizophrenic syndromes. Schizophrenia Research 30, 239–249.

Bebbington P, Wilkins S, Jones P et al. (1993) Life events and psychosis. Initial results from the Camberwell Collaborative Psychosis Study. British Journal of Psychiatry 162, 72–79.

Bell RC, Dudgeon P, McGorry PD, Jackson HJ (1998) The dimensionality of schizophrenia concepts in first-episode psychosis. Acta Psychiatrica Scandinavica 97, 334–342.

Bentall RP, Slade PD (1985) Reality testing and auditory hallucinations: a signal detection analysis. British Journal of Clinical Psychology 24, 159–169.

Bentall RP, Jackson HF, Pilgrim D (1988) Abandoning the concept of 'schizophrenia': some implications of validity arguments for psychological research into psychotic phenomena. British Journal of Clinical Psychology 27, 303–324.

Bentall RP, Claridge GS, Slade PD (1989) The multidimensional nature of schizotypal traits: a factor analytic study with normal subjects. British Journal of Clinical Psychology 28, 363–375.

Bijl RV, van Zessen G, Ravelli A, de Rijk C, Langendoen Y (1998) The Netherlands Mental Health Survey and Incidence Study (NEMESIS): objectives and design. Social Psychiatry and Psychiatric Epidemiology 33, 581–586.

Bilder RM, Mukherjee S, Rieder RO, Pandurangi AK (1985) Symptomatic and neuropsychological components of defect states. Schizophrenia Bulletin 11, 409–419.

Brockington IF, Kendell RE, Wainwright S (1980a) Depressed patients with schizophrenic or paranoid symptoms. Psychological Medicine 10, 665–675.

Brockington IF, Wainwright S, Kendell RE (1980b) Manic patients with schizophrenic or paranoid symptoms. Psychological Medicine 10, 73–83.

Brown AS, van Os J, Driessens C, Hoek HW, Susser ES (1999) Prenatal famine and the spectrum of major psychiatric disorders. Psychiatric Annals 29, 145–150.

Brown KW, White T (1992) Syndromes of chronic schizophrenia and some clinical correlates. British Journal of Psychiatry 161, 317–322.

Burke JG, Murphy BM, Bray JC, Walsh D, Kendler KS (1996) Clinical similarities in siblings with schizophrenia. American Journal of Medical Genetics 67, 239–243.

Butzlaff RL, Hooley JM (1998) Expressed emotion and psychiatric relapse. Archives of General Psychiatry 55, 547–552.

Cardno AG, Holmans PA, Harvey I, Williams MB, Owen MJ, McGuffin P (1997) Factor-derived subsyndromes of schizophrenia and familial morbid risks. Schizophrenia Research 23, 231–238.

Cardno AG, Jones LA, Murphy KC et al. (1999) Dimensions of psychosis in affected sibling pairs. Schizophrenia Bulletin 25, 841–850.

Carpenter WT, Jr (1994) The deficit syndrome [editorial]. American Journal of Psychiatry 151, 327–329.

Carpenter WT, Jr, Bartko JJ, Carpenter CL, Strauss JS (1976) Another view of schizophrenia subtypes. A report from the international pilot study of schizophrenia. Archives of General Psychiatry 33, 508–516.

Carpenter WT, Jr, Strauss JS, Bartko JJ (1980) Diagnostic systems and prognostic validity. Archives of General Psychiatry 37, 228–229.

Castle DJ, Wessely S, Murray RM (1993) Sex and schizophrenia: effects of diagnostic stringency, and associations with premorbid variables. British Journal of Psychiatry 162, 658–664.

Castle DJ, Sham PC, Wessely S, Murray RM (1994) The subtyping of schizophrenia in men and women: a latent class analysis. Psychological Medicine 24, 41–51.

Chapman LJ, Chapman JP, Raulin ML (1976) Scales for physical and social anhedonia. Journal of Abnormal Psychology 85, 374–382.

Chapman LJ, Chapman JP, Raulin ML (1978) Body-image aberration in schizophrenia. Journal of Abnormal Psychology 87, 399–407.

Chapman LJ, Chapman JP, Kwapil TR, Eckblad M, Zinser MC (1994) Putatively psychosis-prone subjects 10 years later. Journal of Abnormal Psychology 103, 171–183.

Chiou NM, Chen CY, Chen CC, Liu CY (1994) [Analysis of psychiatric inpatients in a general hospital.] Chang Keng I Hsueh Tsa Chih 17, 255–263.

Chua SE, Wright IC, Poline JB et al. (1997) Grey matter correlates of syndromes in schizophrenia. A semi-automated analysis of structural magnetic resonance images [see comments]. British Journal of Psychiatry 170, 406–410.

Claridge G (1994) Single indicator of risk for schizophrenia: probable fact or likely myth? Schizophrenia Bulletin 20, 151–168.

Claridge G (1997) Schizotypy. Implications for Illness and Health. Oxford: Oxford University Press.

Claridge G, Broks P (1984) Schizotypy and hemisphere function. I Theoretical considerations and the measurement of schizotypy. Personality and Individual Differences 5, 633–648.

Claridge G, McCreery C, Mason O et al. (1996) The factor structure of 'schizotypal' traits: a large replication study. British Journal of Clinical Psychology 35, 103–115.

Claridge GS (1990) Can a disease model of schizophrenia survive? In: Reconstructing Schizophrenia, Bentall RP, ed. London: Routledge, pp. 87–103.

Cloninger CR, Martin RL, Guze SB, Clayton PJ (1985) Diagnosis and prognosis in schizophrenia. Archives of General Psychiatry 42, 15–25.

Copolov DL, McGorry PD, Singh BS, Proeve M, van Riel R (1990) The influence of gender on the classification of psychotic disorders – a multidiagnostic approach. Acta Psychiatrica Scandinavica 82, 8–13.

Coryell W, Keller M, Lavori P, Endicott J (1990a) Affective syndromes, psychotic features, and prognosis. I. Depression. Archives of General Psychiatry 47, 651–657.

Coryell W, Keller M, Lavori P, Endicott J (1990b) Affective syndromes, psychotic features, and prognosis. II. Mania. Archives of General Psychiatry 47, 658–662.

Costello CG (1992) Research on symptoms versus research on syndromes. Arguments in favour of allocating more research time to the study of symptoms. British Journal of Psychiatry 160, 304–308.

Cox D, Cowling P (1989) Are You Normal? London: Tower Press.

Crow TJ (1985) The two-syndrome concept: origins and current status. Schizophrenia Bulletin 11, 471–486.

Crow TJ (1986) The continuum of psychosis and its implication for the structure of the gene. British Journal of Psychiatry 149, 419–429.

Cuesta MJ, Peralta V (1995) Are positive and negative symptoms relevant to cross-sectional diagnosis of schizophrenic and schizoaffective patients? Comprehensive Psychiatry 36, 353–361.

Cuesta MJ, Peralta V, Caro F (1999) Premorbid personality in psychoses. Schizophrenia Bulletin 25, 801–811.

DeLisi LE, Goldin LR, Maxwell ME, Kazuba DM, Gershon ES (1987) Clinical features of illness in siblings with schizophrenia or schizoaffective disorder. Archives of General Psychiatry 44, 891–896.

Dohrenwend BP, Shrout PE, Link BG, Skodol AE, Stueve A (1995) Life events and other possible psychosocial risk factors for episodes of schizophrenia for episodes and major depression: a case-control study. In: Does Stress Cause Psychiatric Illness? Mazure CM, ed. Washington, DC: American Psychiatric Press, pp. 43–65.

Dworkin RH, Lenzenweger MF (1984) Symptoms and the genetics of schizophrenia: implications for diagnosis. American Journal of Psychiatry 141, 1541–1546.

Eaton WW, Romanoski A, Anthony JC, Nestadt G (1991) Screening for psychosis in the general population with a self-report interview. Journal of Nervous and Mental Disease 179, 689–693.

Ebmeier KP, Blackwood DH, Murray C et al. (1993) Single-photon emission computed tomography with ^{99m}Tc-exametazime in unmedicated schizophrenic patients. Biological Psychiatry 33, 487–495.

Eckman PS, Shean GD (2000) Impairment in test performance and symptom dimensions of schizophrenia. Journal of Psychiatric Research 34, 147–153.

Elkis H, Friedman L, Wise A, Meltzer HY (1995) Meta-analyses of studies of ventricular enlargement and cortical sulcal prominence in mood disorders. Comparisons with controls or patients with schizophrenia [see comments]. Archives of General Psychiatry 52, 735–746.

Erkwoh R, Sabri O, Steinmeyer EM, Bull U, Sass H (1997) Psychopathological and SPECT findings in never-treated schizophrenia. Acta Psychiatrica Scandinavica 96, 51–57.

Erlenmeyer-Kimling L, Adamo UH, Rock D et al. (1997) The New York High Risk Project. Prevalence and comorbidity of axis I disorders in offspring of schizophrenic parents at 25-year follow-up. Archives of General Psychiatry 54, 1096–1102.

Everitt BS, Gourlay AJ, Kendell RE (1971) An attempt at validation of traditional psychiatric syndromes by cluster analysis. British Journal of Psychiatry 119, 399–412.

Farmer AE, McGuffin P, Spitznagel EL (1983) Heterogeneity in schizophrenia: a cluster-analytic approach. Psychiatry Research 8, 1–12.

Fenton WS, McGlashan TH (1991) Natural history of schizophrenia subtypes. II. Positive and negative symptoms and long-term course. Archives of General Psychiatry 48, 978–986.

Fleiss JL, Gurland BJ, Cooper JE (1971) Some contributions to the measurement of psychopathology. British Journal of Psychiatry 119, 647–656.

Galdos PM, van Os JJ, Murray RM (1993) Puberty and the onset of psychosis [see comments]. Schizophrenia Research 10, 7–14.

Garety P, Hemsley DR (1994) Delusions. Investigations into the Psychology of Delusional Reasoning. Maudsley Monographs. Oxford: Oxford University Press.

Goldberg D, Huxley P (1980) Mental Illness in the Community. London: Tavistock Press.

Goldstein JM, Santangelo SL, Simpson JC, Tsuang MT (1990) The role of gender in identifying subtypes of schizophrenia: a latent class analytic approach. Schizophrenia Bulletin 16, 263–275.

Griesinger W (1845) Uber der Pathologie und Therapie der Geisteskranken (Mental Pathology and Therapeutics, 1965). New York: Hafner.

Grossman LS, Harrow M, Goldberg JF, Fichtner CG (1991) Outcome of schizoaffective disorder at two long-term follow-ups: comparisons with outcome of schizophrenia and affective disorders. American Journal of Psychiatry 148, 1359–1365.

Grube BS, Bilder RM, Goldman RS (1998) Meta-analysis of symptom factors in schizophrenia. Schizophrenia Research 31, 113–120.

Gruzelier JH (1996) The factorial structure of schizotypy: Part I. Affinities with syndromes of schizophrenia. Schizophrenia Bulletin 22, 611–620.

Gureje O, Aderibigbe YA, Olley O, Bamidele RW (1994) Premorbid functioning in schizophrenia: a controlled study of Nigerian patients. Comprehensive Psychiatry 35, 437–440.

Häfner H (1988) What is schizophrenia? Changing perspectives in epidemiology. European Archives of Psychiatry and Neurological Sciences 238, 63–72.

Häfner H (1989) [Is schizophrenia a disease? Epidemiologic data and speculative conclusions.] Nervenarzt 60, 191–199.

Harrow M, Grossman LS (1984) Outcome in schizoaffective disorders: a critical review and reevaluation of the literature. Schizophrenia Bulletin 10, 87–108.

Hollis CP (2000) Identifying the best predictors of outcome in adolescent-onset psychoses. Schizophrenia Research 41, 78.

Holthausen EA, Wiersma D, Knegtering RH, van den Bosch RJ (1999) Psychopathology and cognition in schizophrenia spectrum disorders: the role of depressive symptoms. Schizophrenia Research 39, 65–71.

Hwu HG, Wu YC, Lee SF et al. (1997) Concordance of positive and negative symptoms in coaffected sib-pairs with schizophrenia. American Journal of Medical Genetics 74, 1–6.

Jackson MC (1997) Benign schizotypy? The case of spiritual experience. In: Schizotypy. Implications for Illness and Health, Claridge G, ed. Oxford: Oxford University Press, pp. 43–60.

Jaffe SL (1966) Hallucinations in children at a state hospital. Psychiatric Quarterly 40, 88–95.

Johns LC, Nazroo JY, Bebbington P, Kuipers E (2002) Occurrence of hallucinations in a community sample and ethnic variations. British Journal of Psychiatry 180, 174–178.

Johnstone EC, Crow TJ, Frith CD, Owens DG (1988) The Northwick Park 'Functional' Psychosis Study: diagnosis and treatment response. Lancet ii, 119–125.

Johnstone EC, Frith CD, Crow TJ et al. (1992) The Northwick Park 'Functional' Psychosis Study: diagnosis and outcome. Psychological Medicine 22, 331–246.

Jones P, Rodgers B, Murray R, Marmot M (1994) Child developmental risk factors for adult schizophrenia in the British 1946 birth cohort. Lancet 344, 1398–1402.

Kendell RE (1985) Schizophrenia: clinical features. In: Psychiatry, Michels R, Cavenar JO, eds. London: Basic Books, pp. 189–212.

Kendell RE (1989) Clinical validity. Psychological Medicine 19, 45–55.

Kendell RE (1991) The major functional psychoses: are they independent entities or part of a continuum? In: Concepts of Mental Disorder: A Continuing Debate. Kerr A, McClelland H, eds. London: Gaskell, pp. 1–16.

Kendell RE (1993) Diagnosis and Classification. In: Companion to Psychiatric Studies. Kendell RE, Zealley AK, eds. Edinburgh: Churchill Livingstone, pp. 277–294.

Kendell RE, Brockington IF (1980) The identification of disease entities and the relationship between schizophrenic and affective psychoses. British Journal of Psychiatry 137, 324–331.

Kendler KS, Gardner CO (1998) Boundaries of major depression: an evaluation of DSM-IV criteria. American Journal of Psychiatry 155, 172–177.

Kendell RE, Gourlay J (1970) The clinical distinction between the affective psychoses and schizophrenia. British Journal of Psychiatry 117, 261–266.

Kendler KS, Kidd KK (1986) Recurrence risks in an oligogenic threshold model: the effect of alterations in allele frequency. Annals of Human Genetics 50, 83–91.

Kendler KS, Walsh D (1995) Schizotypal personality disorder in parents and the risk for schizophrenia in siblings. Schizophrenia Bulletin 21, 47–52.

Kendler KS, Ochs AL, Gorman AM, Hewitt JK et al. (1991) The structure of schizotypy: a pilot multitrait twin study. Psychiatry Research 36, 19–36.

Kendler KS, McGuire M, Gruenberg AM, O'Hare A, Spellman M, Walsh D (1993a) The Roscommon Family Study. I. Methods, diagnosis of probands, and risk of schizophrenia in relatives [see comments]. Archives of General Psychiatry 50, 527–540.

Kendler KS, McGuire M, Gruenberg AM, O'Hare A, Spellman M, Walsh D (1993b) The Roscommon Family Study. III. Schizophrenia-related personality disorders in relatives. Archives of General Psychiatry 50, 781–8.

Kendler KS, McGuire M, Gruenberg AM, Walsh D (1995) Schizotypal symptoms and signs in the Roscommon Family Study. Their factor structure and familial relationship with psychotic and affective disorders. Archives of General Psychiatry 52, 296–303.

Kendler KS, Gallagher TJ, Abelson JM, Kessler RC (1996) Lifetime prevalence, demographic risk factors, and diagnostic validity of nonaffective psychosis as assessed in a US community sample. The National Comorbidity Survey. Archives of General Psychiatry 53, 1022–1031.

Kendler KS, Karkowski-Shuman L, O'Neill FA, Straub RE, MacLean CJ, Walsh D (1997) Resemblance of psychotic symptoms and syndromes in affected sibling pairs from the Irish Study of High-Density Schizophrenia Families: evidence for possible etiologic heterogeneity. American Journal of Psychiatry 154, 191–198.

Kendler KS, Karkowski LM, Walsh D (1998) The structure of psychosis: latent class analysis of probands from the Roscommon Family Study. Archives of General Psychiatry 55, 492–429.

Kerr A, McClelland H (1991) Concepts of Mental Disorder: A Continuing Debate. London: Gaskell.

Kitamura T, Okazaki Y, Fujinawa A, Yoshino M, Kasahara Y (1995) Symptoms of psychoses. A factor-analytic study. British Journal of Psychiatry 166, 236–240.

Kwapil TR, Miller MB, Zinser MC, Chapman J, Chapman LJ (1997) Magical ideation and social anhedonia as predictors of psychosis proneness: a partial replication. Journal of Abnormal Psychology 106, 491–495.

Launay G, Slade PD (1981) The measurement of hallucinatory predisposition in male and female prisoners. Personality and Individual Differences 2, 221–234.

Lenzenweger MF (1991) Confirming schizotypic personality configurations in hypothetically psychosis-prone university students. Psychiatry Research 37, 81–96.

Liddle PF (1987a) The symptoms of chronic schizophrenia. A re-examination of the positive-negative dichotomy [see comments]. British Journal of Psychiatry 151, 145–151.

Liddle PF (1987b) Schizophrenic syndromes, cognitive performance and neurological dysfunction. Psychological Medicine 17, 49–57.

Liddle PF, Morris DL (1991) Schizophrenic syndromes and frontal lobe performance. British Journal of Psychiatry 158, 340–345.

Liddle PF, Friston KJ, Frith CD, Hirsch SR, Jones T, Frackowiak RS (1992) Patterns of cerebral blood flow in schizophrenia. British Journal of Psychiatry 160, 179–186.

Liddle PF, Barnes TR, Curson DA, Patel M (1993) Depression and the experience of psychological deficits in schizophrenia. Acta Psychiatrica Scandinavica 88, 243–247.

Lindenmayer JP, Bernstein Hyman R, Grochowski S, Bark N (1995a) Psychopathology of schizophrenia: initial validation of a 5-factor model. Psychopathology 28, 22–31.

Lindenmayer JP, Grochowski S, Hyman RB (1995b) Five factor model of schizophrenia: replication across samples. Schizophrenia Research 14, 229–234.

Liu SK, Hwu HG, Chen WJ (1997) Clinical symptom dimensions and deficits on the Continuous Performance Test in schizophrenia. Schizophrenia Research 25, 211–219.

Loftus J, DeLisi LE, Crow TJ (1998) Familial associations of subsyndromes of psychosis in affected sibling pairs with schizophrenia and schizoaffective disorder. Psychiatry Research 80, 101–111.

Loftus J, Delisi LE, Crow TJ (2000) Factor structure and familiality of first-rank symptoms in sibling pairs with schizophrenia and schizoaffective disorder. British Journal of Psychiatry 177, 15–19.

Maher BA (1974) Delusional thinking and perceptual disorder. Journal of Individual Psychology 30, 98–113.

Maher BA (1988) Anomalous experience and delusional thinking: the logic of explanations. In: Delusional Beliefs, Oltmanns TF, Maher BA, eds. New York: Wiley, pp. 15–33.

Mahurin RK, Velligan DI, Miller AL (1998) Executive-frontal lobe cognitive dysfunction in schizophrenia: a symptom subtype analysis. Psychiatry Research 79, 139–149.

Maier W, Lichtermann D, Minges J et al. (1993) Continuity and discontinuity of affective disorders and schizophrenia. Results of a controlled family study. Archives of General Psychiatry 50, 871–883.

Maj M, Perris C (1990) Patterns of course in patients with a cross-sectional diagnosis of schizoaffective disorder. Journal of Affective Disorders 20, 71–77.

Marcelis M, Navarro-Mateu F, Murray R, Selten JP, van Os J (1998) Urbanization and psychosis: a study of 1942–1978 birth cohorts in the Netherlands. Psychological Medicine 28, 871–879.

Marneros A, Deister A, Rohde A, Steinmeyer EM, Junemann H (1989) Long-term outcome of schizoaffective and schizophrenic disorders: a comparative study. I. Definitions, methods, psychopathological and social outcome. European Archives of Psychiatry and Neurological Sciences 238, 118–125.

Marneros A, Deister A, Rohde A (1990) Psychopathological and social status of patients with affective, schizophrenic and schizoaffective disorders after long-term course. Acta Psychiatrica Scandinavica 82, 352–358.

Mason P, Harrison G, Croudace T, Glazebrook C, Medley I (1997) The predictive validity of a diagnosis of schizophrenia. A report from the International Study of Schizophrenia (ISoS) coordinated by the World Health Organization and the Department of Psychiatry, University of Nottingham. British Journal of Psychiatry 170, 321–327.

Maziade M, Roy MA, Martinez M et al. (1995) Negative, psychoticism, and disorganized dimensions in patients with familial schizophrenia or bipolar disorder: continuity and discontinuity between the major psychoses [see comments]. American Journal of Psychiatry 152, 1458–1463.

McCreadie RG, Wilson AO, Burton LL (1983) The Scottish survey of 'new chronic' inpatients. British Journal of Psychiatry 143, 564–571.

McGorry PD, Bell RC, Dudgeon PL, Jackson HJ (1998) The dimensional structure of first episode psychosis: an exploratory factor analysis. Psychological Medicine 28, 935–947.

McKellar P (1968) Experience and Behaviour. Harmondsworth: Penguin Press.

Menninger K, Ellenberger H, Pruyser P, Mayman M (1958) The unitary concept of mental illness. Bulletin of the Menninger Clinic 22, 4–12.

Murray RM (1994) Neurodevelopmental schizophrenia: the rediscovery of dementia praecox. British Journal of Psychiatry Suppl 6–12.

Norman RM, Malla AK, Morrison Stewart SL et al. (1997) Neuropsychological correlates of syndromes in schizophrenia. British Journal of Psychiatry 170, 134–139.

Norman RM, Malla AK, Cortese L et al. (1999) Symptoms and cognition as predictors of community functioning: a prospective analysis. American Journal of Psychiatry 156, 400–405.

O'Grady JC (1990) The prevalence and diagnostic significance of Schneiderian first-rank symptoms in a random sample of acute psychiatric in-patients [see comments]. British Journal of Psychiatry 156, 496–500.

Overall JE, Gorham D (1962) The Brief Psychiatric Rating Scale. Psychological Reports 10, 799–812.

Paykel ES (1978) Contribution of life events to causation of psychiatric illness. Psychological Medicine 8, 245–253.

Peralta V, Cuesta MJ (1999a) Diagnostic significance of Schneider's first-rank symptoms in schizophrenia. Comparative study between schizophrenic and non- schizophrenic psychotic disorders. British Journal of Psychiatry 174, 243–248.

Peralta V, Cuesta MJ (1999b) Dimensional structure of psychotic symptoms: an item-level analysis of SAPS and SANS symptoms in psychotic disorders. Schizophrenia Research 38, 13–26.

Peralta V, de Leon J, Cuesta MJ (1992) Are there more than two syndromes in schizophrenia? A critique of the positive-negative dichotomy. British Journal of Psychiatry 161, 335–343.

Peralta V, Cuesta MJ, de Leon J (1994) An empirical analysis of latent structures underlying schizophrenic symptoms: a four-syndrome model. Biological Psychiatry 36, 726–736.

Peralta V, Cuesta MJ, Farre C (1997) Factor structure of symptoms in functional psychoses. Biological Psychiatry 42, 806–815.

Peters ER, Day S, Garety PA (1996) The Peters et al. Delusions Inventory (PDI): new forms for the 21-item version. Schizophrenia Research 18, 118.

Peters E, Day S, McKenna J, Orbach G (1999a) Delusional ideation in religious and psychotic populations. British Journal of Clinical Psychology 38, 83–96.

Peters ER, Joseph SA, Garety PA (1999b) Measurement of delusional ideation in the normal population: introducing the PDI (Peters et al. Delusions Inventory). Schizophrenia Bulletin 25, 553–576.

Pogue Geile MF (1989) The prognostic significance of negative symptoms in schizophrenia. British Journal of Psychiatry Suppl 155, 123–127.

Pope HG, Jr, Lipinski JF, Jr (1978) Diagnosis in schizophrenia and manic-depressive illness: a reassessment of the specificity of 'schizophrenic' symptoms in the light of current research. Archives of General Psychiatry 35, 811–828.

Posey TB, Losch ME (1983) Auditory hallucinations of hearing voices in 375 normal subjects. Imagination, Cognition and Personality 3, 99–113.

Poulton R, Caspi A, Moffitt TE, Cannon M, Murray R, Harrington H (2000) Children's self-reported psychotic symptoms and adult schizophreniform disorder: a 15–year longitudinal study [in process citation]. Archives of General Psychiatry 57, 1053–1058.

Raine A (1991) The SPQ: a scale for the assessment of schizotypal personality based on DSM-III-R criteria. Schizophrenia Bulletin 17, 555–564.

Raine A, Reynolds C, Lencz T, Scerbo A, Triphon N, Kim D (1994) Cognitive-perceptual, interpersonal, and disorganized features of schizotypal personality. Schizophrenia Bulletin 20, 191–201.

Ratakonda S, Gorman JM, Yale SA, Amador XF (1998) Characterization of psychotic conditions. Use of the domains of psychopathology model. Archives of General Psychiatry 55, 75–81.

Robins E, Guze SB (1970) Establishment of diagnostic validity in psychiatric illness: its application to schizophrenia. American Journal of Psychiatry 126, 983–987.

Robins LN, Helzer JE, Croughan J et al. (1981) NIMH Diagnostic Interview Schedule: Version III. Rockville, MD: National Institute of Mental Health, Division of Biometry and Epidemiology.

Robinson AD (1988) A century of delusions in southwest Scotland. British Journal of Psychiatry 153, 163–167.

Romme MA, Honig A, Noorthoorn EO, Escher AD (1992) Coping with hearing voices: an emancipatory approach. British Journal of Psychiatry 161, 99–103.

Rosa A, van Os J, Fananas L et al. (2000) Developmental instability and schizotypy. Schizophrenia Research 43, 125–134.

Rose G, Barker DJP (1978) What is a case? Dichotomy or continuum. British Medical Journal ii, 873–874.

Rowe EW, Shean G (1997) Card-sort performance and syndromes of schizophrenia. Genetic, Social, and General Psychology Monographs 123, 197–209.

Rust J (1988) The Rust Inventory of Schizotypal Cognitions (RISC). Schizophrenia Bulletin 14, 317–322.

Sackett DL, Richardson WS, Rosenberg W, Haynes RB (1997) Evidence-Based Medicine. New York: Churchill Livingstone.

Salokangas RK (1997) Structure of schizophrenic symptomatology and its changes over time: prospective factor-analytical study. Acta Psychiatrica Scandinavica 95, 32–39.

Samson JA, Simpson JC, Tsuang MT (1988) Outcome studies of schizoaffective disorders. Schizophrenia Bulletin 14, 543–554.

Sham PC, Castle DJ, Wessely S, Farmer AE, Murray RM (1996) Further exploration of a latent class typology of schizophrenia. Schizophrenia Research 20, 105–115.

Sidgewick H, Johnson A, Myers FWH et al. (1894) Report of the census of hallucinations. Proceedings of the Society for Psychical Research 26, 259–394.

Siris SG, Morgan V, Fagerstrom R, Rifkin A, Cooper TB (1987) Adjunctive imipramine in the treatment of postpsychotic depression. A controlled trial. Archives of General Psychiatry 44, 533–539.

Siris SG, Bermanzohn PC, Mason SE, Shuwall MA (1994) Maintenance imipramine therapy for secondary depression in schizophrenia. A controlled trial. Archives of General Psychiatry 51, 109–115.

Soni S, Hollis S, Reed P, Musa S (1992) Syndromes of schizophrenia on factor analysis. British Journal of Psychiatry 161, 860–861.

Spitzer RL, Williams JBW, Gibbon M (1990) User's Guide for the Structured Clinical Interview for DSM-III-R (SCID). Washington, DC: American Psychiatric Association.

Stefanis NC, Hanssen M, Smirnis NK et al. (2002) Evidence that three dimensions of psychosis have a distribution in the general population. Psychological Medicine 32, 347–358.

Strauss JS (1973) Diagnostic models and the nature of psychiatric disorder. Archives of General Psychiatry 29, 445–449.

Susser E, Wanderling J (1994) Epidemiology of nonaffective acute remitting psychosis vs schizophrenia. Sex and sociocultural setting. Archives of General Psychiatry 51, 294–301.

Susser E, Neugebauer R, Hoek HW et al. (1996) Schizophrenia after prenatal famine. Further evidence [see comments]. Archives of General Psychiatry 53, 25–31.

Tien AY (1991) Distributions of hallucinations in the population. Social Psychiatry and Psychiatric Epidemiology 26, 287–292.

Tien AY, Costa PT, Eaton WW (1992) Covariance of personality, neurocognition, and schizophrenia spectrum traits in the community. Schizophrenia Research 7, 149–158.

Tsuang MT, Dempsey GM (1979) Long-term outcome of major psychoses. II. Schizoaffective disorder compared with schizophrenia, affective disorders, and a surgical control group. Archives of General Psychiatry 36, 1302–1304.

UK700 Group (2000) Diagnostic value of the DSM and ICD categories of psychosis: an evidence-based approach. Social Psychiatry and Psychiatry Epidemiology 35, 305–311.

van der Does AJ, Dingemans PM, Linszen DH, Nugter MA, Scholte WF (1993) Symptom dimensions and cognitive and social functioning in recent-onset schizophrenia. Psychological Medicine 23, 745–753.

van der Does AJ, Dingemans PM, Linszen DH, Nugter MA, Scholte WF (1996) Symptoms, cognitive and social functioning in recent-onset schizophrenia: a longitudinal study. Schizophrenia Research 19, 61–71.

van Os J (2000) An default analysis of schizophrenia: comment. Schizophrenia Bulletin 163, 163–166.

van Os J, Fahy TA, Jones P et al. (1996) Psychopathological syndromes in the functional psychoses: associations with course and outcome. Psychological Medicine 26, 161–176.

van Os J, Marcelis M, Sham P, Jones P, Gilvarry K, Murray R (1997a) Psychopathological syndromes and familial morbid risk of psychosis [see comments]. British Journal of Psychiatry 170, 241–246.

van Os J, Jones P, Lewis G, Wadsworth M, Murray R (1997b) Developmental precursors of affective illness in a general population birth cohort. Archives of General Psychiatry 54, 625–631.

van Os J, Jones P, Sham P, Bebbington P, Murray RM (1998) Risk factors for onset and persistence of psychosis. Social Psychiatry and Psychiatric Epidemiology 33, 596–605.

van Os J, Gilvarry C, Bale R et al. (1999a) A comparison of the utility of dimensional and categorical representations of psychosis. UK700 Group [in process citation]. Psychological Medicine 29, 595–606.

van Os J, Gilvarry C, Bale R et al. (1999b) To what extent does symptomatic improvement result in better outcomes in psychotic illness? Psychological Medicine 29, 1183–1195.

van Os J, Verdoux H, Bijl R, Ravelli A (1999c) Psychosis as a continuum of variation in dimensions of psychopathology. In: Search for the Causes of Schizophrenia, Häfner H, Gattaz WF, eds. Berlin: Springer, pp. 59–80.

van Os J, Hanssen M, Bijl RV, Ravelli A (2000) Strauss (1969) revisited: a psychosis continuum in the general population? Schizophrenia Research 45, 11–20.

Venables PH, Rector NA (2000) The content and structure of schizotypy: a study using confirmatory factor analysis [in process citation]. Schizophrenia Bulletin 26, 587–602.

Ventura J, Nuechterlein KH, Subotnik KL, Hardesty JP, Mintz J (2000) Life events can trigger depressive exacerbation in the early course of schizophrenia. Journal of Abnormal Psychology 109, 139–144.

Verdoux H, Maurice-Tison S, Gay B, van Os J, Salamon R, Bourgeois ML (1998a) A survey of delusional ideation in primary-care patients. Psychological Medicine 28, 127–134.

Verdoux H, van Os J, Maurice-Tison S, Gay B, Salamon R, Bourgeois M (1998b) Is early adulthood a critical developmental stage for psychosis proneness? A survey of delusional ideation in normal subjects. Schizophrenia Research 29, 247–254.

Vollema M (1999) Schizotypy: toward the psychological heart of schizophrenia. Groningen: Shaker Publishing.

Vollema MG, Hoijtink H (2000) The multidimensionality of self-report schizotypy in a psychiatric population: an analysis using multidimensional Rasch models [in process citation]. Schizophrenia Bulletin 26, 565–575.

Vollema MG, van den Bosch RJ (1995) The multidimensionality of schizotypy [see comments]. Schizophrenia Bulletin 21, 19–31.

Weich S (1997) Prevention of the common mental disorders: a public health perspective [editorial]. Psychological Medicine 27, 757–764.

Whittington JE, Huppert FA (1996) Changes in the prevalence of psychiatric disorder in a community are related to changes in the mean level of psychiatric symptoms. Psychological Medicine 26, 1253–1260.

Wing JK, Cooper JE, Sartorius N (1974) The Measurement and Classification of Psychiatric Symptoms. London: Cambridge University Press.

World Health Organization (1992) The ICD-10 Classification of Mental and Behavioural Disorders. Geneva: World Health Organization.

Young HF, Bentall RP, Slade PD, Dewey ME (1986) Disposition towards hallucination, gender and EPQ scores: a brief report. Personality and Individual Differences 7, 247–249.

Yuasa S, Kurachi M, Suzuki M et al. (1995) Clinical symptoms and regional cerebral blood flow in schizophrenia. European Archives of Psychiatry and Clinical Neuroscience 246, 7–12.

Zukerman M, Cohen N (1964) Sources of reports of visual and auditory sensations in perceptual-isolation experiments. Psychological Bulletin 62, 1–20.

19

The implications of epidemiology for service planning in schizophrenia

Graham Thornicroft[1] and Michele Tansella[2]

[1]Institute of Psychiatry, King's College London, UK
[2]Department of Medicine and Public Health, University of Verona, Italy

Introduction: the uses of epidemiological data

This chapter addresses the question of how epidemiological data can be used to plan services for people who suffer from schizophrenia. Morris (1975) has described seven uses of epidemiology: (i) assessment of incidence, prevalence, disability and mortality in defined populations; (ii) detailed description of the natural history of specific conditions and completion of the clinical picture of diseases; (iii) delineation of new syndromes and the description of associations between symptoms; (iv) calculation of morbid risk; (v) charting of historical trends; (vi) evaluation of health services in action; and (vii) identification of causal factors. However, what is striking in reviewing the literature on the epidemiology of schizophrenia is that, while both descriptive and analytical epidemiological studies can have direct implications for treatment, for care and for service provision, in fact they are rarely used for these purposes.

In most primary research and review papers on the epidemiology of schizophrenia, there are two points of emphasis: the aetiological implications of the findings and the description of course and outcome of the condition. The more practical consequences of the findings for service delivery are, by contrast, largely discounted. We shall advance the argument here that epidemiological data on schizophrenia should be exploited for their contributions *both* to the longer-term understanding of causation and course, *and* to match services to needs.

This chapter will describe ways in which this form of translation can be made. We consider service planning here to mean the necessary interventions at three levels: the individual patient, the local catchment area and the national/regional general population level. We shall describe the implications of epidemiological findings at each of these levels in turn, but we shall also indicate where findings in this field cannot at present warrant specific interventions.

While the focus of this chapter is upon planning services for people suffering from schizophrenia, this does not imply that we conclude that services should

Table 19.1. Overview of the matrix model

Geographical dimension	Temporal dimension		
	A. Input phase	B. Process phase	C. Outcome phase
1. Country/regional level	1A	1B	1C
2. Local level (catchment area)	2A	2B	2C
3. Patient level	3A	3B	3C

Source: From Thornicroft and Tansella (1999).

usually be planned for schizophrenia patients as a separate group. Later in this chapter we shall describe two overall approaches to this issue: the *segmental* (separate services for distinct categories of patients) and the *systemic* (an integrated array of adult mental health services for defined catchment areas) approaches and shall describe their features.

A conceptual model to structure service planning

A conceptual model can help to formulate service planning, and we have described the 'matrix' model, which has two dimensions: the geographical and the temporal (Thornicroft and Tansella, 1999). The first refers to three geographical levels: (1) country/regional, (2) local and (3) patient. The second dimension refers to three temporal levels: (A) inputs, (B) processes and (C) outcomes. Using these two dimensions we have constructed a 3×3 matrix to bring into focus critical issues for mental health service planning and provision (Table 19.1).

An evidence-based approach to service planning

In relation to the matrix model, planning is the process which intends to transform given inputs into optimum outputs. More specifically, we define planning as 'a linked series of actions designed to achieve a particular goal, and which requires the completion of increasingly specific tasks within a given timescale'. Seven key steps can be identified to plan services (Thornicroft and Tansella, 1999):

1 Establishing service principles
2 Setting boundary conditions
3 Assessing population needs
4 Assessing current provision
5 Formulating a strategic plan for a local system of mental health services
6 Implementing the service components at the local level
7 Monitoring and review cycle.

Table 19.2. Information pathways for planning mental health services

A Epidemiologically based data	B Service provision data
Population characteristics: in terms of the factors associated with psychiatric morbidity	Define categories of service components for primary, secondary and tertiary levels of care
Epidemiological data: morbidity and disability for the particular area by age, sex and social status	Quantify the capacities of the service components
Treated individuals: appropriately/inappropriately	Quality of care of the service sites
Place and type of treatment	Quantitative and qualitative information on staff
Untreated individual: those in need of treatment	Integration and co-ordination of components into a service system
$\rightarrow$	$\downarrow$
$\uparrow$	$\leftarrow$
D Planning process	C Service utilization data
Constitution of a planning group representing a wide range of local interest groups, including expert advisors	Event-based data on clinical contacts by levels of care (inpatient, outpatient, etc.), numbers of events and rates per 10000 population per year
Selective assessment of all data from A, B and C relevant for service planning	Individual-based data on both clinical contacts (as above) and on treatment episodes across different levels of care per year
Setting a medium-term time scale for service plans (3–5 years)	Data on outcomes and costs of different clinical contacts (disaggregated for subgroups of patients) with which to establish substitutability and complementarity of service components in terms of cost-effectiveness
Identify highest priority service needs (both met and unmet)	
Identification of highest priority unmet social needs and information from relevant authorities	
Plan:	
(i) new service functions and necessary facilities	
(ii) extension of capacity of current services	
(iii) disinvestment from lower priority services	
(iv) propose collection of new data necessary for the next planning cycle	

Source: From Thornicroft and Tansella (1999).

For the purposes of this chapter, we shall focus on steps 3 and 4 of this sequence. *Step three* is to assess the service needs of people with schizophrenia. *Step four* is the assessment of current service provision. The combined information from these two steps allows estimates of the gap between need and provision to be calculated. These gaps then have to be assessed for their relative priorities. An information pathway for planning mental health services for schizophrenia is illustrated in Table 19.2, which suggests a sequence for sources which may be useful in service planning: (A) collecting epidemiologically based data; (B) interpreting data on actual service provision, referring both to the quantity and quality of care; (C)

Table 19.3. Epidemiological findings with direct implications at the patient level

Epidemiological findings/risk factors	Service planning implications
Genetic risk	Provide genetic counselling for high-risk individuals
Obstetric complications	Optimize perinatal care for high-risk individuals
Suicide rates highest early in course of disorder	Prioritize suicide prevention measures in early illness career
Symptom severity and social function are inversely correlated	Emphasize continuing treatment for relapse prevention as well as to minimize disability and reduce symptoms
Long-term disability is a relatively common course of illness	Services organized to offer long-term treatment and care if needed
Increased mortality and physical morbidity rates	Health promotion to modify lifestyle, e.g. reducing smoking and improving diet

assessing data on service utilization; and (D) referring to these data in making service plans.

Beyond these broad considerations, there are, in addition, a number of specific findings from research into the epidemiology of schizophrenia that can shape the planning of treatments and services at the patient, local catchment and national/regional levels. This is particularly true in this diagnostic category because of the quality and quantity of relevant research in this area.

Planning services at the level of individual patients

The contributions of epidemiology which have, in our view, the most direct and credible implications for planning services, at the level of individual schizophrenic patients, are summarized in Table 19.3.

Genetic risk

The evidence for the increased risk for schizophrenia among family members of individuals with schizophrenia has been summarized (Gottesman, 1991; Kendler and Diehl, 1995; Warner and de Girolamo, 1995; see also Chs. 10 and 11). Although this knowledge is now commonplace among academics, it is not often brought into the clinical domain. For individual patients, this suggests that they should be offered clear information about the increased risk for relatives, which is highest for the rare cases of children of two schizophrenic parents or for the co-twin of an affected identical twin (lifetime relative risk of about 45) and raised to a lesser extent (7–9 times higher relative risk) in the more common cases of first-degree relatives of probands (Mortensen et al., 1999).

Family members who wish to have this information can be told that for first-degree relatives the risk of schizophrenia is 9.31 (Mortensen et al., 1999). Even so, it is mistaken to think that genetic counselling can impact significantly upon overall incidence rates of schizophrenia, since the population attributable risk is 5.5% for a parent or sibling with schizophrenia (Mortensen et al., 1999). The implication is that, while genetic counselling may be valued by patients and their families (at the individual level), such information must be very carefully communicated to prevent misunderstanding. Nevertheless, such genetic counselling services are not likely to change the incidence or prevalence rates of schizophrenia (at the local or national/regional levels).

Obstetric complications

The overall odds ratio for schizophrenia from obstetric complications is about 2 (Jablensky and Eaton, 1995; Jablensky, 1997; see Ch. 5). At the individual level, the main implication of this finding is the need to inform people with schizophrenia, and their families, about the need for careful perinatal care to minimize hypoxia in the neonate, and to educate obstetric staff of the special need to reduce the risk of possible brain damage in the children of schizophrenic parents (Warner, 1999).

Suicide rates highest early in course of disorder

The overall suicide rate is about nine times higher among people with schizophrenia than in the general adult population (Harris and Barraclough, 1998; see Ch. 15). Rates are highest at the start of treatment, in the early period of hospital admission (Rossau and Mortensen, 1997) and immediately following discharge (Goldacre et al., 1993). There are clear service implications for mental health services in that staff must frequently assess the risk of suicidal behaviour, most especially during the early years of the disorder and during periods of inpatient treatment, and should be most vigilant in the days and weeks following hospital discharge (Appleby et al., 1999). Even so, it is likely that a high-risk strategy alone is less effective than a programmatic approach that improves the detection of suicidality across the range of all psychiatric disorders (Mortensen, 1999). Such a prevention strategy has been proposed by Schaffer and Craft (1999), which addresses the need both to enhance inhibiting factors (such as increasing the availability of social support) and to reduce facilitating factors (such as the availability of drugs that are toxic in overdose).

Symptom severity and social function are inversely correlated

A clear relationship has been described between symptoms and social function, with levels of disability and handicap most pronounced among patients whose primary impairments (symptoms) are most severe (Brier et al., 1991). It follows that good clinical advice to individual patients is to promote treatment with antipsychotic medication and psychological treatments, where this is effective for particular individuals, both for symptomatic relief and to produce lesser disability in the longer term (Eckman et al., 1992; Kemp et al., 1996, Roth and Fonagy, 1996).

Long-term disability is a relatively common course of illness

Although there is not yet a consensus view on the precise long-term course and outcome of schizophrenia (van Os et al., 1997, 1998), Brier et al. (1991) have summarized the overall picture in terms of three phases: early deterioration, a stabilization phase in middle age, and a period of gradual improvement in later life. The proportion of first-onset schizophrenics who become chronically psychotic ranges from 10 to 28% and the small size of this percentage is inconsistent with the old concept of 'inevitable' deterioration (Eaton, 1991).

Nevertheless, one of the most important findings in the epidemiology of schizophrenia (in terms of its service implications) is that a substantial proportion of patients, probably the majority in the first half of their illness careers, suffer from moderate or severe levels of disability and handicap across the range of personal, domestic, family and work activities. The service implications of this are manifold and include providing a range of long-term and integrated interventions, both to prevent relapses and to minimize preventable disability.

Increased mortality and physical morbidity rates

Schizophrenia is associated both with higher standardized mortality ratios and higher rates of physical illness than among the general population (Allebeck, 1989; Harris and Barraclough, 1998; Brown et al., 1999; see Ch. 14). This has also been confirmed for patients who have only been treated in community-based services (Amaddeo et al., 1995). Although rarely put into practice, there are clear implications for planners and practitioners (including psychologists, psychiatrists, psychiatric nurses, health visitors and health educators) to address illness-prevention issues, such as smoking reduction programmes and dietary improvement (McCreadie et al., 1998).

Planning services at the level of the catchment area

The results from epidemiological research which are most relevant for planning and providing services at the local catchment area level are shown in Table 19.4.

Onset in early adulthood

The onset of schizophrenia occurs most commonly in early adulthood (Ch. 7); therefore, clinical services will need to respond in ways that are appropriate to this age group. First, contact with specialist psychiatric staff is likely to be more accessible and acceptable to teenagers and young adults if the settings in which initial

Table 19.4. Epidemiological findings with implications at the catchment area level

Epidemiological findings/risk factors	Service planning implications
Onset in early adulthood, males earlier than females	Organize services to identify prodromes in teenagers and young adults, and related to life cycle problems
Delay of treatment associated with poorer course	Provide easy access to services
High-risk groups: ethnic minorities, prisoners, and dual diagnosis	Targeted services, acceptable to specific high-risk groups
Geographical mobility: immigrants and internal migration	Target services acceptable to immigrants, and organize services to minimize loss to treatment
Urban excess and changes in age/social class structure	Monitor changing population structure and target more resources and staff in urban, poor areas
Increased mortality and physical morbidity rates	Provide services for health promotion and for regular physical health assessment and treatment

assessment takes place are apparently noninstitutional and nonstigmatizing. Similarly, it is important that staff in positions of responsibility for young adults in institutions (such as high schools, training colleges, universities, the military and places of worship) are trained to be able to detect early signs of possible psychosis.

Second, the characteristic age of onset, in the late teens or early adulthood, has implications for the stage of the life cycle. Services will need to recognize, for example, that at this age education is often incomplete and the patient may not have successfully begun or established a working career. In addition, they may not have built a marital relationship or partnership, may still be living with parents and are unlikely to have accumulated material assets or financial savings that would provide a degree of choice in the services available. Indeed the development of social competence prior to onset is one of the most important predictors of outcome (Eaton, 1991).

Delay of treatment is associated with poorer course

The detection of schizophrenia is frequently delayed for 5–7 years (Maurer and Häfner, 1995; Häfner and an der Heiden, 1997; see Ch. 8). There is some evidence that the longer the interval between the onset of the disorder and commencement of treatment, the worse the prognosis (Gift et al., 1981; Johnstone et al., 1986). Although these findings require replication, these results reinforce the clinical imperative to reduce suffering among patients and carers by early intervention in first episodes of psychosis (McGorry and Jackson, 1999).

High-risk groups: ethnic minorities, prisoners, dual diagnosis

There is evidence that the incidence and prevalence of schizophrenia among African–Caribbeans in Britain and among patients from Surinam and the Dutch Antilles treated in the Netherlands are markedly higher than in the White populations in those countries (Jablensky, 1995; see Ch. 4) and these groups may also be subjected more often to compulsory treatment (Davies et al., 1996). In terms of planning, at least in these settings, the specific needs for culturally sensitive treatment and care services will need to be a high priority. A second high-risk group includes remand and sentenced prisoners. The implications for prisons is clear: there needs to be well-trained staff who regularly assess prisoners as a part of the routine health-care services available to prisoners and who can detect and appropriately treat or refer those with schizophrenia (Birmingham et al., 1996).

High rates of alcohol and drug disorders have been found among people with severe mental illnesses such as schizophrenia (Regier et al., 1990; see Ch. 16), and their prevalence appears to be increasing (Cuffel, 1992). Damaging effects from substance abuse in this group include worse clinical and social outcomes than in patients with severe mental illness alone (Lehman et al., 1993), frequent homelessness, heavy inpatient service use and high costs of care (Bartels et al., 1993). A further problem is violence, which is associated with dual diagnosis at higher rates than with psychosis alone (Swanson et al., 1990; see Ch. 17).

In Camberwell, a 1 year prevalence of substance misuse of 36% was found among patients with psychosis treated by the community mental health team (Menezes et al., 1996). Those with dual diagnosis had spent, on average, 1.8 times as many days in hospital as those with psychosis only, with considerable cost implications. A further study in Camberwell indicated that people with dual diagnosis are more than twice as likely to be aggressive or to report having committed a criminal offence as people with psychosis only (Scott et al., 1998). Conventional services have great difficulty engaging this group: generic community mental health and social care professionals lack expertise in substance abuse interventions; addictions services are often inappropriate for people with psychotic illnesses; and patients are often disorganized and poorly compliant with prescribed medication.

Innovative programmes for management of dual diagnosis have been developed in the USA (Drake et al., 1993). There is evidence that these may succeed in engaging patients and in reducing symptoms, social problems, violence, emergency and inpatient service use, and overall treatment cost (Drake et al., 1993; Jerrell et al., 1994). Proven elements in successful programmes are (i) assertive outreach and engagement of people with very erratic service contact; (ii) integration of substance abuse interventions with a comprehensive case management approach; and (iii) using individual and group work to educate about alcohol and drugs, increase motivation, prevent relapse and improve problem-solving skills.

Urban excess of schizophrenia

Higher prevalence rates of schizophrenia among those living in cities have long been described, and were clear to Faris and Dunham working in Chicago in the 1930s (Faris and Dunham, 1939). More recently, it has become clearer that incidence rates are also substantially raised for those born in cities (Lewis et al., 1992; see Ch. 4). Moreover, Pedersen and Mortensen (2001) have been able to discriminate the effect of urbanicity at birth from the effect of urbanicity during upbringing and to prove the dose–response relationship between urbanicity during upbringing and schizophrenia risk. In Denmark, the relative risk for schizophrenia in those born in urban areas is 2.40 compared with those living in rural areas. Although the level of relative risk here is far lower than for a family history of schizophrenia in a first-degree relative, the population attributable risk in the latter group is 5.5%, compared with 34.6% for city dwellers (Mortensen et al., 1999). In England, by comparison, the overall annual period prevalence rate of all psychotic disorders is 0.4%, masking a range of 0.2% in rural areas to 0.9% in the most socially deprived urban areas (Mason and Wilkinson, 1996). The implications for service planning are to target more resources and staff in urban, poorer areas.

In a longitudinal perspective it is also important to recognize that secular population trends may have important implications for the predictable demands for services to treat schizophrenia (Kramer, 1976). Changes in the age structure will mean variations in the age group at risk for onset of illness, while selective in- and out-migration may also serve to increase or reduce the concentration of schizophrenic patients in particular areas, including the operation of local economic conditions in the housing and labour markets (Lesage and Tansella, 1989; Dauncey et al., 1993). In addition to higher rates of prevalence in urban areas than in rural areas, there is some evidence that urban schizophrenic patients are also more disabled than their rural counterparts (McCreadie et al., 1997; Shepherd et al., 1997), which further reinforces the need to organize services to recognize the greater pressure of morbidity in city areas. The implications of this at the catchment area level include the recognition that the prevalence of schizophrenia will vary by a factor of about four between affluent and impoverished parts of a wider catchment area, and that services will need to be distributed accordingly, rather than on a strict per capita basis.

Increased mortality and physical morbidity rates

The epidemiological findings of increased mortality and physical morbidity rates in schizophrenic individuals are summarized in the previous section. In terms of detecting and treating established physical disease, the necessary service arrangements will vary according to the setting, and in many economically developed countries this will necessitate agreements between the general health sector (most

Table 19.5. Epidemiological findings with implications at the national/regional level

Epidemiological findings/risk factors	Service planning implications
Urban excess of schizophrenia	Funding formula adjusted for urbanicity and social deprivation
High unemployment rates	Specific programme for vocational rehabilitation
Fluctuating course of relapses and remissions	Change pension and disability social security payment systems to allow more flexible movement into and out of the 'disabled' category

often provided by primary care practitioners) and the specialist mental health treatment services that have responsibility for providing physical health care to people with schizophrenia (Kendrick et al., 1991; Ustun and Sartorius, 1995).

Planning services at the national/regional level

The implications for service planning at national/regional levels that arise from the epidemiological knowledge base are fewer and less specific than those at the individual or local levels. Table 19.5 indicates the most important issues.

Urban excess of schizophrenia

The higher prevalence rates in urban areas already discussed indicate that the formulae used to allocate funds to local health services across a region or nation may need to reflect prevalence rates of 'severe mental illness'. In so far as schizophrenia accounts for about half of the total prevalence of all psychotic disorders, its prevalence rates are a reasonable proxy for severe mental illness and can be used to guide resource allocation (Thornicroft, 1991; Jarman and Hirsch, 1992). The first implication at the regional/national level is that this information needs to be communicated by researchers and clinicians to politicians and officials so that they can take account of variations in morbidity in constructing resource allocation formulae. Second, decisions at national and regional levels, based upon such scientific evidence, will impact upon the financial resources available to the local level. This may, in turn, prevent the need for uninformed local debates about which areas deserve greater mental health service investment.

High unemployment rates

In many economically 'developed' countries, the levels of unemployment among people with schizophrenia are frequently above 85% and reflect the fact such people cannot compete in the labour market and are, therefore, excluded from the many benefits of the workplace (Warr, 1987). The implications are that mental health services may need to develop dedicated activities to support the entry into and the survival of people with schizophrenia in the mainstream labour market. In parallel, supported, nontraditional cooperatives may provide opportunities for patients to work in a mixed workforce, as is the case in several regions in Italy (Tansella et al., 1998; Warner, 1999).

Fluctuating course of relapses and remissions

Although a common course of schizophrenia is to follow a chronically relapsing and remitting pattern, it is rare for pension and social security systems to work in a way that reflects these changing levels of disability, or to provide incentives for periods of work between relapses. Indeed the opposite is more often the case, in that people with a diagnosis of schizophrenia need to declare themselves permanently disabled to qualify for some welfare benefits entitlements, with unknown consequences for their self-image and self-esteem. The implication of this at the national/regional level is to promote change to policies and procedures so that pension and social security disability payment systems allow more flexible movement into and out of the 'disabled' category, according to clinical status, and increase the allowable earned income levels within disability pension schemes (Warner, 1999).

Conclusions

Although most epidemiological research in the field of schizophrenia has been directed towards understanding the aetiology, onset, course and outcome of the condition, nevertheless some of these results may also be used to improve mental health services. In this chapter, we have selected the results of epidemiological work that have at present the most clear service consequences. At the same time, there are well-established results that do not have such clear consequences for how treatment and care are delivered. For example, sex differences in the age of onset are now well known but are of little practical significance for service planners (Angermeyer and Kuhn, 1988; Piccinelli and Gomez Homen, 1997).

One primary conclusion from this review is that a 'two way street' should be further developed between epidemiological studies and services planning. On one hand, services should be planned to benefit from the best available evidence on the occurrence of schizophrenia and the needs of those whom it affects. On the other hand, services should also offer the best possible conditions to support the conduct of research, especially large-scale, collaborative epidemiologically based studies.

In this final section, we wish to return to an issue we raised earlier in this chapter: should services be separately organized for patients with a diagnosis of schizophrenia, or should such patients be treated alongside others with severe mental disorders in general adult community-based mental health services? Here we can distinguish mental health *service component* planning, from mental health *system planning*. The first type of planning is *segmental,* in the sense that it takes the needs of individual institutions or particular diagnoses one at a time without putting these needs in a general framework of the other services available in the same area. By comparison, *system planning* is often population based and aims to organize for defined populations a system of care that underlines the connections between different components, and even the relationships with other health sector services as well as social and private services in the same area. In other words, system planning is the practical consequence of taking a public health approach to assessing the mental health needs of a population, with all that such an approach implies (Thornicroft and Tansella, 1999).

Within this public health orientation, we would emphasize the compatibility between the need for integrated services for local populations and the need for specialized treatments and other interventions dedicated to patients suffering from schizophrenia and their carers. One practical example of this need is the organization of psycho-educational programmes for relatives of patients suffering from schizophrenia. The advantages of these programmes have now been well established (Hogarty et al., 1991; McFarlane et al., 1991, 1995; Mari and Streiner, 1996), and they should be considered as an integral part of a local service for schizophrenic patients.

We wish to make one further point. In addition to the results stemming from dedicated health service research and epidemiological studies, the findings of other studies, including those intended to enhance aetiological understanding (Andreasen, 1999), may also have important implications for planning and delivering services to people with schizophrenia and should, therefore, in future be fully exploited for these purposes.

REFERENCES

Allebeck P (1989) Schizophrenia: a life-shortening disease. Schizophrenia Bulletin 15, 81–89.

Amaddeo F, Bisoffi G, Bonizzato P, Micciolo R, Tansella M (1995) Mortality among patients with psychiatric illness. A ten-year case register study in an area with a community-based system of care. British Journal of Psychiatry 166, 783–788.

Andreasen NC (1999) Understanding the causes of schizophrenia. New England Journal of Medicine 340, 645–647.

Angermeyer M, Kuhn L (1988) Gender difference in age at onset of schizophrenia. European Archives of Psychiatry and Neurological Sciences 237, 351–364.

Appleby L, Shaw J, Amos T et al. (1999) Suicide within 12 months of contact with mental health services: national clinical survey. British Medical Journal 318, 1235–1239.

Bartels SJ, Teague GB, Drake RE et al. (1993) Service utilization and costs associated with substance use disorder among severely mentally ill patients. Journal of Nervous and Mental Disease 181, 227–232

Birmingham D, Mason D, Grubin D (1996) Prevalence of mental disorders in remand prisoners: consecutive case study. British Medical Journal 313, 1521–1524.

Breakey W (1996) Integrated Mental Health Services. Oxford: Oxford University Press.

Brier A, Schreiber J, Dyer J, Pickar D (1991) National Institute of Mental Health longitudinal study of chronic schizophrenia. Prognosis and predictors of outcome. Archives of General Psychiatry 48, 239–246.

Brown S, Birtwhistle J, Roe L, Thompson C (1999) The unhealthy lifestyle of people with schizophrenia. Psychological Medicine 29, 697–701.

Cuffel B (1992) Prevalence estimates of substance abuse in schizophrenia and their correlates. Journal of Nervous and Mental Disease 180, 589–592.

Dauncey K, Giggs J, Baker K, Harrison G (1993) Schizophrenia in Nottingham: lifelong residential mobility of a cohort. British Journal of Psychiatry 163, 613–619.

Davies S, Thornicroft G, Higginbotham A, Leese M, Phelan M (1996) Ethnic differences in the risk of compulsory psychiatric admission among representative cases of psychosis in London. The PRiSM study of psychosis in South London. British Medical Journal 312, 533–537.

Drake RE, McHugo GJ, Noordsy DL (1993) Treatment of alcoholism among schizophrenic outpatients: 4-year outcomes. American Journal of Psychiatry 150, 328–329.

Eaton WW (1991) Update on the epidemiology of schizophrenia. Epidemiologic Reviews 13, 320–328.

Eckman TA, Wirshing WC, Marder SR et al. (1992) Techniques for training schizophrenic patients in illness self-management: a controlled trial. American Journal of Psychiatry 149, 1545–1549.

Faris RE, Dunham W (1939) Mental Disorders in Urban Areas. An Ecological Study of Schizophrenia and other Psychoses. Chicago: University of Chicago Press.

Gift TE, Strauss JS, Harder DW, Kokes RF, Ritzler BA (1981) Established chronicity of psychotic symptoms in first-admission schizophrenic patients. American Journal of Psychiatry 138, 779–784.

Goldacre M, Seagrott V, Hawton K (1993) Suicide after discharge from psychiatric in-patient care. Lancet 342, 283–286.

Gottesman I (1991) Schizophrenia Genesis: The Origins of Madness. New York: Freeman.

Häfner H, an der Heiden W (1997) Epidemiology of schizophrenia. Canadian Journal of Psychiatry 42, 139–151.

Harris E, Barraclough B (1998) Excess mortality of mental disorder. British Journal of Psychiatry 173, 11–53.

Hogarty GE, Anderson CM, Reiss DJ et al. (1991) Family psychoeducation, social skills training, and maintenance chemotherapy in the aftercare treatment of schizophrenia. II. Two-year effects of a controlled study on relapse and adjustment. Environmental–Personal Indicators in the Course of Schizophrenia (EPICS) Research Group. Archives of General Psychiatry 48, 340–347.

Jablensky A (1995) Schizophrenia: recent epidemiological issues. Epidemiologic Reviews 17, 10–20.

Jablensky A (1997) The 100-year epidemiology of schizophrenia. Schizophrenia Research 28, 111–1225.

Jablensky A, Eaton W (1995) Schizophrenia. In: Epidemiological Psychiatry, Jablensky A, ed. London: Ballière Tindall, pp. 283–306.

Jarman B, Hirsch S (1992) Statistical models to predict district psychiatric morbidity. In: Measuring Mental Health Needs, Thornicroft G, Brewin C, Wing JK, eds. Gaskell Press: Royal College of Psychiatrists, pp. 62–80.

Jerrell JM, Hu T, Ridgely MS (1994) Cost-effectiveness of substance disorder interventions for the severely mentally ill. Journal of Mental Health Administration 21, 281–295.

Johnstone EC, Crow TJ, Johnson AL, MacMillan JF (1986) The Northwick Park Study of first episodes of schizophrenia. I. Presentation of the illness and problems relating to admission. British Journal of Psychiatry 148, 115–120.

Kemp R, Hayward P, Applewhaite G, Everitt B, David A (1996) Compliance therapy in psychotic patients: a randomized controlled trial. British Medical Journal 312, 345–349.

Kendler K, Diehl S (1995) Schizophrenia: genetics. In: Comprehensive Textbook of Psychiatry, 6th edn., Vol. 1, Kaplan H, Saddock B, eds. Baltimore, MD: Williams & Wilkins, pp. 942–957.

Kendrick A, Sibbald B, Burns T, Freeling P (1991) Role of general practitioners in care of long term mentally ill patients. British Medical Journal 302, 508–511.

Kramer M (1976) Issues in the development of statistical and epidemiological data for mental health services research. Psychological Medicine 6, 185–215.

Lehman AF, Myers CP, Thompson JW et al. (1993) Implications of mental and substance use disorders: a comparison of single and dual diagnosis patients. Journal of Nervous and Mental Diseases 181, 365–370.

Lesage A, Tansella M (1989) Mobility of schizophrenic patients, nonpsychotic patients and the general population in a case register area. Social Psychiatry and Psychiatric Epidemiology 24, 271–274.

Lewis G, David A, Andreasson S, Allebeck P (1992) Schizophrenia and city life. Lancet 340, 137–140.

Mari JJ, Streiner D (1996) Family intervention for those with schizophrenia. In: Schizophrenia Module of The Cochrane Database of Systematic Reviews, Adams C, Annderson J, Mari JJ, eds. updated 10 September 1996. Available in The Cochrane Library database on disk and CDROM. The Cochrane Collaboration, Issue 3. Oxford: Update Software; 1996. Updated quarterly. London: British Medical Journal Publishing Group.

Mason P, Wilkinson G (1996) The prevalence of psychiatric morbidity. OPCS survey of psychiatric morbidity in Great Britain. British Journal of Psychiatry 168, 1–3.

Maurer K, Häfner H (1995) Methodological aspects of onset assessment in schizophrenia. Schizophrenia Research 15, 165–176.

McCreadie R, Leese M, Tilak-Singh D, Loftus L, Macewan T, Thornicroft G (1997) Nithsdale, Nunhead and Norwood: similarities and differences in prevalence of schizophrenia and utilisation of services in rural and urban areas. British Journal of Psychiatry 170, 31–36.

McCreadie R, Macdonald E, Blacklock C et al. (1998) Dietary intake of schizophrenic patients in Nithsdale, Scotland: case-control study. British Medical Journal 317, 784–785.

McFarlane WR, Ranz JR, Horen BA (1991) Creating a supportive environment using staff psychoeducation in a supervised residence. Hospital and Community Psychiatry 42, 1154–1159.

McFarlane WR, Lukens E, Link B et al. (1995) Multiple family groups and psychoeducation in the treatment of schizophrenia. Archives of General Psychiatry 52, 679–687.

McGorry P, Jackson HJ (1999) The Recognition and Management of Early Psychosis: A Preventive Approach. Cambridge: Cambridge University Press.

Menezes P, Johnson S, Thornicroft G et al. (1996) Drug and alcohol problems among individuals with severe mental illness in South London. British Journal of Psychiatry 168, 612–619.

Morris J (1975) The Uses of Epidemiology, 3rd edn. Edinburgh: Churchill Livingstone.

Mortensen P (1999) Can suicide research lead to suicide prevention? Acta Psychiatrica Scandinavica 99, 397–398.

Mortensen P, Pedersen C, Westergaard T et al. (1999) Effects of family history and place and season of birth on the risk of schizophrenia. New England Journal of Medicine 340, 603–608.

Pedersen CB, Mortensen PB (2001) Evidence of a dose–response relationship between urbanicity during upbringing and schizophrenia risk. Archives of General Psychiatry 58, 1039–1046.

Piccinelli M, Gomez Homen F (1997) Gender Differences in the Epidemiology of Affective Disorders and Schizophrenia. Geneva: World Health Organization.

Regier DA, Farmer ME, Rae DS et al. (1990) Comorbidity of mental disorders with alcohol and other substances: results from the Epidemiological Catchment Area. Journal of the American Medical Association 164, 2511–2518.

Rossau C, Mortensen P (1997) Risk factors for suicide in schizophrenic patients. A nested case control study. British Journal of Psychiatry 171, 355–359.

Roth A, Fonagy P (1996) What Works for Whom? A Critical Review of Psychotherapy Research. New York: Guilford Press.

Schaffer D, Craft L (1999) Methods of adolescent suicide prevention. Journal of Clinical Psychiatry 60, 70–74.

Scott H, Johnson S, Menezes P et al. (1998) Substance misuse and risk of aggression and offending. British Journal of Psychiatry 172, 345–350.

Shepherd G, Beardsmore A, Moore C, Hardy P, Muijen M (1997) Relation between bed use, social deprivation, and overall bed availability in acute adult psychiatric units, and alternative residential options: a cross sectional survey, one day census data, and staff interviews. British Medical Journal 314, 262.

Swanson J, Holzer C, Ganju V (1990) Violence and psychiatric disorder in the community: evidence from the Epidemiological Catchment Area Survey. Hospital and Community Psychiatry 41, 761–770.

Tansella M, Amaddeo F, Burti L, Garzotto N, Ruggeri M (1998) Community-based mental health care in Verona, Italy. In: Mental Health in Our Future Cities, Goldberg D, Thornicroft G, eds. Hove: Psychology Press, pp. 239–262.

Thornicroft G (1991) Social deprivation and rates of treated mental disorder: developing statistical models to predict psychiatric service utilisation. British Journal of Psychiatry 158, 475–484.

Thornicroft G, Tansella M (1999) The Mental Health Matrix. A Manual to Improve Services. Cambridge: Cambridge University Press.

Ustun B, Sartorius N (1995) Mental Illness in General Health Care. An International Study. Chichester: Wiley.

van Os J, Wright P, Murray R (1997) Follow-up studies of schizophrenia I: natural history and nonpsychopathological predictors of outcome. European Psychiatry 12(Suppl. 5), S327–S341.

van Os J, Jones P, Sham P, Bebbington P, Murray R (1998) Risk factors for onset and persistence of psychosis. Social Psychiatry and Psychiatric Epidemiology 33, 596–605.

Warner R (1999) Schizophrenia and the environment: speculative interventions. Epidemiologia e Psichiatria Sociale 8, 19–34.

Warner R, de Girolamo G (1995) Schizophrenia. Geneva: World Health Organization.

Warr P (1987) Work, Unemployment and Mental Health. Oxford: Oxford University Press.

20

Prevention of schizophrenia – not an impossible dream

John McGrath

Queensland Centre for Schizophrenia Research, Wolston Park Hospital, Wacol, Australia

Introduction

In arguing for increased research funding, attention is often drawn to the finding that schizophrenia accounts for 2.3% of the total burden of disease (disability adjusted life years, DALYs) in established market economies (Murray and Lopez, 1996). How is it that, despite 1.4–2.8% of national health care being devoted to the direct costs of schizophrenia, the burden of disability is still so high? What would the burden of schizophrenia be if funds were unlimited and optimal treatments (medication, psychosocial interventions, service mix, etc.) were delivered consistently? Most commentators would concede that the burden would still be inevitable. In other words, a substantial proportion of the DALYs associated with schizophrenia are 'unavertable' in terms of secondary and tertiary prevention. An alternative, and more ambitious, approach to averting DALYs is to reduce the incidence of a disorder. This chapter will discuss issues related to primary prevention in general and then speculate on directions for future research related to schizophrenia.

The science of prevention

In its simplest form, primary prevention aims to reduce the incidence of a disease. Prevention strategies can be directed at different target populations (Gordon, 1983; Mrazek and Haggerty, 1994): (i) universal preventive interventions are aimed at the general population regardless of risk status/susceptibility status; (ii) selective preventive interventions target particular population subgroups, who may be more susceptible to a disorder but who are still symptom free; (iii) indicated prevention is targeted at individuals who have the early features or subclinical manifestations of a disorder.

Universal interventions have strengths and weakness that relate to the features of both the exposure (the risk-modifying variable, be it genetic, epigenetic or an interaction between the two) and the disorder. This approach alleviates the need to identify a minority of individuals who are 'high-risk' – the focus of much current research in the prevention of schizophrenia. If we can identify such individuals, and if we can reduce their risk, then this is a highly desirable goal. However, if we cannot identify high-risk individuals, we need to consider alternative strategies.

Geoffrey Rose (1992) has emphasized that population-based interventions are best suited to risks that are distributed throughout the population, albeit not in equal measure. Those at high risk of disease, seemingly an obvious target for preventative action, may in fact be relatively rare. Those at medium risk may be more common and, therefore, may account for a much higher proportion of disease. For example, if a large proportion of the community is exposed to a small risk, then population-based interventions may avert more illness (greater number of cases prevented) than interventions based on the rare, high-risk individuals. Rose (1992) then introduced the concept of the 'prevention paradox' – a preventive measure that brings large benefits to the community but which offers little to the majority who are, themselves, at low risk. Indeed, the intervention may mean that such individuals have to give up something; hence the paradox. For example, many population-based interventions (e.g. vaccination, wearing a seatbelt) bring little direct benefit to the individual, but individuals are willing to accept them because they cause little inconvenience. Inconvenience is weighed against the frequency of the undesirable outcome and its severity.

Risk factors and causes

In order to develop a framework for primary prevention, it is important to understand terminology surrounding risk factors and causes (Susser, 1991; Kraemer et al., 1997). A risk factor can be anything that is, statistically, associated with disease. As such, risk factors may point us towards causes but are not necessarily involved in producing an outcome or disease. Variables that correlate with outcomes but do not precede them should not be labelled risk factors, but rather sequelae, consequences or concomitants. When considering risk factors, it is also important to understand that there are risk indicators that can be epiphenomena or proxy markers of an underlying risk-modifying factor that is closely allied with cause. A major problem with a brain disease like schizophrenia is that the current knowledge base is limited and, therefore, we cannot confidently predict if a risk factor is causally related or whether it is a proxy marker.

As a result, the term 'risk-modifying factor' should be reserved for factors that appear to operate within the causal chain (contribute to the outcome). If factors that truly modify risk could be reduced, then so should the incidence of the resultant disorder. In neurodevelopmental models of schizophrenia, we are looking for distal or 'upstream' risk-modifying variables. Also, these factors may operate directly or indirectly (sometimes referred to as first- or second-order effects). Risk-modifying factors can be fixed (e.g. sex) or variable (drug abuse). They can, of course, also be protective or adverse.

In order to reduce the incidence of schizophrenia, we need to identify candidate risk-modifying variables that can themselves be modified. Ideally, the interventions should have a number of characteristics. They should be effective, in that they should reduce or eliminate the risk-modifying variable. They must be safe and acceptable to the community or susceptible individual. This involves the balance of risk and benefit, together with convenience. Finally, they must be cost effective and, ideally, cheap, especially if applied universally.

Barriers to the primary prevention of schizophrenia

A major factor that has eroded confidence in primary prevention of schizophrenia has been a perception that we have made little progress in our understanding of the aetiology of conditions of this type. We know about many risk factors but cannot yet identify those that are powerful modifiers of risk except, perhaps, genetic influences, which we do not yet understand. The slow progress has engendered a feeling of nihilistic despair. The other factor that has hindered progress is the debate about when to start primary prevention research. Should we wait until every minute detail about aetiology and pathogenesis is unravelled before primary prevention attempts are made, or should we trust inconclusive but suggestive data? In the past, there have been some spectacular applications of primary prevention, based on either incorrect or incomplete assumptions. The miasma theory of ill health (that brackish, impure water and soil gave off noxious emanations) led to the call for improved sanitation long before microorganisms were suspected or discovered. The consumption of limes on long sea voyages was found to prevent scurvy without the benefit of an understanding of ascorbic acid.

Another problem that impedes primary prevention research in schizophrenia is the lag time between the window for intervention (e.g. during brain development) and the assessment of outcome (e.g. the onset of schizophrenia). The effectiveness of some interventions can be assessed at birth (e.g. folate supplements to reduce spinal tube closure defects; rubella vaccination to reduce congenital rubella). If the presence or absence of schizophrenia is defined as the main outcome variable, and the intervention occurs prenatally, then the intervening period must reflect the age-incidence curve. By age 30, only 33% of women and 51% of men destined to develop schizophrenia during their lifetime would have developed the illness (Welham et al., 2000). Surrogate or interim endpoints related to known antecedents of schizophrenia (see below) may be a solution.

Over the 20th century, the prevention of psychosis has not been a focus of study. One notable exception is the Mauritius study (Mednick et al., 1981). Based on an hypothesis linking autonomic skin responsivity to a vulnerability to schizophrenia,

1800 3-year-old children were screened using a psychophysiological measure and allocated to low- and high-risk groups. Blind to group status, a portion of these children were provided with a package of interventions including nursery school education and diet. While the investigators now concede that their original marker of vulnerability lacks validity, it will still be of considerable interest to follow up this cohort with respect to psychosis and a broad range of educational and social outcomes (Raine et al., 1997).

Possible preventive strategies in schizophrenia

Selective prevention

While this chapter will focus on the universal prevention of schizophrenia, it is important to note ideas and potential strategies for selective and indicated prevention that are also in development. For example, if we could identify individuals at high risk of developing schizophrenia, then selective prevention measures might be recommended. Apart from the increased risk of psychosis in those with a positive family history, our ability to identify individuals prior to the onset of schizophrenia is still poor. The positive predictive value may be improved by combining risk factors such as those derived from longitudinal cohort studies (e.g. cognitive, behavioural and psychosocial antecedents of schizophrenia), psychophysiological measures (e.g. smooth pursuit eye movement, P300, etc.), the presence of minor physical anomalies or obstetric complications.

Selective intervention relies on efficient means of identifying those at increased risk (via single or multistage screening). The sensitivity and specificity of the screens must be balanced with the safety and efficacy of any proposed intervention. While avoidance of illicit substances and stress management may seem to be reasonable and safe selective interventions, we lack a sufficient evidence base to guide us. The use of antipsychotic medications in prepsychotic individuals is an ethically complex issue, and one that, as yet, lacks an evidence base (Tsuang et al., 2000). Individuals thought to be at increased risk may be a target for careful review and prompt treatment if psychosis is noted to arise, but such follow-up, however well intentioned, is not a benign intervention.

Indicated prevention

For individuals with early features of psychosis, there is a growing body of evidence showing that integrated treatments (low-dose medication, psycho-education and cognitively oriented psychological treatments) improve outcomes (McGorry and Jackson, 1999): an example of indicated prevention. Prompt treatment for those in the earliest phases of schizophrenia should improve a range of short-term outcomes, and there is much hope that indicated prevention may also translate to improved long-term outcome. Future research should help to clarify this issue (McGrath and McGlashan, 1999).

Universal interventions: the search for risk factors

Unlike the search for susceptibility genes for schizophrenia, those interested in nongenetic risk factors are not able to map the environment systematically. However, research has identified a number of pre- and perinatal candidate risk factors for schizophrenia. These include family history, season of birth, place of birth, obstetric complications, prenatal exposure to viruses and prenatal famine (see Ch. 5). Other risk factors have been identified that are more proximal to the onset of illness (e.g. head injury, substance abuse, life events).

When assessing risk factors, it is important to consider the strength of the evidence (consistency, design rigour), the effect size associated with the exposure (odds ratios or relative risks), and the population attributable risk (PAR). The PAR is an estimate of how many cases could be prevented if a particular risk factor were eliminated (assuming that the risk factor is causally related to the outcome; Last, 1988). It should be noted that the PAR is a problematic concept. For example, the total PAR values for various risk factors could total more than 100% because of possible additive or competing effects: the measure does not take into account interactions between different risk factors. However, PAR does serve to rank order risk factors in a manner of interest to prevention research. It emphasizes the fact that small risk factors, if widely distributed among the community, may 'cause' more cases than rarer, but larger, risk factors. It also has to assume that risk factors are true, risk-modifying factors with causal effect.

Genetic factors

Of the currently known risk factors for schizophrenia, family history is by far the most robust (see Ch. 10). However, Mortensen and colleagues (1999) reported that the PAR of having one or both parents affected was only 3.8%. While the interaction between genetic and nongenetic risk factors is almost certainly more complicated than these figures suggest, the finding reinforces the fact that, while risk factors with large odds ratios are attractive targets, their real effect on the population may be small (see Chs. 10 and 11).

Current evidence suggests that many different genes, each of small effect, contribute to the risk of schizophrenia. If we could identify individuals with these genes, then it may be feasible to deliver some type of selective intervention to those identified as susceptible. The timing of this intervention could be prenatal, early life, or around the time of maximal risk. However, it is entirely plausible that the genes that contribute to susceptibility are relatively common, and that most individuals with these genes are unaffected. Genetic risk factors may not readily translate into universal interventions. Despite the ever-increasing pace of discovery in molecular biology, gene therapy seems a distant hope at the moment.

Season and place of birth

People born in winter and spring tend to have a slightly increased relative risk of developing schizophrenia compared with those born in autumn and summer. Mortensen and colleagues (1999) reported a very small effect size (1.11) for season of birth in their Danish sample. However, as a substantial fraction of the population are exposed (i.e. born during winter/spring), the attributable risk was substantial (10.5%). Season of birth is a risk indicator and thus can only serve to generate candidate risk-modifying variables. Currently, candidate exposures that may be related to the season of birth effect include perinatal viral exposures (Torrey et al., 1997) and low prenatal vitamin D (McGrath, 1999). While the season of birth effect in the northern hemisphere population is robust (Torrey et al., 1997), a meta-analysis of data from southern hemisphere studies did not support an effect (McGrath and Welham, 1999). This north–south difference may help clarify the nature of the underlying risk-modifying factors.

People born in the city tend to have a greater risk of developing schizophrenia than those born in rural regions (Marcelis et al., 1998; Mortensen et al., 1999; see Ch. 4). The relative risk of developing schizophrenia when born in the city versus being born in the country is about 2.4. However, because exposure to urban birth was relatively frequent in both the Danish and Dutch studies, the PAR for this variable was substantial (in the order of 30 to 35%). Place of birth, once again, appears to be a proxy marker for a risk-modifying variable such as viral infection, nutrition, low vitamin D and unspecified toxic exposures (Mortensen, 2000).

Place and season of birth should provide fertile domains for the generation of candidate exposures. However, until we can identify risk-modifying variables responsible for these effects, prevention research is not feasible.

Pregnancy and birth complications

Links between pregnancy and birth complications and an increased risk of schizophrenia have been examined over many decades (see Ch. 5). While the data are not entirely consistent, the weight of the evidence supports a modest increased risk of schizophrenia in those exposed to a variety of obstetric complications. The PAR related to these exposures is not clear but is probably modest (5–10%). There is an extensive literature on how to improve perinatal outcomes, much of it based on randomized controlled trials. Intervention at a population level (all pregnant women) could include general options related to improving antenatal care and more specific options such as smoking cessation. One attractive feature of this type of intervention is that disorders other than schizophrenia could be averted, and pregnant women tend to be more receptive to health promotion than the general community. This is another example of an intervention with low prevention paradox.

One group may derive additional benefit from optimal antenatal care – women with schizophrenia. Women with schizophrenia tend to experience more obstetric complications at delivery (Sacker et al., 1996; Bennedsen, 1998). It has also been suggested that the effect of family history together with obstetric complications amplifies the subsequent risk of schizophrenia in the offspring (Mednick et al., 1987). If this is true, it follows that optimizing antenatal care to women who have a 'high-risk' fetus may be a suitable avenue for selective prevention.

Prenatal infection

A range of prenatal infective agents can impact on brain development. While influenza was the focus of much research during the 1990s, the strength of the evidence of prenatal exposure to influenza is weak and inconsistent (McGrath and Castle, 1995). Other candidate viruses include rubella (Susser et al., 1999), coxsackievirus B (Rantakillio et al., 1997) and Borna virus (Salvatore et al., 1997) (see Ch. 5).

There are no robust data yet to either support or reject the theory that pre- or perinatal exposure to infection increases the risk of schizophrenia. However, until there are convincing data from well-designed and adequately powered studies, the viral theory should remain as a candidate risk factor. From the perspective of universal interventions, viral illness can be prevented by vaccinations, and there are now examples of public health interventions where mass vaccinations have eliminated certain viruses completely. This is another area where the intervention cannot confidently be put forward for schizophrenia, but it has many other beneficial effects.

Nutritional factors

There has been considerable interest in recent years about the impact of prenatal nutrition and various adult-onset disorders such as diabetes, cardiovascular disease and hypertension (Barker, 1992). Prenatal nutritional factors are biologically plausible risk-modifying factors for neurodevelopmental disorders (Brown et al., 1996). Susser and colleagues (1996) identified increased risk of schizophrenia in the offspring of women who were pregnant during a famine in the Netherlands during World War II. While studies of the incidence of schizophrenia in developing nations (where poor nutrition is more prevalent) do not show higher rates, there remains the possibility that deficits in specific micronutrients may play a role. In a population-based study from Finland (Wahlbeck et al., 2001), the offspring of women with low late-pregnancy body mass index had an increased risk of schizophrenia. While we cannot assume that this variable was causally related to risk of schizophrenia in the offspring, it does open a window for possible intervention.

Even in the absence of deficits, supplementing prenatal nutrition warrants consideration. For example, supplementing folate to women periconceptually is associated with a reduction in the incidence of neural tube defects in their offspring (Scott et al., 1994). Recent evidence from a randomized controlled trial of nutritional supplements for preterm infants found not only that cognitive outcomes (measured at age 7 years) were superior in the group allocated the enriched infant formulae but also this group had less cerebral palsy (Lucas et al., 1998). This study suggested that suboptimal nutrition during a critical period of brain growth could impair functional compensation in those sustaining an earlier brain insult.

In summary, while the evidence implicating prenatal nutrition as a risk factor in schizophrenia is scant, it is another attractive candidate for universal intervention. Better maternal nutrition is safe, relatively cheap and could feasibly impact on a range of health outcomes.

Developmental risk factors: from infancy to onset

The Copenhagen High Risk Cohort (Schulsinger et al., 1987) reported that high-risk individuals (offspring of mothers with schizophrenia) who had had periods of institutionalization were more likely to develop schizophrenia than those high-risk individuals without episodes of institutional care. It is difficult to determine if the exposure of these high-risk children to institutional rearing is a true risk modifier (operating directly to increase the penetrance of the underlying genetic factor) or an epiphenomenon related to the temperament of the preschizophrenic child. Tienari and colleagues (1994) examined carefully the families who had adopted high-risk children (i.e. offspring of mothers with schizophrenia). While members of the cohort are still to pass through much of their period of morbid risk, early results suggest that those high-risk children adopted into the highest functioning families appear to be 'protected'. These findings suggest that a modifying effect of the environment in high-risk children should be given added scrutiny. Further work is needed on how to identify susceptible children, and on how to identify the particular protective features of the environment.

There is now robust evidence that children who go on to develop schizophrenia display subtle neurodevelopmental deviations (Tarrant and Jones, 1999; see Ch. 6). As a group, these children tend to have abnormalities of social functioning, delayed motor milestones, speech problems and impaired cognitive/educational abilities. While it is not clear if these features operate within the causal chain (contribute to an increased risk of developing schizophrenia) or are passive risk indicators (markers of the underlying schizophrenia or the process that may modify risk), the findings suggest directions for primary prevention research. However, several key issues need consideration in order to develop this type of research. Are interventions available that could ameliorate features associated with increased risk of developing schizophrenia? Are these interventions safe, cheap and acceptable? Are the interventions associated with a broad range of positive outcomes other than reduced risk of schizophrenia, such as better school achievements, improved self-esteem, etc?

Research has found a significant excess of life events in the 6 months prior to the onset of psychosis, and that this association persisted when life events that may have been secondary to being psychotic were excluded (Bebbington et al., 1993; van Os et al., 1994). It is not clear how this finding could be translated to primary prevention. The effect may be mediated through individual vulnerability. This, then, would be a possible target for either primary or secondary intervention, with the aim of that intervention being reduction in vulnerability in some way or protection from life events insofar as that is possible.

Future directions: what type of research do we need?

There is an urgent need for strategic research designed to generate and rigorously test candidate nongenetic, risk-modifying factors for schizophrenia. A framework for the primary prevention of schizophrenia can be built on this type of research. While we have some broad clues in the form of risk indicators (urban birth, season of birth, pregnancy and birth complications), we need to 'fine map' these domains. We should continue to try to identify novel domains from which to generate candidate exposures. One way to look for clues is to identify disease gradients and then search for clues to explain these gradients. These gradients can be across time (season of birth, between-year variability) and across space (neighbourhood variation, urban–rural gradient and latitude gradients in prevalence). Within medical epidemiology, migrant studies have played an important role in generating candidate exposures. They can vary the environmental factors while 'holding' ethnicity constant (and, it is assumed, a degree of genetic variability) (Hennekens and Buring, 1987). The cause of the increased risk of psychosis in second-generation African–Caribbeans born in the UK is still unclear. These studies of schizophrenia in migrant groups may help to generate awareness of novel candidate exposures (Harrison et al., 1997; McDonald and Murray, 2000; see Ch. 4).

It is essential that the data used to address this problem are derived from epidemiologically informed sampling frames. Sample sizes need to be representative of the underlying population so the PAR values that guide public health planning can be generated. Links between candidate exposures and genetic epidemiology will also be crucial for future research.

Just as candidate genes are ranked according to various rules (e.g. are they located in a 'hot spot', how many introns/exons within the gene, biological plausibility, etc.?), those interested in exposures need sorting rules. When rank-ordering candidate exposures for more intense scrutiny, there is a case to prioritise those with universal public health potential (e.g. vaccinations for infectious agents, nutritional supplements). If the exposure is already associated with disorders other than schizophrenia, then this makes it a more attractive candidate from a public health perspective (single interventions could lead to improvements in multiple outcomes).

Epidemiological research can serve to 'sharpen the focus', allowing candidate risk factors to be identified. However, history has shown that risk factor epidemiology can sometimes enter cycles of uninformative replications ('circular epidemiology': Kuller, 1999). Season of birth has been studied as a risk factor for 80 years with little real progress in identifying the underlying risk-modifying exposure. In reaction to this, some research groups are looking to developments in the neurosciences in order to test the impact of candidate exposures on neuronal development, both in vitro and in whole animal studies. Such analyses range from gene expression profiling through to cognitive psychology techniques such as prepulse inhibition.

These techniques are removed from the schizophrenia phenotype, but nevertheless can provide valuable evidence about the biological plausibility of candidate risk factors. Dialogue between those involved in risk factor epidemiology and those in developmental neurobiology can provide new clues about the potential timing of exposures (e.g. vulnerable periods of brain development) and broad classes of exposure (e.g. exposures that may impact on neural apoptosis, migration, etc.). Such scientific cross-fertilization can be informative for basic neuroscience as well. Clues from epidemiology linked vitamin A and increased risk of craniofacial abnormality, which then led to the discovery of the role of retinoic acid in brain development and ultimately to its nomination as a potential risk factor for schizophrenia (LaMantia, 1999).

Animal models for schizophrenia based on developmental interventions include lesions in selected brain areas (Lipska et al., 1993) prenatal exposure to specific viruses such as influenza (Fatemi et al., 1999) and Borna virus (Hornig et al., 1999), and prenatal hypoxic/ischaemic insults (Mallard et al., 1999). The potential to extend this type of research with the use of genetic knock-out mice (to test gene–environment interactions) and gene expression profiling (cross-referencing altered gene expression in animal experiments with gene expression studies in schizophrenia) offers powerful new tools to the neuroscience community. This type of research may galvanize the search for novel nongenetic risk factors for schizophrenia.

Sartorius and Henderson (1992) proposed three options for the research community interested in the primary prevention of mental illness. The first option was to forget about primary prevention completely and concentrate on better treatments and cures. The second option was to fund more research in order to discover the causes of serious psychiatric illness and then commence primary prevention.

The final option was to start primary prevention based on existing knowledge, albeit imperfect. Clearly, we need a balance of all three approaches. Basic strategic research needs to go hand in hand with attempts at primary prevention. The nihilism and despair of the past needs to be replaced by a sense of determination and urgency. The dream of making the primary prevention of schizophrenia a reality may be quixotic, but it is certainly not impossible.

Acknowledgement

The project described in this chapter was supported by the Stanley Foundation.

REFERENCES

Barker DJP (1992) Fetal and Infant Origins of Adult Disease. London: British Medical Journal.

Bebbington P, Wilkins S, Jones P et al. (1993) Life events and psychosis: initital results from the Camberwell Collaborative Psychosis Study. British Journal of Psychiatry 162, 72–79.

Bennedsen BE (1998) Adverse pregnancy outcome in schizophrenic women: occurence and risk factors. Schizophrenia Research 33, 1–26.

Brown AS, Susser ES, Butler PD, Richardson AR, Kaufmann CA, Gorman JM (1996) Neurobiological plausibility of prenatal nutritional deprivation as a risk factor for schizophrenia. Journal of Nervous and Mental Disease 184, 71–85.

Fatemi SH, Emamian ES, Kist D et al. (1999) Defective corticogenesis and reduction in Reelin immunoreactivity in cortex and hippocampus of prenatally infected neonatal mice. Molecular Psychiatry 4, 145–154.

Gordon R (1983) An operational classification of disease prevention. Public Health Reports 98, 271–282.

Harrison G, Glazebrook C, Brewin J et al. (1997) Increased incidence of psychotic disorders in migrants from the Caribbean to the United Kingdom. Psychological Medicine 27, 799–806.

Hennekens CH, Buring JE (1987) Epidemiology in Medicine. Boston, MA: Little, Brown.

Hornig M, Weissenbock H, Horscroft N, Lipkin WI (1999) An infection-based model of neuro-developmental damage. Proceedings of the National Academy of Sciences of the USA 96, 12102–12107.

Kraemer HC, Kazdin AE, Offord DR, Kkessler RC, Jensen PS, Kupfer DJ (1997) Coming to terms with the terms of risk. Archives of General Psychiatry 54, 337–343.

Kuller LH (1999) Circular epidemiology [see comments]. American Journal of Epidemiology 150, 897–903.

LaMantia A (1999) Forebrain induction, retinoic acid, and vulnerability to schizophrenia: insights from molecular and genetic analysis in developing mice. Biological Psychiatry 46, 19–30.

Last JM (1988) A Dictionary of Epidemiology. New York: Oxford University Press.

Lipska BK, Jaskiw GE, Weinberger DR (1993) Postpubertal emergence of hyperresponsiveness to stress and to amphetamine after neonatal excitotoxic hippocampal damage: a potential animal model of schizophrenia. Neuropsychopharmacology 9, 67–75.

Lucas A, Morley R, Cole TJ (1998) Randomised trial of early diet in preterm babies and later intelligence quotient. British Medical Journal 317, 1481–1487.

Mallard EC, Rehn A, Rees S, Tolcos M, Copolov D (1999) Ventriculomegaly and reduced hippocampal volume following intrauterine growth-restriction: implications for the aetiology of schizophrenia. Schizophrenia Research 40, 11–21.

Marcelis M, Navarro-Mateu F, Murray R, Selten J-P, van Os J (1998) Urbanization and psychosis: a study of 1942–1978 birth cohorts in the Netherlands. Psychological Medicine 28, 871–879.

McDonald C, Murray RM (2000) Early and late environmental risk factors for schizophrenia. Brain Research Reviews 31, 130–137.

McGorry PD, Jackson HJ (1999) The Recognition and Management of Early Psychosis: a Preventive Approach. Cambridge: Cambridge University Press.

McGrath JJ (1999) Hypothesis: is low prenatal vitamin D a risk-modifying factor for schizophrenia? Schizophrenia Research 40, 173–177.

McGrath J, Castle D (1995) Does influenza cause schizophrenia? A five year review. Australian and New Zealand Journal of Psychiatry 29, 23–31.

McGrath J, McGlashan TH (1999) Improving outcomes for recent-onset psychoses: disentangling hope, speculation and evidence. Acta Psychiatrica Scandinavica 100, 83–84.

McGrath JJ, Welham JL (1999) Season of birth and schizophrenia: a systematic review and meta-analysis of data from the Southern Hemisphere. Schizophrenia Research 35, 237–242.

Mednick SA, Schulsinger F, Venables PH (1981) The Mauritius Project. In: Prospective Longitudinal Research: An Empirical Basis for the Primary Prevention of Psychosocial Disorders, Mednick SA, Baert A, eds. Oxford: Oxford University Press, pp. 314–316.

Mednick SA, Parnas J, Schulsinger F (1987) The Copenhagen High-Risk Project, 1962–86. Schizophrenia Bulletin 13, 485–495.

Mortensen PB (2000) Urban–rural differences in the risk for schizophrenia. International Journal of Mental Health 29, 101–110.

Mortensen PB, Pedersen CB, Westergaard T et al. (1999) Effects of family history and place and season of birth on the risk of schizophrenia. New England Journal of Medicine 340, 603–608.

Mrazek PJ, Haggerty RJ (1994) Reducing Risk for Mental Disorders: Frontiers for Preventive Intervention Research. Washington, DC: National Academic Press.

Murray CJ, Lopez AD (1996) The Global Burden of Disease. Boston, MA: Harvard School of Public Health.

Raine A, Venables PH, Mednick SA (1997) Low resting heart rate at age 3 years predisposes to aggression at age 11 years: evidence from the Mauritius Child Health Project. Journal of the American Academy of Child and Adolescent Psychiatry 36, 1457–1464.

Rantakallio P, Jones P, Moring J, von Wendt, L (1997) Associations between central nervous system infections during childhood and adult onset schizophrenia and other psychoses: A 28-year follow-up. International Review of Epidemiology 26, 837–843.

Rose G (1992) The Strategy of Preventive Medicine. Oxford: Oxford University Press.

Sacker A, Done DJ, Crow TJ (1996) Obstetric complications in children born to parents with schizophrenia: a meta-analysis of case-control studies. Psychological Medicine 26, 279–287.

Salvatore M, Morzunov S, Schwemmle M, Lipkin WI (1997) Borna disease virus in brains of North American and European people with schizophrenia and bipolar disorder. Bornavirus Study Group. Lancet 349, 1813–1814.

Sartorius N, Henderson AS (1992) The neglect of prevention in psychiatry. Australian and New Zealand Journal of Psychiatry 26, 550–553.

Schulsinger F, Parnas J, Mednick S, Teasdale TW, Schulsinger H (1987) Heredity–environment interaction and schizophrenia. Journal of Psychiatric Research 21, 431–436.

Scott JM, Weir DG, Molloy A, McPartlin J, Daly L, Kirke P (1994) Folic Acid Metabolism and Mechanisms of Neural Tube Defect. Chichester, UK: Wiley.

Susser E, Neugebauer R, Hoek H et al. (1996) Schizophrenia after prenatal famine: further evidence. Archives of General Psychiatry 53, 25–31.

Susser EB, Brown A, Matte TD (1999) Prenatal factors and adult mental and physical health. Canadian Journal of Psychiatry 44, 326–334.

Susser M (1991) What is a cause and how do we know one? A grammar for pragmatic epidemiology. American Journal of Epidemiology 133, 635–648.

Tarrant CJ, Jones PB (1999) Precursors to schizophrenia: do biological markers have specificity? Canadian Journal of Psychiatry 44, 335–349.

Tienari P, Wynne LC, Moring J et al. (1994) The Finnish Adoptive Family Study of schizophrenia. Implications for family research. British Journal of Psychiatry Suppl. 20–26.

Torrey EF, Miller J, Rawlings R, Yolken RH (1997) Seasonality of births in schizophrenia and bipolar disorder: a review of the literature. Schizophrenia Research 28, 1–38.

Tsuang MT, Stone WS, Faraone SV (2000) Towards the prevention of schizophrenia. Biological Psychiatry 48, 349–356.

van Os J, Fahy TA, Bebbington P et al. (1994) The influence of life events on the subsequent course of psychotic illness. A prospective follow-up of the Camberwell Collaborative Psychosis Study. Psychological Medicine 24, 503–513.

Wahlbeck K, Forsen T, Osmond C, Barker DJ, Eriksson JG (2001) Association of schizophrenia with low maternal body mass index, small size at birth, and thinness during childhood. Archives of General Psychiatry 58, 48–52.

Welham J, McLachlan G, Davies G, McGrath J (2000) Heterogeneity in schizophrenia; mixture modelling of age-at-first-admission, gender and diagnosis. Acta Psychiatrica Scandinavica 101, 312–317.

Glossary of epidemiological terms

Adjusted/controlled Confounding variables have been taken into account. Specific methods for the evaluation and control of confounders include restriction of the study population, matching, randomization of exposures, stratification and multivariate analysis.

Allele One of several forms of a gene.

Association Statistical dependence between two or more events, characteristics or other variables. The association between two variables is described as positive when the occurrence of higher values of one variable is associated with the occurrence of higher values of another variable. In a negative association, the occurrence of higher values of one variable is associated with lower values of the other variable. The presence of an association does not necessarily imply a causal relationship. The terms 'association' and 'relationship' are used interchangeably.

Association studies (genetic) Comparison of the rates of marker alleles in cases and controls.

Bias Any trend in the collection, analysis, interpretation, publication or review of data that can lead to conclusions that are systematically different from the truth.

Case-control study A study that starts with the identification of persons with the disease (or outcome of interest) and a suitable control or comparison group of persons without the disease. The relationship of an attribute to the disease is examined by comparing the cases and controls with regard to how frequently the attribute is present or, if quantitative, the levels of the attribute in each of the groups.

Cohort study In the classic cohort study, the investigator defines at the outset two or more groups of people that are free of disease and that differ according to the extent of their exposure to a potential cause of the disease. These groups are referred to as the study cohorts (from the Latin word for one of the 10 divisions of a Roman legion). A cohort study may also begin with a single cohort (i.e. a birth cohort) that is heterogeneous with respect to exposure history. Comparisons of disease experience are made within the cohort across subgroups defined by one or more exposures. The alternative terms for a cohort study (follow-up, longitudinal or prospective study) describe an essential feature of the method, which is observation of the population for a sufficient number of person-years to generate reliable incidence or mortality rates in the population subsets. This generally implies study of a large population, study for a prolonged period or both. In *retrospective cohort studies* all the relevant events (exposure and outcome) have already occurred when the study is initiated. In *prospective cohort studies*, the relevant studies may or may not have occurred at the time the study has begun, but the outcomes have not yet occurred.

Confounder   A variable that is associated with the exposure and independently affects the risk of developing the disease. Such a variable must be controlled or adjusted for in order to obtain an undistorted estimate of the study factor under risk (see *Adjusted*).

Confounding   An observed association (or lack of one) may be caused by a mixing of effects between the exposure, the disease and a third factor, a confounder (see *Confounder*). A measure of the effect of an exposure on risk is distorted because of the association of the exposure with other factor(s) that influence that outcome under study.

Ecological fallacy   The bias that may occur because an association observed between variables on an aggregate level does not necessarily represent the association that exists at an individual level.

Ecological study   A study in which the units of analysis are populations or groups of people rather than individuals.

Effect   The objective of most epidemiological studies is to detect and estimate effects. The term 'effect' can be used in two senses. Effect can be used to mean the endpoint of a causal mechanism or, more usually, in a quantitative sense to indicate the amount of change in a population's disease frequency caused by a specific factor.

Endophenotypes   Biological markers of underlying genetic susceptibility to a particular disorder.

Exposure   A supposed cause of a disease or outcome.

Gene–environment interaction   Different effects of a genotype on disease risk in persons with different environmental exposures or vice versa. There are several mechanisms by which genotype and environment can co-influence disease outcome.

Heritability   The degree to which variability in the manifestation of the disorder (the phenotype) is influenced by genetic factors.

Individual patient data meta-analysis   A type of meta-analysis where the investigators do not rely on published data but ask each author for their full dataset. This allows adjustment for confounders and more accurate estimation of effects.

Linkage   The tendency of two alleles at different loci on the same chromosome to be inherited together. The greater the physical proximity, the smaller the probability of genetic recombination occurring between them and, therefore, the greater the probability that they will be co-inherited.

Meta-analysis   The process of using statistical methods to combine the results of different studies. Meta-analysis has a qualitative component (i.e. application of predetermined criteria of quality) and a quantitative component (i.e. integration of the numerical information).

Nested case-control study   A study in which both the cases and controls are drawn from within a cohort, rather than including the entire cohort population in the study. Such studies can be conducted at a fraction of the cost and yet produce the same findings with nearly the same level of precision. Case-control studies can also be nested within other study designs such as cross-sectional studies, though this is less common.

Odds ratio   The odds ratio for case-control studies (also known as the *exposure-odds ratio*) is the ratio of the odds in favour of exposure among the cases to the odds in favour of exposure among noncases. The odds ratio for a cohort study (or *risk-odds ratio*) is the ratio of the odds in favour of getting the disease, if exposed, to the risk of getting the disease if not exposed.

Phenotype   The observable characteristics of an individual, determined by genetic and environmental factors.

Population attributable fraction   (See *Population attributable risk percent*).

Population attributable risk percent   The proportion of a disease in the study population that is attributable to the exposure and, therefore, could be eliminated if the exposure were eliminated. Also known as the *Population attributable fraction*.

Population stratification   Spurious association with marker alleles in genetic association studies may arise from the confounding effect of differences in the racial and ethnic composition between the case and control groups.

Proxy variable   Use of a single variable (i.e. social class) to represent (often inadequately) a diverse range of underlying factors both known and unknown.

Publication bias   An editorial preference for publishing particular findings (i.e. positive results), which leads to the failure of the authors to submit negative findings for publication or failure of journal editors to accept and publish reports with negative findings. This can distort the results of meta-analyses based on published data.

Recall bias   Systematic error caused by differences in accuracy or recall to memory of prior events or experiences. For example, mothers whose children have schizophrenia may be more likely than mothers of healthy children to remember details of birth complications or developmental delays.

Relative risk   The ratio of the risk of disease among the exposed compared with the risk in the unexposed (also known as risk ratio). For rare diseases, the relative risk approximates to the odds ratio (see *Odds ratio*).

Residual confounding   Adjustment does not fully remove the effect of a confounder, often because of inadequate information on the confounder or close correlation or interaction between variables.

Risk factor   An attribute or exposure that is associated with an increased probability of a specified outcome; not necessarily causal.

Segregation analysis   A mathematical modelling procedure applied to family study data with the goal of determining the mode of genetic transmission.

Selection bias   Error resulting from systematic differences in characteristics between those who are selected for study and those who are not. Examples include use of hospital cases, thus excluding those who are not sick enough to require hospital care or those excluded by distance, cost or other factors. This can be a particular problem in case-control studies where presence or absence of the exposure may influence which particular individuals are entered into the study. Selection bias also invalidates generalizable conclusions from surveys that include only volunteers from a healthy population.

SMR   See *Standardized mortality (morbidity) ratio.*

Standardized mortality (morbidity) ratio   The ratio of the number of deaths observed in the study population to the number that would be expected if the study population had the same specific death rates as the standard population, multiplied by 100.

REFERENCES

Hennekens CH, Buring JE (1987) Epidemiology in Medicine. Toronto: Little, Brown.

Last JM (1988) A Dictionary of Epidemiology. New York: Oxford University Press.

Rothman K, Greenlander S (1998) Modern Epidemiology, 2nd edn. Philadelphia, PA: Lippincott-Raven.

Tsuang MT, Tohen M, Zahner GEP (1995) Textbook in Psychiatric Epidemiology, New York: Wiley-Liss.

Index